ADOLESCENT MEDICINE SECRETS

ADOLESCENT MEDICINE SECRETS

Cynthia Holland-Hall, MD, MPH
Assistant Professor of Clinical Pediatrics
The Ohio State University College of Medicine and
    Public Health
Children's Hospital
Columbus, Ohio

Robert T. Brown, MD
Professor of Clinical Pediatrics and Clinical Obstetrics
    and Gynecology
The Ohio State University College of Medicine and
    Public Health
Chief, Section of Adolescent Health
Children's Hospital
Columbus, Ohio

HANLEY & BELFUS, INC. / Philadelphia

Publisher: HANLEY & BELFUS, INC.
                  Medical Publishers
                  210 South 13th Street
                  Philadelphia, PA 19107
                  (215) 546-7293; 800-962-1892
                  FAX (215) 790-9330
                  Web site: http://www.hanleyandbelfus.com

Note to the reader: Although the information in this book has been carefully reviewed for correctness of dosage and indications, neither the authors nor the editor nor the publisher can accept any legal responsibility for any errors or omissions that may be made. Neither the publisher nor the editor makes any warranty, expressed or implied, with respect to the material contained herein. Before prescribing any drug, the reader must review the manufacturer's current product information (package inserts) for accepted indications, absolute dosage recommendations, and other information pertinent to the safe and effective use of the product described.

Library of Congress Control Number: 2002107072

ADOLESCENT MEDICINE SECRETS   ISBN 1-56053-501-6

Last digit is the print number: 9   8   7   6   5   4   3   2   1

DEDICATION

To my parents, Robert and Barbara Holland.

CHH

To Sally, for all your support and for listening to all the bad puns.

RTB

CONTENTS

III. REPRODUCTIVE HEALTH

IV. MENTAL HEALTH AND PSYCHOSOCIAL CONCERNS

CONTRIBUTORS

Joan F. Atkin, M.D.
Clinical Associate Professor of Pediatrics, Division of Molecular and Human Genetics, The Ohio State University College of Medicine and Public Health; Children's Hospital, Columbus, Ohio

Caroline J. Barangan, M.D.
Division of Adolescent Medicine, Department of Pediatrics, Albert Einstein College of Medicine of Yeshiva University; Montefiore Medical Center, Bronx, New York

Mark Allen Bechtel, M.D.
Assistant Clinical Professor of Medicine, Division of Dermatology, The Ohio State University College of Medicine and Public Health; Chief of Dermatology, Children's Hospital, Columbus, Ohio

John T. Beetar, Ph.D.
Clinical Assistant Professor, Department of Pediatrics, The Ohio State University College of Medicine and Public Health; Pediatric Neuropsychologist, Children's Hospital, Columbus, Ohio

Robert T. Brown, M.D.
Professor of Clinical Pediatrics and Clinical Obstetrics and Gynecology, The Ohio State University College of Medicine and Public Health; Chief, Section of Adolescent Health, Children's Hospital, Columbus, Ohio

Catherine L. Butz, Ph.D.
Clinical Assistant Professor, Division of Psychology, Department of Pediatrics, The Ohio State University College of Medicine and Public Health; Children's Hospital, Columbus, Ohio

Marcel J. Casavant, M.D., FACEP, FACMT
Associate Professor, Departments of Pediatrics and Emergency Medicine, The Ohio State University College of Medicine and Public Health; Medical Director, Central Ohio Poison Center, Columbus, Ohio

Maurice S. Clifton, M.D.
Assistant Professor, Department of Pediatrics, University of Pittsburgh School of Medicine; Children's Hospital of Pittsburgh, Pittsburgh, Pennsylvania

Andrew N. Colvin, Ph.D.
Clinical Assistant Professor, Department of Pediatrics, The Ohio State University College of Medicine and Public Health; Pediatric Neuropsychologist, Children's Hospital, Columbus, Ohio

Stephen C. Cook, M.D.
Division of Pediatric Cardiology, Children's Hospital, Columbus, Ohio

Susan M. Coupey, M.D.
Professor of Pediatrics, Division of Adolescent Medicine, Department of Pediatrics, Albert Einstein College of Medicine of Yeshiva University; Montefiore Medical Center, Bronx, New York

Wallace V. Crandall, M.D.
Assistant Clinical Professor, Department of Pediatrics, The Ohio State University College of Medicine and Public Health; Children's Hospital, Columbus, Ohio

Curt J. Daniels, M.D.
Assistant Professor of Clinical Internal Medicine and Pediatrics, Department of Cardiology, The Ohio State University College of Medicine and Public Health; Children's Hospital, Columbus, Ohio

Martin Fisher, M.D.
Professor of Clinical Pediatrics, New York University School of Medicine, New York, New York; Chief, Division of Adolescent Medicine, Department of Pediatrics, North Shore University Hospital, North Shore–Long Island Jewish Health System, Manhasset, New York

Roger A. Friedman, M.D.
Clinical Professor of Allergy, Immunology, and Pediatrics, Department of Pediatrics, The Ohio State University College of Medicine and Public Health; Children's Hospital, Columbus, Ohio

John A. Germak, M.D.
Associate Professor of Clinical Pediatrics, Department of Pediatrics, The Ohio State University College of Medicine and Public Health; Director of Pediatric Endocrinology, Children's Hospital, Columbus, Ohio

Melanie A. Gold, D.O.
Associate Professor of Pediatrics, Division of Adolescent Medicine, Department of Pediatrics, University of Pittsburgh School of Medicine; Director of Family Planning Services, Children's Hospital of Pittsburgh, Pittsburgh, Pennsylvania

Geri D. Hewitt, M.D.
Assistant Professor, Departments of Obstetrics and Gynecology and Pediatrics, The Ohio State University College of Medicine and Public Health; Section Chief of Obstetrics and Gynecology, Children's Hospital, Columbus, Ohio

Gloria C. Higgins, Ph.D., M.D.
Associate Professor, Department of Pediatrics, The Ohio State University College of Medicine and Public Health; Division of Rheumatology, Children's Hospital, Columbus, Ohio

Cynthia Holland-Hall, M.D., M.P.H.
Assistant Professor of Clinical Pediatrics, The Ohio State University College of Medicine and Public Health; Adolescent Medicine Section, Children's Hospital, Columbus, Ohio

Jeffrey D. Hord, M.D.
Associate Professor of Pediatrics, Northeastern Ohio Universities College of Medicine, Rootstown, Ohio; Director of Pediatric Hematology-Oncology, Children's Hospital Medical Center, Akron, Ohio

S. Anne Joseph, M.D.
Assistant Clinical Professor of Pediatrics, Department of Child Neurology, The Ohio State University College of Medicine and Public Health; Children's Hospital, Columbus, Ohio

Katalin I. Koranyi, M.D.
Professor of Clinical Pediatrics, Section of Infectious Diseases, Department of Pediatrics, The Ohio State University College of Medicine and Public Health; Children's Hospital, Columbus, Ohio

Kathleen L. Lemanek, Ph.D.
Clinical Associate Professor, Division of Psychology, Department of Pediatrics, The Ohio State University College of Medicine and Public Health; Children's Hospital, Columbus, Ohio

Barbara J. Long, M.D., M.P.H.
Assistant Clinical Professor, Division of Adolescent Medicine, Department of Pediatrics, University of California, San Francisco, School of Medicine, San Francisco, California

John D. Mahan, M.D.
Professor, Department of Pediatrics, The Ohio State University College of Medicine and Public Health; Division Director, Pediatric Nephrology, Children's Hospital, Columbus, Ohio

Ann Pakalnis, M.D.
Associate Professor of Clinical Pediatrics and Neurology, Department of Pediatrics, The Ohio State University College of Medicine and Public Health; Children's Hospital, Columbus, Ohio

Juliann M. Paolicchi, M.A., M.D.
Assistant Professor of Clinical Pediatrics and Neurology, Department of Pediatrics; Director, Clinical Neurophysiology Fellowship, The Ohio State University College of Medicine and Public Health; Director, Comprehensive Epilepsy Program, Children's Hospital, Columbus, Ohio

Lynda S. Peel, M.A., R.D., L.D.
Program Manager, Clinical Nutrition; Lactation Program, Children's Hospital, Columbus, Ohio

Vaughn I. Rickert, Psy.D.
Professor of Clinical Population and Family Health, Center for Community Health and Education, Heilbrun Department of Population and Family Health, Mailman School of Public Health, Columbia University, New York, New York

Peter D. Rogers, M.D., M.P.H.
Clinical Associate Professor of Pediatrics, Department of Pediatrics, The Ohio State University College of Medicine and Public Health; Section of Adolescent Health, Children's Hospital, Columbus, Ohio

Patricia S. Simmons, M.D.
Associate Professor, Department of Pediatrics, Mayo Medical School; Mayo Clinic, Rochester, Minnesota

Kym A. Smith, B.S.
Clinical Research Coordinator, Department of Adolescent Medicine, Children's Hospital of Pittsburgh, Pittsburgh, Pennsylvania

Victor C. Strasburger, M.D.
Professor of Pediatrics; Professor of Family and Community Medicine; Chief, Division of Adolescent Medicine, Department of Pediatrics, University of New Mexico School of Medicine, Albuquerque, New Mexico

Diane M. Straub, M.D., M.P.H.
Division of Adolescent Medicine, Department of Pediatrics, University of California, San Francisco, School of Medicine, San Francisco, California

Tahniat S. Syed, M.D.
Department of Adolescent Medicine, Children's Hospital of Pittsburgh, Pittsburgh, Pennsylvania

Martin A. Turman, M.D., Ph.D.
Associate Professor, Department of Pediatric Nephrology, University of Oklahoma Health Sciences Center; Children's Hospital, Oklahoma City, Oklahoma

Constance M. Wiemann, Ph.D.
Associate Professor, Section of Adolescent Medicine and Sports Medicine, Department of Pediatrics, Baylor College of Medicine; Texas Children's Hospital, Houston, Texas

Keith Owen Yeates, Ph.D.
Associate Professor, Department of Pediatrics, The Ohio State University College of Medicine and Public Health; Director of Pediatric Neuropsychology, Children's Hospital, Columbus, Ohio

PREFACE

Adolescent Medicine Secrets, the newest addition to The Secrets Series®, provides a convenient reference for active clinicians and trainees in many disciplines, particularly the primary care specialties. The information is presented in the easy-to-use Secrets question-and-answer format, and the topics are divided into four major areas: General Adolescent Health, Physical Disorders Affecting Adolescents, Reproductive Health, and Mental Health and Psychosocial Concerns. It is our hope that this text will be used regularly by clinicians who see adolescents in the course of their daily practices and by students and residents seeking to increase their knowledge and comfort in caring for adolescent patients.

We would like to offer our thanks to Carole Clark for her secretarial support, to Linda Belfus and Cecelia Bayruns of Hanley & Belfus for their patience and editorial help, and especially to our contributing authors, whose expertise has enabled us to publish a text of such high quality.

Cynthia Holland-Hall, MD, MPH
Robert T. Brown, MD

I. *General Adolescent Health*

1. ADOLESCENT HEALTH STATISTICS

Cynthia Holland-Hall, M.D., M.P.H.

1. How many teenagers are there in the United States?

According to U.S. census data, there were over 32,000,000 people between the ages of 13 and 20 years old in 2000. They represent about 11.5% of the total population. Although the adolescent population is growing, it is declining as a percentage of the total U.S. population.

2. Is the adolescent population more or less ethnically diverse than the general population?

The adolescent population in the U.S. is somewhat more diverse than the general population. For example, African Americans and Hispanics account for 12% and 11%, respectively, of the U.S. population overall. Among persons 10–19 years old, however, 16% are African American and 15% are Hispanic. These adolescent minority populations, as well as the Asian/Pacific Islander population, continue to grow at a faster rate than the white, non-Hispanic population of teens.

3. How many teens do not live at home with their families?

Data are limited, but it is estimated that as many as 300,000 teens live in foster care or other substitute care. On any given day, about 100,000 persons are detained or incarcerated in the juvenile justice system. It is difficult to estimate the number of homeless and runaway youth. Some data indicate that as many as 2 million teens and young adults (many of whom may be over 18 years old) live primarily on the streets. These out-of-home young people have disproportionate numbers of unmet physical and mental health needs.

4. How many teens are living in poverty?

In 1998, 17% of all adolescents lived in families with incomes below the federal poverty line (FPL). In the African American and Hispanic populations, nearly one-third of all children and adolescents lived below the FPL. Those who live in single-parent households are much more likely to live in poverty.

5. How many adolescents lack health insurance?

In 1997, 17% of adolescents had no health insurance, including one-third of those living in families whose incomes were below the FPL. Many of these teens were eligible for Medicaid but were not enrolled. Teens are more likely than younger children to lack insurance. Not surprisingly, uninsured teens are more likely to have unmet health needs.

6. What are the most common reasons that adolescents go to emergency departments?

Teens account for over 10 million emergency department visits per year, approximately half of which are for injuries. The most common noninjury reasons for emergency department visits are asthma, upper respiratory infections, and gastrointestinal/abdominal symptoms.

7. What is the mortality rate for American teenagers? Is it increasing or decreasing?

The mortality rate is decreasing steadily. In 1999 the mortality rate for 15–19-year-olds was 70/100,000. The mortality rate for teenaged boys is about twice that of teenaged girls. A decline in deaths from firearm injuries has contributed to the overall decrease over the past decade.

8. What are the leading causes of death for American teens?

The three leading causes of death for persons 15–19 years old of all races are (1) accidents (unintentional injuries), (2) homicide, and (3) suicide. For persons 10–14 years old, they are (1) accidents, (2) malignancies, and (3) homicide. About three-quarters of all deaths in these age groups are preventable.

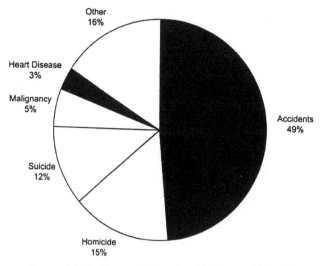

Causes of death, all races, both genders, 15–19 years old in 1999.

9. What is the leading cause of death for young black men in the United States?

Homicide is responsible for nearly half of all deaths in black men 15–19 years old and 20–24 years old.

10. What unintentional injury is the most common cause of death among 10–24 year olds?

Motor vehicle accidents account for about one-third of all deaths in 10–24 year olds. This is not surprising given that 33% of high school students surveyed in 1999 stated that they rode with a drinking driver in the past month, and 16% stated that they rarely or never use safety belts. The good news is that both percentages have declined over the past decade.

11. How many high school students are sexually active?

About one-half. By the time they graduate, about two-thirds of students have had sex, and about one in five students has had four or more different sexual partners.

12. Is the birth rate for adolescent girls increasing?

No. The teen birth rate has been falling, and the birth rate to 15–17-year-old girls is now the lowest it has been in the past few decades. Decreases in sexual activity, increases in condom use, and the availability of more effective contraceptive methods may contribute to this decline.

13. Are teens getting fewer sexually transmitted infections (STIs) as well?

Although the rates of certain infections, such as gonorrhea, have decreased over the past decade, STIs remain quite prevalent among sexually active adolescents. The reported rates of chlamydial and gonococcal infections are higher for girls 15–19 years old than for any other demographic group. Infection with *Trichomonas vaginalis*, herpes simplex virus, and human papillomavirus, although they are not reportable, are even more common. About one of four adolescents will be diagnosed with a STI before graduating from high school.

14. What proportion of persons with acquired immunodeficiency syndrome (AIDS) are adolescents?

Among males, less than 1% of patients with AIDS are adolescents; among females, 1% of patients with AIDS are adolescents. Keep in mind, however, that the time from contracting human immunodeficiency virus (HIV) to the time of onset of AIDS is generally 8–10 years. Young adults in their twenties account for 17% of AIDS cases in males and 22% of cases in females. Many of these patients were infected as teens.

15. Which teens are most likely to smoke cigarettes?

Smoking among teens is increasing. White non-Hispanic males and females are the most likely to smoke; black non-Hispanic males and females are the least likely.

16. How many adolescents are expected to die of tobacco-related illness?

The Centers for Disease Control and Prevention estimates that approximately 5 million persons who were under 17 years old in 1995 will die prematurely of tobacco-related illness.

17. How many adolescents have attempted or considered suicide?

In 1999, 25% of female high school students and 14% of male high school students stated they had attempted or seriously considered suicide in the past 12 months. This measure reflects the overall mental health of American high school students.

18. How many adolescents drop out of high school?

In 1998, 4 of 100 students aged 15–19 years in grades 10–12 dropped out of school. Teens from low income families were four times more likely to drop out than teens from high income families.

19. Do most older adolescents have jobs?

In 1999, over one-half of adolescents 16–19 years old worked during the summer, and about two-fifths were employed during the school year. Several more engage in "freelance" jobs such as babysitting and yard work. The most common jobs for teens include working in restaurants and the fast-food industry, in retail stores, and on farms.

20. Are adolescents who work at risk for negative consequences?

Occupational injuries in teens accounted for over 250,000 visits to emergency departments in 1998. Adolescents are less likely than adults to have experience in the workplace and often receive little or no training in injury prevention. A reduction in the incidence of adolescent work injuries is included in the Healthy People 2010 objectives. In addition, teens who work, particularly those who work more than 20 hours per week, are more likely to have problems in school, and they have less time for extracurricular school and peer activities.

21. What is the prevalence of overweight among American teens?

Ten percent of adolescents have a body mass index (BMI) at or above the 95th percentile for their age and gender, and another 16% have a BMI between the 85th and 95th percentile (i.e., they are at risk for becoming overweight).

22. How many teens get enough fruits and vegetables in their diets?

Only 24% of high school students eat five or more servings of fruits and vegetables per day (the recommended daily intake).

23. Are American teens getting enough physical activity?

No. Seventy-three percent of high school students stated that they did not participate in even moderate physical activity on five or more of the past seven days. Only 56% were enrolled in physical education class, and of those, 24% stated that they exercised less than 20 minutes during an average class.

24. Because of injuries, pregnancy, STIs, and mental and behavioral problems, adolescents make frequent visits to the doctor. True or false?

False. Despite their needs, adolescents have lower rates of health care utilization than either younger children or adults. Older (i.e., 18–19-year-old) female adolescents are the most likely to have had a health care visit within the past year; older male adolescents are the least likely.

BIBLIOGRAPHY

1. Centers for Disease Control and Prevention: Youth Risk Behavior Surveillance—United States, 1999. MMWR 49(SS-5):1–96, 2000.
2. MacKay AP, Fingerhut LA, Duran CR: Adolescent Health Chartbook. Health, United States, 2000. Hyattsville, MD, National Center for Health Statistics, 2000.
3. National Vital Statistics Report, vol. 49, no. 11, October 12, 2001.
4. Ozer EM, Brindis CD, et al: America's Adolescents: Are They Healthy? San Francisco, University of California–San Francisco, National Adolescent Health Information Center, 1998.

2. INTERVIEWING ADOLESCENTS

Caroline J. Barangan, M.D., and Susan M. Coupey, M.D.

INTERVIEWING AIDS FOR THE CLINICIAN

1. How does the HEADSSS system assist in interviewing adolescents?

HEADSSS is an acronym developed by Berman in 1972 to organize the psychosocial history. It allows coverage of various topics about the adolescent's life, relationships, and activities during the interview: home, education, activities, drugs, safety, sexuality, and suicide/depression.

2. What are the five boxes?

The five boxes is another interviewing method that achieves the same results as HEADSS. Pertinent questions in each "box" or area (medical, home, school/work, peers, romance) elicit a full health history.

3. What is the GAPS questionnaire?

The GAPS questionnaire is essentially the HEADSSS interview in questionnaire form. GAPS stands for **G**uidelines for **A**dolescent **P**reventive **S**ervices, which was issued by the American Medical Association in 1992. It describes the recommended annual preventive service visits for adolescents aged 11–21 years old. Although the questionnaire allows the clinician to utilize time with the adolescent more efficiently, it should not take the place of one-to-one interviewing. The form may not be filled out accurately, and important information may be missed because the right questions were not asked. Furthermore, rapport and trust can be developed only through direct interaction.

SETTING THE STAGE FOR THE ADOLESCENT VISIT

4. At what age should private interviews with a pediatric patient be initiated?

Adolescence is generally considered to span the ages of 11–21 years. It is appropriate for the clinician to spend a portion of the office visit interviewing the adolescent alone beginning at 11 years old. Clinicians can begin to spend some time interviewing the preadolescent (8–10 years of age) alone in preparation for future visits as an adolescent. In the preadolescent and early adolescent years, this private time may occur during the physical exam, unless, of course, the patient wants the parent or guardian to be in the room during the examination. Sensitive topics and general topics about the patient's interests, activities, and relationships can be discussed during this time. Private time is important in building the rapport and trust needed for a good clinician-patient relationship. Your confidentiality policy should be discussed with both patient and parent before spending this time alone with the patient.

5. How is an adolescent's developmental level assessed early in an interview?

It is often said that adolescents should be interviewed in a developmentally appropriate manner. There are no straightforward measures for assessing an adolescent's developmental level. The clinician needs to make a judgment/assessment about the adolescent's experience and understanding regarding various topics, such as relationships, sexual activity, and substance use. Early in the interview, the clinician should make general conversation about neutral topics (sports, music, and movies), ask basic questions about more sensitive topics (relationship with family members and peers, dating, sexual activity), and encourage questions from the adolescent. The responses to the clinician's questions and the questions that are

5

asked by the adolescent give the interviewer a sense of the developmental level. This assessment guides the clinician through the remainder of the interview: what questions to ask, how to ask them, how much time to spend on one topic as opposed to another, and the extent of the education to be done.

6. How does the clinician use the developmental assessment to guide the remainder of the interview?

Suppose a 14-year-old girl presents for a check-up. During the private interview, the clinician can ask whether her friends have boyfriends and what the couples do together (hold hands, kiss, hug, heavy petting, sexual intercourse). Then the clinician can ask if the adolescent has a boyfriend or would like to have one and what she thinks is a sexual relationship. Subsequent questions can ask about what the patient and her boyfriend do together. Further questions and anticipatory guidance depend on the adolescent's responses. If she is not interested in sexual experimentation, the clinician should give positive feedback on abstinence and a brief introduction to safe sex, encouraging the adolescent to ask questions. If she is interested in sexual experimentation, a basic talk on contraception options and the importance of contraception should be done. If she has already had sexual intercourse, a more extensive and detailed counseling session should be done, and questions should be asked about her experiences (types of sex, contraception used, good experience vs. bad experience).

7. How do you explain confidentiality to an adolescent?

Confidentiality should be explained to adolescents at the beginning of the first visit. After the introductions are made, let them know that what they discuss with you is confidential and ask what "confidential" means to them. Explain that whatever they talk about is not told to anyone else, including parent(s), unless they give you permission to do so. This principle applies even if a parent asks you directly about what was discussed during the visit. Explain that the only exception to this rule is when the clinician believes that the adolescent is in danger or is a danger to himself/herself or others (e.g., suicidal or homicidal ideation, abuse). In this case, the appropriate persons must be informed, including parent(s), so that the adolescent can get the necessary help. Encourage good communication with parents about all issues discussed during the visit.

8. How is interviewing an adolescent with a chronic illness different from interviewing a healthy adolescent?

The same questions asked of an adolescent without a chronic illness should be asked of the adolescent with a chronic illness. The interview should not be focused on the chronic illness. It should always be focused on the adolescent. However, the clinician should be sensitive to various factors common to adolescents with chronic illnesses and disabilities. Adolescents with chronic illnesses may have a developmental age that lags behind their chronologic age, and this observation should guide the interview.

Chronically ill adolescents may have delayed growth and pubertal development. Such delays may be concerns for adolescent patients, making them feel self-conscious. Providing the adolescent with reassurance and a forum to voice these concerns is important.

Sexual activity is a particularly important topic to discuss in detail with chronically ill adolescents. Although some adolescents with chronic illness initiate sexual intercourse later than healthy counterparts, others initiate sexual intercourse earlier. Most are thinking about sexuality, regardless of their illness. Some adolescents with chronic illness are concerned about fertility and think that they cannot get pregnant or make their partner pregnant. This concern has important implications for the adolescent's use of contraception. Most chronic illnesses do not affect fertility, and pregnancy poses a significant health threat to many adolescent girls who are chronically ill. Adolescents who are mentally retarded or handicapped are at increased risk of sexual assault. Asking adolescents whether they have had this experience and determining whether they are at risk are therefore important.

9. What roles should the clinician avoid during an interview?

1. The clinician should avoid the surrogate parent role. Adolescents do not respond to a clinician who is judgmental, does not listen to their views and opinions, and only tells them what to do. It is also unhealthy for adolescents to view the clinician as the parent that they have always wanted.

2. The clinician should avoid playing the role of the adolescent. Adolescents should look to the clinician as a role model and a mature resource—not as their buddy.

3. The clinician should avoid taking sides in disagreements between parent and child. Taking sides will only come back to haunt the clinician. Either side (parent or adolescent) may use the words of the clinician against the other. Instead, the clinician should be a mediator to facilitate communication between both parties.

10. What is the difference between explicit and implicit barriers to communication in an interview?

Explicit barriers to communication are obvious blocks to productive communication, such as the hostile and angry adolescent who does not want to respond to questions or the adolescent who responds to questions with one- or two-word answers.

Implicit barriers to communication are subtle, but they also undermine productive communication. Examples are cognitive dissonance, unexpected resistance, verbal/nonverbal mismatch, and interviewer discomfort. **Cognitive dissonance** is the interviewer's difficulty in relating to the adolescent who makes statements that contradict each other or common sense. **Unexpected resistance** occurs when the adolescent suddenly and without reason refuses to talk about a topic after previously dicussing it freely. **Verbal/nonverbal mismatch** occurs when the adolescent's facial expression, tone of voice, or body gestures do not match verbal statements. **Interviewer discomfort** occurs when the clinician has an unexpected emotional reaction related to his or her own past experiences or provocation by the adolescent.

WORKING WITH PARENTS

11. How do you explain confidentiality to a parent?

Parents should be told about the need for confidentiality between physician and adolescent at the beginning of the initial visit. The concept should be explained in a way that will not cause the parents to feel that their child and the doctor will be hiding things from them. The clinician should explain to parents that the majority of the visit will be spent with the adolescent alone. Privacy allows the clinician and the adolescent to talk about topics that the adolescent may be embarrassed to discuss in front of the parent. The confidentiality policy allows adolescents to talk freely about themselves and their life. Whatever is discussed between clinician and adolescent will not be revealed to anyone else without the adolescent's permission. The exception to this policy is adolescents who are in danger or pose a danger to themselves or others. In this case, the appropriate persons, including parents, will be informed of the situation. Without the confidentiality policy, the likelihood that the adolescent will be open and honest with the clinician is lower because of fear that a parent will be told. As much information as possible must be obtained from adolescents to provide them with the best care. Reassuring the parent that the clinician's goal is to ensure the adolescent's well-being and not to undermine the parent's relationship or authority is extremely important. The clinician also should reassure the parent that the adolescent will be encouraged to talk with his or her parents about what is discussed in private during the visit.

12. How do you involve the caregiver in the initial adolescent visit/interview?

It is important to involve the parent in the adolescent's health care. Doing so prevents the parent from feeling alienated and facilitates good communication between all parties. At the beginning of the initial visit, adolescents and parents should be interviewed for a brief time together. After the clinician introduces him- or herself to the adolescent and parent, the clinician should explain confidentiality, as previously described. The clinician also should explain how the visit will be structured: (1) interview with the adolescent and parent together, (2) interview with the adolescent alone, (3) physical exam, (4) discussion of plan with the adolescent, and (5) closing session with adolescent and parent together. After a personal medical history and family history are obtained from both adolescent and parent, the parent should be asked about any additional concerns or questions. Once this dialogue is completed, the parent is asked to step out of the room. The parent should be given the opportunity to speak confidentially with the clinician at each annual visit and at any other pertinent time. Parents may have concerns that they are reluctant to voice in the company of their children. At the end of the visit the parent is included in a summary session. Any further questions are answered at this time.

PUTTING THE ADOLESCENT AT EASE

13. How can a clinician increase the likelihood that an adolescent will respond to questions more honestly and less anxiously?
- Ask questions about psychosocial issues in a direct manner.
- Explain the concept of confidentiality, and ensure the adolescent of its application to all meetings between clinician and adolescent.
- Let adolescents know that you are sincerely interested in their feelings and views.
- Avoid lecturing and being judgmental.
- Do not rush through the visit
- Focus on the adolescent patient rather than the parent(s).
- Try to keep a neutral facial expression during the interview. The adolescent may misinterpret facial expressions as negative.
- Be sympathetic, supportive, and reassuring.

14. At the initial adolescent visit/interview, what techniques help to establish rapport with the adolescent?
- Keep the focus on the adolescent. For example, allow adolescents to make introductions between you and anyone who accompanies them.
- Avoid talking down to adolescents.
- Start with neutral topics.
- Try to find common ground; for example, the fact that both clinician and adolescent may be fans of the same sports team
- Do not talk about the adolescent with others as if the adolescent were not in the room.
- Be yourself. Adolescents can sense when an adult is putting up a front.

15. How does the clinician communicate professional expertise to the adolescent? Why is this issue important?
Clinicians communicate professional expertise in their professional attire and demeanor; ability to converse in a clear, confident, and grammatically correct manner; encouragement of questions; willingness to spend time providing explanations or clarifications; and ability to convey comfort in caring for adolescents. Adolescents look to clinicians as role models and resources. If adolescents view the clinician as a professional and an expert, they are more likely to trust the clinician and the clinician-patient relationship can develop, leading to adolescent (patient) satisfaction. Adolescents are also more likely to adhere to medical plans and medication if they are satisfied with the medical care that they receive.

SPECIFIC INTERVIEWING TECHNIQUES

16. Why is interviewing technique particularly important with adolescents?
Interviewing adolescents is a complex task requiring unique technique and skills. Adolescents are neither children nor adults and cannot be approached as either. The psychosocial

history constitutes a major portion of the adolescent interview. Obtaining the psychosocial history is an extensive process because many sensitive and potentially embarrassing topics are discussed. This process is even more difficult because adolescents have a limited ability to think abstractly and because each adolescent differs in level of understanding and experience. The interviewing clinician needs to have a fair amount of flexibility because different approaches are required for different adolescents. In addition, establishing rapport with and gaining the trust of an adolescent require effort and patience.

17. How should you address nonverbal cues during an interview?

It is important to take note of adolescents' facial expressions, body gestures, and tone of voice and to assess the context in which they occur during the interview. These nonverbal cues are indicators of what the adolescent is feeling or thinking. These feelings or thoughts may be in contradiction to what the adolescent says verbally. Such cues should always be acknowledged and explored. For example, if an adolescent girl keeps her eyes directed downward and her tone of voice soft and quiet, the clinician should make a verbal observation of this behavior, such as "You seem quiet and a little sad." The adolescent can subsequently confirm your assessment and answer questions or correct your assessment and elaborate. Addressing nonverbal cues may lead to information that you would not otherwise have obtained. It also shows adolescents that you are paying attention and interested in their feelings and thoughts.

18. Why are direct questions, such as "Are you having sex?" or "Are you sexually active?," not the best way to ask about the adolescent's sexual history?

"Having sex" and "sexually active" are subjective terms that are interpreted differently by different adolescents. Some adolescents believe that having sex means intercourse with penile-vaginal penetration only. They may not perceive oral or anal activity as having sex. Some adolescents may not know what sexual activity means. They may interpret the term "sexual activity" as the amount of physical movement made by a participant during intercourse. Do not assume that the adolescent understands a phrase or question in the same manner that the speaker intends. Adolescents, especially early adolescents, are still concrete thinkers. A better approach is to ask whether the adolescent has ever had a sexual relationship with another person. Regardless of the response, the clinician should inquire about what the adolescent thinks that a sexual relationship entails. If the adolescent acknowledges a sexual relationship, the clinician should inquire as to what types of sexual practices the adolescent has experienced and the gender of the person(s) with whom the adolescent has had sex.

19. What are some effective ways to close the interview?

Each clinician should create his or her own style of interview closure. Possibilities include the following:
- Ask adolescents for a "weather forecast" of their life.
- Ask for feedback from the adolescent about the visit.
- Ask adolescents what they considered the most important aspect of the visit.
- Ask the adolescent to summarize the main issues that were discussed and the subsequent plan that was decided upon; offer assistance as needed.

The last few minutes of a visit should include an opportunity for the adolescent and his or her parents to ask any final questions. The clinician can give a summary of the visit with confirmation of any plans and follow-up.

20. What is the "reflection response" technique?

Reflection response is a technique for encouraging adolescents to elaborate on a statement that they have made by repeating the statement to the adolescent in a question form.

Adolescent: I can't stand my mom.

MD: You can't stand your mom?

Adolescent: Yeah. She can't stay out of my business. It's like she doesn't trust me or something.

21. What is active listening?

One technique of active listening is called facilitation. It is a method of encouraging adolescents to continue telling their story by using questions such as, "And then what happened?," "And then what did she say?," or " And then what did you do?" An efficient method of taking a history from adolescents is to encourage them to tell the story in their own words with minimal interruption and with active listening by the clinician.

22. Educating adolescents should be an active process rather than a passive process. How is this goal accomplished during an interview?

A didactic lecture at the end of an interview, with the adolescent passively listening, is the least effective method of educating adolescents. They are probably only partially listening and are even more likely to forget or ignore what is said. Education should take place during the interview in an active and interactive manner. With each topic that is discussed, adolescents should be encouraged to voice their thoughts, knowledge, and beliefs. The clinician should build on the adolescent's knowledge, fill in the gaps, and modify misconceptions. Providing education in this manner makes more of an impact on adolescents because they are actively participating in the process.

23. What do you do with the patient who gives limited (one- or two-word) responses?

Adolescents who give limited responses are usually anxious, nervous, or shy. They should be approached gently. The clinician should try to engage them by asking benign questions about neutral topics such as movies, television, sports, or music. Hopefully, the adolescent will be more talkative once he or she is more comfortable. The clinician should continue to encourage adolescents to elaborate on their limited responses. If the adolescent continues to give limited responses, the clinician should not be discouraged. The clinician should proceed with the visit as outlined and bring the adolescent back for another visit in the near future. Most adolescents will be less apprehensive during the second visit.

APPROACHING SENSITIVE TOPICS

24. Why is the quality of the patient's relationships with members of the household important?

It is important to ask adolescents about who lives in their home, what their relationships with these persons are like, and whether there have been any recent changes in the household (e.g., moves, deaths, births, divorces or separations, persons moving in or moving out). Adolescents look to household members to provide support as they deal with the process of accomplishing the tasks of adolescence. They expect the home to be stable and safe. If the home is a source of stress because of changes in the household or conflicts between members of the household, adolescents are at risk for participation in high-risk behaviors, influence by adverse peer pressures, and depression. When adolescents are unable to trust any household member or do not have anyone at home in whom to confide, they are likely to develop other psychosocial difficulties.

25. Why is it important to ask adolescents about their school experience in some detail?

Questions about school or college experience should be specific and detailed. The adolescent should not be asked, "How is school?" because the likely answer is "okay." Examples of specific questions include the following:

- What grades have you received?
- What are your best and worst subjects?
- Are your grades better or worse than they were last quarter, semester, or year?
- How are your relationships with your classmates and teachers?
- Have you ever repeated a grade?
- Are you in special classes?

- Do you make it to school all the time, most of the time, or some of the time?
- How many days have you missed this semester?

Depending on the answers to these questions, further questions should be asked to elaborate or clarify the responses. Important information, such as a learning disability, problems at home that may cause absenteeism or poor grades, abuse by classmates, depression, delinquency, or poor grades caused by substance use, will be missed if this aspect of the interview is neglected.

26. What is the greatest impediment to obtaining a complete sexual history?

The greatest impediment is not the embarrassed adolescent or the overprotective parent. The greatest impediment is not asking the appropriate questions in the appropriate manner.

27. At what age should you begin to ask about the adolescent's sexual activity?

Ask about the adolescent's sexual activity at the first adolescent visit (12 years of age). Questions about sexual activity can be asked even earlier during the pre-adolescent years. How these questions are asked and how extensive the questioning should be depend on the patient's level of experience and understanding.

28. How should you question the adolescent about sexual orientation?

Never assume that all adolescents are heterosexual. Some adolescents are sure that they are homosexual, some are unsure about their sexual orientation, and most are sure that they are heterosexual. Because an adolescent may not have had previous sexual experiences, asking about sexual behavior will not give the information that you are seeking. Reassuring the adolescent that many adolescents think about sex and their own sexuality helps to put him or her at ease. Then the clinician should ask whether the adolescent finds himself or herself attracted to males, females, or both. Asking such questions in a direct and matter-of-fact manner shows the adolescent that the clinician will not be judgmental regardless of the response.

29. When is it appropriate to ask about past or ongoing sexual abuse?

During an adolescent interview it is always appropriate to inquire about sexual abuse. As with many sensitive topics, if the questions are not asked, the adolescent is not likely to tell, especially since adolescents may feel embarrassed or guilty about sexual abuse. They may have been intimidated into not revealing such information to anyone.

30. How should you ask about past or ongoing sexual abuse?

While asking questions regarding sexual history, the clinician should inquire about sexual abuse, both past and present. Adolescents should be asked whether anyone has ever touched them anywhere on their body without their permission or if anyone has ever touched them anywhere on their body in a way that made them uncomfortable. As an alternative approach, the clinician may ask, "Have you had any uncomfortable sexual experiences?" The clinician should be sensitive to the cues, verbal and nonverbal, that adolescents may give to indicate that they have been sexually abused. For example, a patient may become visibly uncomfortable when talking about her mother's current live-in boyfriend.

31. Is it appropriate to ask direct questions about suicidal ideation?

During an interview with an adolescent it is definitely appropriate to ask direct questions about suicidal ideation. It may be the only way to elicit whether the adolescent is at risk for suicide. Contrary to belief, asking questions about suicide does not cause the adolescent to attempt or commit suicide.

BIBLIOGRAPHY

1. Charting the journey through adolescence: A guide to the transitional interview. Adolesc Health Update 1:1–7, 1988.

2. Cole SA, Bird J: The Medical Interview: The Three-Function Approach, 2nd ed. St. Louis, Mosby, 2000.
3. Coupey SM: Interviewing adolescents. Pediatr Clin North Am 44:1349–1364, 1997.
4. Coupey SM: Primary Care of Adolescent Girls. Philadelphia, Hanley & Belfus, 2000.
5. Elster AB, Kuzsets N: AMA Guidelines for Adolescent Preventive Services (GAPS). Baltimore, Williams & Wilkins, 1993.
6. Goldenring JM, Cohen E: Getting into adolescent HEADS. Contemp Pediatr 5:75–90, 1988.
7. Green M (ed): Bright Futures: Guidelines for Health Supervision of Infants, Children, and Adolescents. Arlington, VA, National Center for Education in Maternal and Child Health, 1994.
8. Marks A: How to make the most of an adolescent's first visit. Pediatr Manage Dec:97–101, 1992.

3. SCREENING AND PREVENTION

Martin Fisher, M.D.

1. What national guidelines are available to guide pediatricians in providing preventive services for adolescents?

Five sets of guidelines developed in the United States during the 1990s outline the preventive health services that should be provided to adolescent patients in clinical settings: (1) Guidelines for Adolescent Preventive Services (GAPS), developed by the Division of Adolescent Health of the American Medical Association (AMA); (2) Bright Futures Guidelines for Health Supervision of Infants, Children, and Adolescents, sponsored by the Maternal and Child Health Bureau of the Health Resources and Services Administration and the Medicaid Bureau of the Health Care Financing Administration; (3) Recommendations for Pediatric Preventive Health Care, of the American Academy of Pediatrics (AAP); (4) Age Charts for Periodic Health Examinations of the American Academy of Family Practice (AAFP); and (5) Guide to Clinical Preventive Services, a report of the U.S. Preventive Services Task Force (USPSTF), developed by the U.S. Department of Health and Human Services. Details of the recommendations specific to adolescents have been reviewed by Jenkins and Saxena in 1995, Elster in 1998, and Fisher in 1999. In general, these guidelines represent consensus statements by panels of experts based on the best cost-benefit analyses available in the medical literature.

2. What principles are used to determine the appropriateness of screening tests and procedures?

Screening tests and procedures are used to detect problems before they would otherwise become apparent in order to initiate treatment that can alter the course and consequences of an illness. For screening to be worthwhile, the illness must be (1) important and/or serious, (2) relatively prevalent in the population, (3) treatable or preventable. In addition, there should be an advantage to early detection, diagnosis and treatment. Screening tests must be acceptable (simple, convenient, relatively painless, inexpensive) to all involved (patient, parents, practitioners, technicians), yield reliable results (interobserver, split sample, test–retest), and be valid (i.e., sensitive and specific).

3. Which routine immunizations are required for all adolescents?

Three sets of immunizations, covering six different infections, are appropriate for all adolescents:

1. **Diphtheria and tetanus (dT)**. Adolescents who received a full set of vaccinations (including at least three dT immunizations) during childhood require booster immunizations at 10-year intervals. Those without documented evidence of childhood immunizations require a primary series of three dT immunizations.

2. **Polio**. Adolescents who received a complete set of at least 3–4 polio vaccinations do not need additional immunizations unless they travel to an endemic region. Those who require a primary series should receive inactivated polio vaccine as a series of three immunizations.

3. **Measles, mumps, and rubella (MMR)**. All adolescents require documentation of two measles vaccinations (unless there is a history of illness or documented seroconversion) and at least one immunization against mumps and rubella. Most children and adolescents receive two MMR vaccinations as the best way of meeting these requirements. Since the recommendation for two measles vaccines (initiated because an initial vaccine does not provide immunity in all people) is now over 10 years old, most adolescents will have received two MMR vaccines in childhood, but some adolescents still require a second MMR to complete their series.

4. How about hepatitis B?

The hepatitis B series is now recommended for all children and adolescents. The series consists of three vaccinations, with the second shot given 1 month and the third shot given 6–12 months after the first. One recent regimen called for a two-shot series, using vaccines from specific companies in those who are 11–15 years of age. It is now accepted that a time delay in completing the two- or three-shot series does not pose a problem.

5. Should teenagers be immunized against varicella?

Immunization against varicella is recommended for adolescents who have not had clinical evidence of chicken pox. One shot is required for those who are 12 years of age and younger; two shots given at least 1 month apart are required for those who are 13 years of age and older. Some clinicians choose to test for immunity and give the vaccine only to adolescents who are seronegative, because there is a reasonable chance of immunity even in those who are unaware of previous exposure.

6. Which additional immunizations should adolescents with chronic illness receive?

As recommended in a recent statement by the AAP, the Centers for Disease Control and Prevention (CDC), and several other national organizations, pneumococcal and influenza vaccines are recommended for adolescents with specific chronic illnesses. Pneumococcal polysaccharide vaccine is recommended as a single shot for adolescents with the following conditions:

- Anatomic or functional asplenia (including sickle cell disease)
- Nephrotic syndrome
- Cerebrospinal fluid leaks
- Conditions associated with immunosuppression (including HIV).

Influenza vaccine is recommended annually for the following adolescents:

- Those who have chronic cardiac or pulmonary disease (including asthma)
- Those who live in facilities with others who have chronic illnesses
- Those who have required care during the preceding year because of a chronic metabolic disease (including diabetes mellitus), renal dysfunction, hemoglobinopathy, or immunosuppression
- Those who receive long-term aspirin therapy and therefore might be at risk for the development of Reye syndrome after influenza

7. Should adolescents be immunized against meningococcal meningitis?

Because of sporadic outbreaks of meningococcal meningitis on some college campuses and the potential fatal consequences and public health implications of the illness, the AAP recommends that all college students, especially first-year students living away from home, receive one dose of meningococcal vaccine. Currently available immunizations cover types A, C, Y, and W, which are responsible for approximately one-half of all cases, but do not cover type B, which is responsible for the remaining half. Immunizations are given either as part of the pre-entry physical examination or during mass immunization efforts on campus. The CDC has agreed that consideration should be given to this approach, although there is some concern about the financial implications.

8. Which adolescents should be immunized against hepatitis A?

Hepatitis A vaccine (HAV) was first licensed in the United States in 1995. It is given as two or three shots, depending on formulation, and has been recommended by the CDC for (1) those traveling to an endemic region internationally; (2) those living in communities with high rates of hepatitis A and periodic outbreaks nationally; (3) gay males; (4) users of illicit injection drugs; (5) those working closely with nonhuman primates; (6) those with chronic liver disease; and (7) those with clotting factor disorders. More recently, the CDC has recommended routine HAV for children and adolescents who live in states where the incidence of hepatitis A is twice the national average of ≥ 10 cases per 100,000 population (Arizona, Alaska, Oregon, New Mexico, Utah, Washington, Oklahoma, South Dakota, Idaho, Nevada, California) and consideration of routine immunization of children and adolescents in states with an incidence of 10–20 cases per 100,000 population (Missouri, Texas, Colorado, Arkansas, Montana, Wyoming). The CDC acknowledges that various strategies may be needed to accomplish widespread vaccination in all of these states. The CDC also recommends routine immunization in communities during specific outbreaks.

9. When and how should adolescents be screened for tuberculosis (TB)?

A recent report from the CDC and the American Thoracic Society (ATS) recommends that tuberculin skin testing should not be performed routinely in low-risk people but should be reserved for those with specific risk factors. Adolescents at risk include the following:
- Those who are close contacts of persons with active TB disease
- Those who live in or come from an area with a high prevalence of disease
- Those who live or work in institutional settings (e.g., prisons, homeless shelters, hospitals, and chronic care facilities)
- Those who have conditions associated with progression of tuberculosis (e.g., HIV infection, injection drug use, chronic illnesses that lead to immunocompromise, or prolonged steroid and other immunosuppressive therapy)

Routine testing of adolescents may still be performed in some settings. For example, many colleges still require routine TB testing before admission, and some clinicians still perform routine testing in their clinics and practices. All testing is performed using purified protein derivative (PPD); the multipronged tine test is no longer considered an appropriate screening test.

10. How should a positive tuberculin test be interpreted and evaluated?

The CDC and ATS recommend that a PPD test be read as positive based on specific risk criteria. A PPD ≥ 5 mm is considered positive in people with HIV, recent exposure to a person with active TB, evidence of old disease on x-ray, a history of organ transplantation, or other immunocompromised conditions. People with other risk factors (listed in question 9) should be considered positive with a PPD ≥ 10 mm, whereas those who are at low risk should be considered positive only if the PPD is ≥ 15 mm. A medical examination and chest x-ray are required for those with a positive PPD; prophylactic medication (generally isoniazid) is prescribed for those with a negative chest x-ray, whereas multidrug therapy is required for those with active disease.

11. How often should adolescents be seen for routine preventive health care?

Most authorities recommend that adolescents be seen yearly for a routine preventive health visit. The GAPS, AAP, and Bright Futures guidelines make this recommendation explicitly, citing the need to evaluate the changes that take place in adolescents annually, especially in the psychosocial realm. The USPSTF and AAFP do not make specific recommendations, citing the need for more research to determine the optimal interval for preventive visits and screening procedures. The GAPS guidelines recommend performing a physical examination only three times during adolescence but continue to recommend a screening visit annually. This recommendation has met with opposition from parents, physicians, and insurance companies.

12. What laboratory tests should be performed routinely in all adolescents?

Few laboratory tests are recommended for all adolescents as part of routine health screening. In fact, most of the official guidelines include no routine laboratory testing at all, although the AAP continues to recommend a routine hemoglobin and urinalysis once during the adolescent years. Some tests are recommended for adolescents with specific risk factors (such as those who are sexually active or at risk for hyperlipidemia, as described below), and many clinicians will undoubtedly continue to perform simple tests (such as hemoglobin determinations and urinalysis). Nonetheless, most routine tests, including some tests performed previously (such as sickle cell screening), do not have an appropriate cost-benefit ratio that warrants their continuation.

13. How should screening for obesity and eating disorders be performed?

Weight and height should be recorded and plotted on a growth chart at all adolescent preventive health visits. Unexplained weight loss in any adolescent or failure to achieve appropriate increases in weight or height in growing children and early adolescents should cause concern about a possible eating disorder. Conversely, undue increases in weight should cause concern about obesity. Questions about eating habits and body image should be asked of all adolescents, especially those in whom the growth curve reveals a cause for concern. Measurement of body mass index (BMI = wt in kg/[ht in m]^2), can help in the evaluation and monitoring of both eating disorders and obesity.

14. Which screening tests are recommended for sexually active adolescents?

A pelvic examination and Pap smear are recommended annually for all sexually active females. Annual screening for chlamydial and gonococcal infection is also recommended. Chlamydia and gonorrhea testing are performed using endocervical specimens in girls; screening for urethritis may be performed using urinary leukocyte esterase in boys. Newly available ligase chain reaction (LCR) testing is recommended by some authorities, using either urine or cervical samples, but these tests are expensive. Visual inspection for herpes and human papillomavirus is recommended in all sexually active adolescents, and a serologic test for syphilis is recommended for those considered at risk (i.e., living in an endemic area, history of another STI, more than one sexual partner in past 6 months, gay males, those who have exchanged sex for money).

15. Should cholesterol screening be performed routinely in all adolescents?

Official guidelines recommend that cholesterol screening should not be performed in all adolescents (universal screening) but should be reserved instead for those with specific risk factors (selected screening). The National Cholesterol Education Program Expert Panel on Blood Cholesterol Levels in Children and Adolescents has recommended obtaining a nonfasting cholesterol level in adolescents who have a history of (1) cardiovascular disease at less than 55 years of age in a parent or grandparent; (2) hyperlipidemia in a parent; or (3) smoking, hypertension, physical inactivity, obesity, or diabetes mellitus (at the discretion of the practitioner). Universal screening of one cholesterol value is recommended in early adulthood, and a fasting lipid profile is indicated for all adolescents and young adults with an elevated cholesterol value on nonfasting screening.

16. What risk factors should prompt a clinician to test adolescents for HIV?

As recommended by GAPS, adolescents at risk for HIV infection should be offered confidential HIV screening with the enzyme-linked immunosorbent assay (ELISA) and confirmatory test. Adolescents considered at risk are those who have used intravenous drugs, had an STI, lived in an area with a high prevalence of STIs and HIV, had more than one sexual partner in the past six months, exchanged sex for drugs, are males who have engaged in sex with other males, or have a partner at risk for HIV infection. Appropriate pretest and posttest counseling must be available for all adolescents who receive HIV testing.

17. Should adolescents have routine vision and hearing tests?

Despite lack of agreement in the official recommendations from national organizations, it is generally recommended that all adolescents be evaluated for myopia, because adolescence is the age at which onset is most likely. Additional vision testing (strabismus, color) is not recommended routinely. Routine hearing tests are recommended only for adolescents with regular exposure to loud noises (rock concerts, occupational exposure or firearms). The congenital and infectious causes of decreased hearing found in children are not generally applicable to adolescents.

18. What factors in adolescents are important in the prevention of cardiovascular disease in adulthood?

Risk factors for cardiovascular disease in adults that may be apparent during the adolescent years include:

- A positive family history of early-onset cardiovascular disease or hyperlipidemia
- Hypertension, as determined by comparison with age-appropriate parameters
- Elevated total cholesterol levels (more specifically, increased low-density lipoprotein levels and/or decreased high-density lipoprotein levels)
- Obesity, as determined on weight and height curves or by body mass index calculations
- Diabetes mellitus (either type 1 or type 2)
- Smoking
- Lack of physical exercise
- Emotional stress (although the exact level of risk caused by emotional factors is still to be fully elucidated)

Therefore, all teens should have annual blood pressure and BMI evaluations, receive counseling about the benefits of a healthy diet and regular physical activity, and be assisted with smoking cessation.

19. Should a breast examination be performed in and taught to all female adolescents?

Although breast examination is included in the physical examination of most adolescent females, the GAPS guidelines do not specifically advocate its performance as part of the routine health care visit. GAPS cites lack of evidence that the breast examination in adolescent females is beneficial, since development of breast cancer during adolescence is so rare. Teaching of the breast examination to female adolescents, which was once a mainstay of health education efforts, has now been given less importance by most authorities. Research shows that most adolescents do not follow through on the teaching, that it leads to increased anxiety in those who do, and that those who find a mass are most likely to detect a benign lesion, which leads to unnecessary surgery in most cases. Of late, questions have even been raised about the teaching of the breast examination to adult women for the same reasons.

20. Should a testicular examination be performed on and taught to all adolescent males?

Because testicular cancer is most common in the adolescent and young adult age group, performing and teaching these examinations to adolescent males are more appropriate than breast examination in adolescent females. The AAP, AAFP, Bright Futures, and USPSPF include testicular examination in their recommendations. GAPS does not specifically recommend testicular examination or teaching as part of the routine health visit.

21. Should all adolescents be screened for scoliosis?

As is the case for breast and testicular screening, GAPS does not include scoliosis screening in its recommendations. GAPS bases its opinion on a lack of evidence that the cost of screening, including the evaluation of large numbers of adolescents with positive findings, is worth the savings achieved for the few adolescents who are spared surgery. However, most clinicians believe that scoliosis screening should be included in the annual physical examination. The screening should begin in childhood, preferably before the adolescent growth spurt. The use of a scoliometer, a device that looks like a carpenter's plane and measures the angle of trunk rotation, can help prevent unnecessary x-rays and orthopedic referrals. An angle of less than 5° on the scoliometer implies a minimal chance of having an angle of 20° or more on x-ray, for which bracing would be recommended.

22. What topics should be included in the health guidance provided to adolescents during a routine health visit?

Health guidance may be provided through discussions with physicians and other clinical staff or the use of appropriate questionnaires, computer programs, and/or literature. Topics that should be included in the health guidance provided to adolescents include the following:

1. **Sexuality education**, including the advantages of abstinence, the use of condoms and other methods of birth control, and counseling about protection from STIs, HIV, and sexual exploitation.

2. **Substance use counseling**. The avoidance or cessation of use of cigarettes, alcohol, other abusable substances, and anabolic steroids should be discussed, encouraged, and implemented.

3. **Injury prevention**. Topics of discussion include use of seat belts, bicycle/motorcycle helmets, and athletic protective equipment; avoidance of alcohol and other substances while using motor vehicles, playing sports or swimming; and avoidance of weapon use, promotion of weapon safety, and resolution of conflicts without violence.

4. **Nutrition and exercise**. Guidance should be provided about the use of a healthy diet, appropriate weight management, and regular exercise.

5. **General health care**. Ensuring that adolescents receive regular dental care, use sun protection, and are aware of normal physical and emotional development is recommended by national guidelines.

23. What is known about the success of smoking prevention and smoking cessation programs offered to adolescents?

Smoking prevention programs have generally been offered to children and adolescents in school-based settings, most commonly in junior high school classes. Data have shown that these programs have short-term effects in delaying the onset of smoking for some people but minimal effects on lowering the numbers of adolescents who begin smoking over the long term. In contrast to prevention programs, most smoking cessation programs are offered in office- and clinic-based settings.

24. Are drug and alcohol prevention programs effective in adolescents?

Drug and alcohol prevention programs for adolescents have been available for over 30 years. Evidence indicates that initial programs, which were based purely on education, did not have beneficial effects (and at times may have actually increased drug use in the targeted populations). More recent programs, based on skills training and social influence models, have had varying success, depending on the follow-up period, experimental design, adolescents' risk status, and which substances are studied.

BIBLIOGRAPHY

1. American Academy of Family Physicians: Age charts for periodic health examinations. Kansas City, MO, American Academy of Family Physicians, 1994.
2. American Adacemy of Pediatrics, Committee on Infectious Diseases: Immunizations of adolescents: Recommendations of the Advisory Committee on Immunization Practices, the American Academy of Pediatrics, the American Academy of Family Physicians, and the American Medical Association. Pediatrics 99:479–487, 1997.
3. American Academy of Pediatrics, Committee on Infectious Diseases: Meningococcal disease prevention and control strategies for practice-based physicians [Addendum: Recommendations for college students]. Pediatrics 106:1500–1504, 2000.
4. American Academy of Pediatrics: Report of the Committee on Infectious Diseases. Elk Grove Village, IL, American Academy of Pediatrics, 2000.
5. American Academy of Pediatrics, Committee on Psychosocial Aspects of Child and Family Health 1995–1996: Guidelines for Health Supervision III. Elk Grove Village, IL, American Academy of Pediatrics, 1997.
6. American Thoracic Society and Centers for Disease Control and Prevention: Targeted tuberculin testing and treatment of latent tuberculosis infection. Am J Respir Crit Care Med 1161:S221–S247, 2000.

7. Botvin GJ, Botvin EM: Adolescent tobacco, alcohol, and drug abuse: Prevention strategies, empirical findings, and assessment issues. J Devel Behav Pediatr 13:290–301, 1992.

8. Bruvold WH: A meta-analysis of adolescent smoking prevention programs. Am J Public Health 83:872–880, 1993.

9. Centers for Disease Control and Prevention: Meningococcal disease and college students: Recommendations of the Advisory Committee on Immunization Practices (ACIP). MMWR 49: 11–20, 2000.

10. Centers for Disease Control and Prevention: Prevention of hepatitis A through active or positive immunization: Recommendations of the Advisory Committee on Immunization Practices (ACIP). MMWR 48:1–37, 1999.

11. Elster AB: Comparison of recommendations for adolescent clinical preventive services developed by national organizations. Arch Pediatr Adolesc Med 152:193–198, 1998.

12. Elster AB, Kuznets NJ: Guidelines for Adolescent Preventive Services (GAPS): Recommendations and Rationale. Baltimore, William & Wilkins, 1992.

13. Fisher M: Adolescent health assessment and promotion in office and school settings. Adolesc Med State Art Rev 10:71–86, 1999.

14. Goldbloom RB: Self-examination by adolescents. Pediatrics 76:126–128, 1985.

15. Green M (ed): Bright Futures: Guidelines for Health Supervision of Infants, Children and Adolescents. Arlington, VA, National Center for Education in Maternal and Child Health, 1994.

16. Greydanus DE, Patel DR, Rimsza ME: Contraception in the adolescent: An update. Pediatrics 107:562–573, 2001.

17. Jenkins RR, Saxena SB: Keeping adolescents healthy. Contemp Pediatr 12:76–89, 1995.

18. Kautz SM, Skaggs DL: Getting an angle on spinal deformities. Contemp Pediatr 15:111–127, 1998.

19. Marks A, Fisher M: Health assessment and screening during adolescence. Pediatrics 80:133–158, 1987.

20. National Cholesterol Education Program: Highlights of the Report of the Expert Panel on Blood Cholesterol Levels in Children and Adolescents. Pediatrics 89:495–501, 1992.

21. National High Blood Pressure Education Program Working Group on Hypertension Control in Children and Adolescents: Update on the 1987 Task Force Report on high blood pressure in children and adolescents: A Working Group report from the National High Blood Pressure Education Program. Pediatrics 98:649–658, 1996.

22. Poland GA: Adolescent hepatitis B immunization: Making it simpler. Pediatrics 107:771–772, 2001.

23. U.S. Preventive Services Task Force: Guide to Clinical Preventive Services, 2nd ed. Baltimore, Williams & Wilkins, 1996.

24. U.S. Peventive Services Task Force: Screening for adolescent idiopathic scoliosis: Review article. JAMA 269:2667–2672, 1993.

25. Windle M, Windle RC: Adolescent tobacco, alcohol and drug use: Current findings. Adoles Med State Art Rev 10:153–164, 1999.

4. ADOLESCENT GROWTH AND DEVELOPMENT

Robert T. Brown, M.D.

1. What is unique about growth and development during adolescence?

Growth and development during adolescence, composed of physical, cognitive, and psychosocial aspects, occurs more rapidly and in more ways than at any other time in extrauterine life.

2. What are the components of growth and development?

Growth and development include pubertal changes and physical growth, cognitive development, and psychosocial development.

3. Define puberty.

Puberty is the period of biologic development in which the body of the child is transformed into that of an adult with the attendant growth in size and development of reproductive capability.

4. How long does puberty last?

The entire process of puberty can take as little as 3–4 years or as much as 4–7 years. Reproductive capability can be achieved within 2–3 years after the onset of puberty. Puberty should progress from Tanner stage 2 to stage 5 (see question 9 for explanation of Tanner stages) in boys in approximately 4 years, the same time within which girls must progress from Tanner stage 2 to menarche.

5. How early and how late can puberty start and still be normal?

Puberty can begin as early as 6 or 7 years of age in girls, particularly African-American girls, and as late as 13 years. In boys, puberty can start as early as 8 years and as late as 13.5 years of age.

6. What makes puberty begin?

No one knows exactly what instigates the changes of puberty at any particular time, but we do know that puberty starts with a desensitization of the arcuate nucleus of the hypothalamus to circulating gonadal steroid (estrogen and testosterone) levels.

7. What gonadal hormonal changes occur during puberty?

Estrogen and testosterone rise to adult levels with stimulation from the pituitary gonadotropins, luteinizing hormone (LH) and follicle-stimulating hormone (FSH), which in turn are stimulated by the gonadotropin-releasing hormone (GnRH) from the hypothalamus, also known as luteinizing hormone-releasing hormone (LHRH). (See figure, next page.)

8. Which comes first: height growth or development of secondary sex characteristics?

Desensitization of the hypothalamus to circulating gonadal steroids with consequent rise in levels of gonadal steroids (estrogen or testosterone) precedes increase in height growth velocity, as is evident from the fact that puberty begins before the period of peak height velocity.

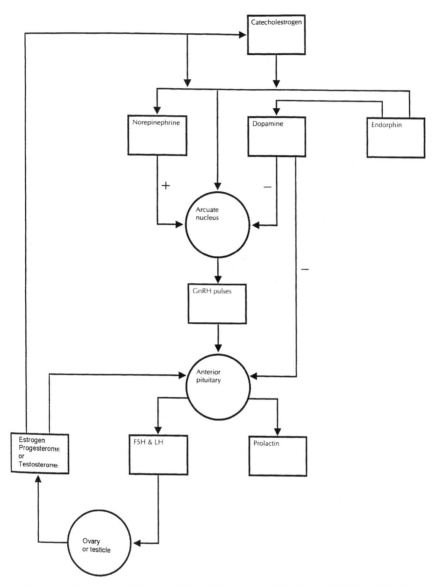

Hypothalamic-pituitary-gonadal axis. (Adapted from Speroff L, Glass RH, Kase NG: Neuroendocrinology. In Clinical Gynecologic Endocrinology and Infertility. Baltimore, Williams & Wilkins, 1994, p 159.)

9. What are Tanner stages? Why are they used to describe pubertal changes?

J.M. Tanner, an English pediatric endocrinologist, first described a system of documenting progress through puberty using the physical configurations of secondary sex characteristics. This system is more accurate than chronologic age in timing pubertal changes and correlates to a large degree with skeletal maturation. Tanner described the configurational changes of the breast and pubic hair pattern in girls and of the genital and pubic hair configuration in boys. He assigned to each gender 5 stages of development, with stage 1 being childlike and stage 5 being adult.

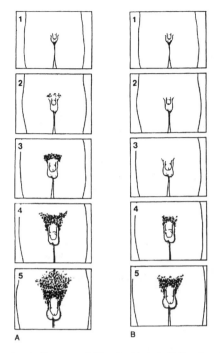

Sexual maturity stages. *A*, Boys' pubic hair. *B*, Boys' genitalia.

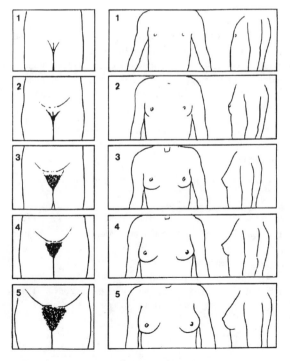

Sexual maturity stages. *A*, Girls' pubic hair. *B*, Girls' breasts.

10. When is puberty precocious?

Puberty is considered to be precocious or to have begun too early if it begins before age 6 in African-American girls or age 7 in Caucasian girls. In boys, precocious puberty is defined as testicular and genital enlargement before age 8.

11. What is the period of peak height velocity?

The period of peak height velocity, also known as the pubertal growth spurt, is the period during puberty when the growth rate accelerates from about 5 cm/year during childhood to possibly 15 cm or more in just a few months. After the growth spurt, adolescents' growth rates decline rapidly, and growth stops 2 or 3 years later.

12. How does puberty differ between boys and girls?

Puberty, on average, occurs about 2 years earlier in girls than in boys. During puberty, girls go through the period of peak height velocity earlier (Tanner stage 2–3), than boys (Tanner stage 3–4).

13. When during puberty does menarche occur?

Menarche, or the first menstrual period, usually occurs when a girl has reached Tanner stage 3–4 breast development. In some girls menarche can occur as late as Tanner stage 4–5.

14. At what age is menarche considered delayed?

If a girl has not had her first period by 4 years after her breasts begin to develop, she is considered to have primary amenorrhea.

15. What defines delayed puberty?

Puberty is considered to be delayed if it has not begun by 12.5 years in girls or 13.5 years in boys.

16. What functions can knowledge of Tanner stages serve?

Knowledge of Tanner stages can allow a physician to gauge more accurately the progress of physical development in an adolescent. Tanner stages also can be used to provide adolescents with an easy way to follow their own development. Tanner stages correlate with other changes, such as laboratory tests (e.g., hematocrits/hemoglobins and serum alkaline phosphatase). Knowledge of Tanner stages also can assist in diagnosis of certain pathologic developmentally related conditions, such as slipped capital femoral epiphysis, Osgood-Schlatter syndrome, and scoliosis.

17. How are the Tanner stages defined in girls and boys?

Tanner stage secondary sex characteristics are depicted in the figures in question 9. Explanations are given in the tables below.

Classification of Genital Maturity Stages in Boys (Tanner Ratings)

STAGE	PUBIC HAIR	PENIS	TESTES
1	None	Preadolescent	Preadolescent
2	Scanty, long, slightly pigmented	Slight enlargement	Enlarged scrotum, pink, texture changed
3	Darker, begins to curl, small amount	Longer	Larger
4	Resembles adult type, but less in quantity; coarse curly	Larger; glans and breadth increase in size	Larger; scrotum darker
5	Adult distribution, spread to medial thighs	Adult	Adult

Adapted from Daniel WA Jr: Adolescents in Health and Disease. St. Louis, Mosby, 1977.

Classification of Genital Maturity Stages in Girls (Tanner Ratings)

STAGE	PUBIC HAIR	BREASTS
1	Preadolescent	Preadolescent
2	Sparse, slightly pigmented, straight, at medial border of labia	Breast and papilla elevated as small mound, areolar diameter increased
3	Darker, beginning to curl, increased amount	Breast and areola enlarged, without contour separation
4	Coarse, curly, abundant, but amount less than in adult	Areola and papilla form secondary mound
5	Adult feminine triangle, spread to medial surface of thighs	Mature, nipple projects, areola part of general breast contour

Adapted from Daniel WA Jr: Adolescents in Health and Disease. St. Louis, Mosby, 1977.

18. Is breast development normal in boys?

In 50–65% of adolescent boys, there is some breast enlargement or gynecomastia, usually in Tanner stages 3–4. The enlargement is bilateral in about one-half to two-thirds of cases and usually resolves by Tanner stage 5 or within 3 years of onset. Free testosterone levels may be slightly lower in such boys.

19. What is cognitive development?

Cognitive development is the progession of thinking abilities from the characteristics of a child's mind to those of an adult. According to Piaget and his followers, the mind can progress through distinct stages of thinking capabilities during childhood and into adulthood. These stages are characterized by the incorporation of behavior patterns into thinking patterns and may synchronize with observable (on positron-emission tomography scans) changes of the adolescent brain to the adult brain.

20. What cognitive stages are important to adolescents?

Children from 7–12 years old are said to think in a concrete manner. They can consider mentally only things with which they have direct contact or knowledge. At about the age of 12, the child begins to be able to think in what Piaget calls a formal operational manner. The characteristics of formal operational thought include the ability to generate abstractions and hypotheses; to consider contrary-to-fact situations; to generate all possibilities from a specific situation; to approach a problem in a systematic fashion; and to use combinatory logic.

21. Does an adolescent necessarily proceed from concrete to abstract thinking?

No. If the potential for formal thought is not nurtured, it does not develop well, and the person may remain a concrete thinker for life. In some cognitive areas an adolescent may become more adept as a formal thinker than in others (e.g., academic subjects vs. social situations).

22. How can adolescents be helped to think like adults?

Stimulation by schoolwork and by conversations and intellectual challenges at home and at school can help an adolescent to develop formal operational thinking skills.

23. Why is understanding of cognitive development important to clinicians?

Clinicians must tailor their questions, explanations, and instructions to the cognitive developmental level of patients if they are to be understood. A concrete thinker cannot understand a clinician who uses abstract, formal operational concepts when asking questions or giving explanations and instructions.

24. What is psychosocial development? What are its tasks?

Psychosocial development is the development of the ability to understand the self, its relation to others, and its place in the overall scheme of things. Development in this arena can be viewed as the achieving of competency in four tasks:

1. Developing independence
2. Developing mature sexuality
3. Developing a realistic vocational goal
4. Developing a mature and positive self-image

25. How can independence best be fostered?
Parents can best foster independence by giving adolescents responsibilities commensurate with their maturational levels and by allowing them to take measured risks. This process really begins in childhood.

26. What are the hallmarks of developing independence in early, middle, and late adolescence?
Early adolescence, which can be defined as ages 10–13, is marked by alternation of a gut-level striving for independence in same-sex peer groups without much thought and a desire for parental support and nurturance. Middle adolescence (14–16 years) is characterized by associating with mixed-sex peer groups and intellectual challenging of parents. Late adolescence (17–21 years) is characterized by shedding the need for peer group support and striving to achieve adult status while realizing that parents are colleagues and friends to be valued.

27. Define sexuality.
Sexuality can be defined as the physical characteristics of and capacities for specific sex behaviors, together with psychosocial values, norms, attitudes, and learning processes that influence such behaviors. It also includes a sense of gender identity and related concepts, behaviors, and attitudes about the self and others as women and men in the context of society.

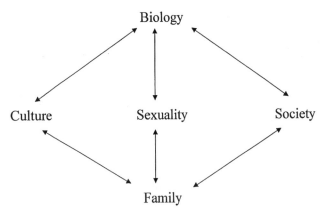

Factors influencing development of sexuality. (Adapted from Brown RT, Cromer BA: Adolescent sexuality. In Sanfilippo JS, Muram D, Lee PA, et al (eds): Pediatric and Adolescent Gynecology. Philadelphia, W.B. Saunders, 1994, p 278.

28. What factors define sexuality?
Biology (both genotype and phenotype), family, culture, and society define sexuality. Biology via genotype and phenotype defines basic sexuality, which is modified by family role models for male and female behaviors, the culture within whose norms families function, and society, which informs each of its cultures with common influences.

29. What are the hallmarks of developing sexuality in early, middle, and late adolescence?
Early adolescent sexuality is characterized by thoughts and feelings usually about the opposite gender with little activity. Middle adolescents enter mixed-sex peer groups and begin to have short, intense "love" relationships characterized by trying to find the ideal partner. Late

adolescents enter into more permanent relationships in which each partner begins to care as much about the other partner as about the self.

30. What problems can result from defining sexuality?

An adolescent may discover that he or she cares more for the same gender sexually. Realizing and beginning to act on feelings for the same sex engenders a series of potential problems not faced by heterosexual youth. On the other hand, heterosexual girls can have problems exploring their sexuality safely if they do not have an effective father figure against whom they can safely express their sexuality with no fear of inappropriate response. They then may seek an older partner who will be more prone to involve them in risky sexual behavior.

31. What are the behavioral markers of developing sexuality?

Dating, exploring physical sexual activity, and spending more time with a romantic partner are hallmarks of developing sexuality.

32. How many adolescents experience sexual intercourse?

Less than 50% of adolescents have had sexual intercourse by the time they are seniors in high school. This is a significant decrease from the rates in the early 1990's.

33. Can adolescents who are virgins participate in sexual behaviors?

Adolescents who have yet to experience vaginal sexual intercourse may nevertheless be involved in sexual activity such as mutual masturbation, fellatio, cunnilingus, and anal intercourse. Therefore, adolescents need to be counseled about risks of these behaviors as well as the risks of vaginal intercourse.

34. Do adolescents who have sexual intercourse protect themselves against negative consequences?

Approximately three-fourths of sexually active adolescents use contraception. Rates of condom use at last intercourse are as high as 70%, particularly when intercourse is with a new or casual partner.

35. How is choosing a vocation a psychosocial task?

Choosing a vocation that fits one's desires and abilities requires self-knowledge that can be obtained only with significant cognitive development. In our society, adolescents must be on the road to a career area, but not a specific job, before they can be said to be leaving adolescence.

36. What kind of self-image best correlates with personal efficacy?

A realistic and positive self-image best correlates with personal efficacy. This self-image can be difficult to obtain and may be a goal toward which one strives throughout life.

37. How is a positive self-image best fostered?

A positive self-image in an adolescent is best fostered with unconditional parental love and praise for jobs well done and by allowing children and adolescents to take on challenges and to risk failure.

BIBLIOGRAPHY

1. Brown RT: Adolescent sexuality at the dawn of the 21st century. Adolesc Med State Art Revs 11:19, 2000.
2. Campbell FA, Pungello EP, Miller-Johnson S, et al: The development of cognitive and academic abilities: Growth curves from an early childhood educational experiment. Dev Psychol 37:231–242, 2001.
3. Kulin HE, Müller J: The biological basis of puberty. Pediatr Rev 17:75, 1996.
4. Luna B, Thulborn KR, Munoz DP, et al: Maturation of widely distributed brain function subserves cognitive development. Neuroimage 13:786–793, 2001.

5. Piaget J: Science of Education and the Psychology of the Child (translated by D. Coltman). New York, Orion Press, 1970.
6. Sowell ER, Delis D, Stiles J, Jernigan TL: Improved memory functioning and frontal lobe maturation between childhood and adolescence: A structural MRI study. J Int Neuropsychol Soc 7:312–322, 2001.
7. Strasburger VC, Brown RT: Adolescent Medicine: A Practical Guide, 2nd ed. Philadelphia, Lippincott-Raven, 1998, pp 1–11.
8. Tanner JM: Growth at Adolescence, 2nd ed. Oxford, Blackwell Scientific, 1962.

5. ADOLESCENTS WITH CHRONIC CONDITIONS

Robert T. Brown, M.D., and Cynthia Holland-Hall, M.D., M.P.H.

1. What makes a condition chronic?

A chronic condition is one that will not resolve in the foreseeable future.

2. How many adolescents have chronic health conditions?

According to best estimates, approximately 35% of adolescents have at least one chronic disorder (of at least 3 months' duration).

3. What are the most common chronic health conditions among adolescents?

The most common chronic health conditions in adolescents are respiratory allergies, asthma, and recurrent and severe headaches. Atopic dermatitis and other skin allergies, frequent ear infections, digestive allergies, and musculoskeletal impairments are the next most common entities.

4. What are the most common chronic health conditions associated with significant disability?

The most common chronic health conditions with significant morbidity are asthma and musculoskeletal impairments, followed by heart disease, significant hearing impairment, and significant vision impairment.

5. Are there demographic differences in rates of significant chronic health conditions?

Yes. Adolescents who are poor have higher rates of serious chronic health conditions.

6. What factors can affect the health status of adolescents with chronic health conditions?

- When in the patient's life the problem was acquired (during adolescence is more difficult)
- Whether the problem was congenital or acquired after birth
- If acquired during adolescence, in which psychosocial stage it was acquired (effect of acquiring the condition varies based on the tasks of the stage of development)
- Whether the problem is progressive or static (static is easier to deal with)
- Whether the problem is constantly present or episodic; if episodic, whether the occurrences are predictable or not (unpredictable is more difficult to cope with)
- The degree of difficulty imposed on daily life by the actual mechanics of coping with the chronic problem
- Whether the problem is visible and, if it is, to what degree the problem is disfiguring (not visible may be more difficult because it is easier to deny)
- The attitudes of parents, siblings, and peers
- The way in which society views this particular type of condition
- The coping mechanisms that the adolescent uses to deal with the problem (denial, projection, regression, anger, adjustment, acceptance)
- The degree of medical care needed for the condition

7. What role do parents play in the adjustment of adolescents to a chronic health condition?

The attitude and behaviors of parents are critical in helping an adolescent with a chronic health condition to adapt adequately. Parents can feel anxiety, guilt, anger, and depression.

They can use denial as a coping mechanism. With good preventive counseling, parents can learn to recognize their reactions and not to allow natural emotions to have a detrimental effect on the adolescent's ability to cope with the condition.

8. Why do parents of adolescents with health problems feel guilt?

Guilt is a normal emotion in any parent whose child has a chronic health condition. Sometimes feelings of guilt are generated by perceived or actual behaviors or events, and sometimes guilt arises simply because the parents wonder whether they could have done anything to prevent the child's problems. Counseling about the normalcy of guilt and how to overcome it without letting it hurt the child is critical to good parental adjustment and effective coping with the child's condition.

9. Does guilt have negative consequences?

Unresolved guilt can lead to anger at the child and to consequent overcompensation in the form of being overly attentive to the child's needs or distancing from the child emotionally or even physically. The child of a parent who feels guilty can be made to feel as if his or her problem is more important than the child itself.

10. What does transition mean for adolescents with chronic health conditions?

Transition is the passage from the dependency of adolescence to the self-responsibility of adulthood. For an adolescent with a chronic health condition this passage includes switching from child health care clinicians to adult health care clinicians; from being asexual to becoming a person who can express his or her sexuality; from being financially and vocationally dependent to becoming independent in these spheres; and from dependent living to independent living.

11. What can clinicians do to help these transitions?

Clinicians can help by recognizing that adolescents with chronic health conditions have certain rights:
- The right to sexual expression
- The right to privacy
- The right to be informed
- The right to access needed services
- The right to choose marital status
- The right to choose whether to have children
- The right to develop their fullest potential

12. What are the health care goals for adolescents with a chronic health condition?
- Possession of enough information to understand their chronic condition
- Opportunity to associate with nonhandicapped persons of the same age
- Opportunity to have some experience of living on their own
- Opportunity to learn about different occupations and careers
- Chance to talk with someone about a personal problem
- Work experience
- Opportunity to participate in an educational program at the appropriate level
- Opportunity to do household tasks
- Chance to talk with someone about physical abilities and disabilities
- Opportunity to learn social graces
- Opportunity to earn money
- Opportunity to develop a hobby
- Availability of a comprehensive sex education program

CHRONIC FATIGUE

13. When is fatigue considered chronic?
The definition of chronic fatigue syndrome (CFS) requires 6 months of unremitting fatigue. Adolescents who are tired without relief for 3 or more months can be said to be chronically fatigued without having the syndrome.

14. What conditions can lead to chronic fatigue in adolescents?
Lack of sleep, anemia, poor diet, lack of fluid intake, hypothyroidism, chronic illness, and postviral chronic fatigue of adolescence.

15. How does chronic fatigue in adolescents differ from CFS in adults?
Chronic fatigue in adolescents can be of shorter duration and frequently does not meet all of the criteria of CFS. It is also much more likely to resolve.

Centers for Disease Control and Prevention Case Definition of Chronic Fatigue Syndrome

1. CFS is characterized by fatigue that is:
   - Medically unexplained
   - Of new onset
   - Of at least 6 months' duration
   - Not the result of ongoing exertion
   - Not substantially relieved by rest
   - Causes substantial reduction in previous levels of occupational, educational, social or personal activities

2. In addition, there must be four or more of the following symptoms:
   - Impaired memory or concentration
   - Sore throat
   - Tender neck (cervical) or armpit (axillary) lymph nodes
   - Muscle pain (myalgia)
   - Headaches of a new type, pattern, or severity
   - Unrefreshing sleep
   - Postexertional malaise (lasting more than 24 hours)
   - Multijoint pain (arthralgia without swelling or redness)

Conditions that exclude a diagnosis of CFS include other medical disorders known to cause fatigue, major depressive illness, medication that causes fatigue as a side effect, and alcohol or substance abuse

From Fukuda F, et al: The chronic fatigue syndrome: A comprehensive approach to its definition and study. Ann Intern Med 121:953–959, 1994, with permission.

16. If common medical problems are ruled out, what else may cause chronic fatigue?
Experts are unsure, but the condition in adolescents frequently seems to follow a viral infection such as influenza or infectious mononucleosis. Whether the problem is a consequence of an aberrant immune reaction to the infection or whether there are behavioral cues after a viral infection remains to be determined.

17. What is the most common cause of fatigue in adolescents?
The most common cause of fatigue in adolescents is lack of sleep. Adolescents need 8–10 hours of sleep each night for optimal rest.

18. How should the diagnostic work-up proceed with a chronically fatigued adolescent?
The first step is a complete history, including activities of daily living such as sleep patterns, eating patterns, stressors, and quality of sleep. The history should point the clinician toward a probable cause. A physical examination can help to confirm the initial impression, and laboratory tests can further the clinician's confidence in the diagnosis.

19. Do adolescents with chronic fatigue improve?

Yes. Over 80% of adolescents who meet the criteria for CFS improve within 4 years. For chronic fatigue of adolescence, few good data are available, but clinicians in the field have the impression that almost all chronically fatigued adolescents return to previous levels of functioning within 2–3 years.

20. How can a clinician assist the recovery of the adolescent with chronic fatigue?

The clinician can first reassure the family that no serious illness, such as cancer, is present. Then the clinician can inform the family of the time-limited nature of the condition and of the things that can be done to help symptoms resolve. Examples include a supervised, slowly increasing exercise/conditioning program, learning to deal with stress more effectively, drinking plenty of fluids, and eating a well-balanced diet.

DEVELOPMENTAL DISABILITIES

21. What is the most important point to remember about an adolescent with a developmental disability?

He or she is still a teenager. Most adolescents with developmental disabilities, particularly those with mild-to-moderate mental retardation, undergo the majority of the developmental tasks that cognitively normal adolescents experience. They go through puberty, have sexual feelings, desire independence and peer affiliation, and begin to make more of their own decisions. They may, however, experience these changes in different ways, and the final outcomes may be different from those achieved by developmentally normal adolescents.

22. What special challenges can adolescence present for people with developmental disabilities?

The adolescent's desire for independence may be countered by the reality that he or she must remain dependent on parents or others to meet certain needs. The capacity for abstract or symbolic thinking may be limited. Physical differences may limit the ability to conform and fit in with peer groups, and acceptance by the peer group may be limited. The capacity to form intimate relationships also may be different from that of peers.

23. How do you take a psychosocial history from an adolescent with a developmental disability?

The biggest mistake that a clinician can make is to assume that an adolescent with a developmental disability is not engaging in potentially risky behaviors. Adolescents who spend time with developmentally normal peers are commonly exposed to drugs and alcohol, may witness or engage in sexual talk and behaviors, and often have challenging interpersonal relationships with peers that may be exacerbated by their differences. Furthermore, their understanding of such situations may be limited, potentially placing them at even greater risk. Ask questions in simple, straightforward language, remembering that adolescents with a developmental disability are typically concrete thinkers. Ask questions both with and without the parent present to get the best yield. This process may be enlightening to a parent who never considered the child with special needs to be at risk.

24. Can adolescents with developmental disabilities experience depression?

Certainly. Patients with mild-to-moderate mental retardation may be keenly aware of the differences between themselves and developmentally normal peers. Some patients—for example, those with Down syndrome—may have physical differences as well as differences in cognitive abilities. The desire to conform and to be accepted by peers is a normal developmental task of adolescence. An adolescent who realizes that he or she will never be just like peers or will never be able to participate fully in certain activities in which peers engage may develop depressive symptoms. Asking the adolescent whether he or she is usually a happy or a sad person and what makes him or her happy or sad may help uncover mood symptoms.

25. How do you talk to an adolescent with a developmental disability about sex?

Begin by determining the adolescent's concept of sex. Ask what the words "boyfriend" and "girlfriend" mean. Ask what the adolescent thinks boyfriends and girlfriends do when they are alone together. Find out if the adolescent is interested in a romantic relationship and whether he or she sees sex as an important part of this relationship. Determine sexual experiences by asking explicitly about kissing, touching, and other sexual behaviors.

Remember that cognitively limited adolescents need explicit, directed education and information about sexuality. They are less likely to experience "incidental learning" about sex from peers and the media, as many adolescents do. They need to learn specific skills to protect themselves from sexual exploitation, to which they are vulnerable.

26. How can you help patients with a developmental disability to avoid sexual abuse or exploitation?

Discuss "public" vs. "private" body parts with the patient, and review which people in the patient's life (e.g., mother, physician) may have legitimate reasons to see or touch the "private" parts and which people do not (e.g., teachers, coaches, schoolmates). Use role playing to explore reactions to inappropriate sexual advances and teach appropriate responses. Model this technique to caregivers so that they can continue such teaching on a regular basis at home, since repetition is critical. Discuss the importance of supervision with the caregivers as well.

27. How should you respond to a parent who says, "You don't need to talk about sex with him. He's not interested in it"?

Discuss and, if appropriate, validate the parent's reasons for believing that the child is not interested in sex. Inform parents that after puberty most adolescents have some biologic sex drive and that it is important to help them manage feelings and urges in ways that are safe for themselves and others. Explore the family's views on masturbation, and explain that from a medical standpoint, masturbation performed in private can be an appropriate and safe outlet for sexual feelings. Again, by modeling candid discussions about sex with the patient in front of the parent, you may help the parent understand that the adolescent can have sexual feelings and how to respond to them.

28. What areas of reproductive health care should you address with patients with a developmental disability and their family?

Adolescents with developmental disabilities may experience delayed or precocious puberty; thus, it is important to review the timing of pubertal changes. Discuss menstrual abnormalities that may occur in girls. Assess the need for contraception, and explore contraceptive options when appropriate. Explain that sexually active adolescents need to be tested for sexually transmitted infections (STIs) and that young adult women need Pap smears periodically. Discuss various options for meeting these needs. Sexually active young men should be screened for STIs, and they and their parents should be taught testicular examination.

29. What menstrual problems may occur in girls with developmental disabilities?

Menorrhagia and premenstrual syndrome are common in girls with Down syndrome. Girls with more profound mental retardation may have worsening aggressive behaviors or seizure activity during menses. Menstrual hygiene may present a challenge in some girls. Hormonal contraception may be appropriate treatment in many cases, including the use of continuous oral contraceptive pills to reduce the frequency of menses.

30. List some tips for performing a gynecologic exam in a young woman with a developmental disability.

- Take your time. Young women with a developmental disability require patience, simple explanations of procedures, and flexibility on the part of the provider.
- Be concrete with your explanations. Use pictures or anatomic dolls if available.

- Allow the patient time to practice. Give her a gown to take home so that she and her mother can practice positioning and review the parts of the exam.
- Be flexible with positioning. Some patients do better on their sides or in frog-leg position than in the traditional lithotomy position.
- Use less-invasive means for STI testing, such as urine testing, when available.
- Consider using ultrasound to evaluate for pelvic pathology if the patient cannot tolerate a bimanual exam.
- Perform a finger-guided Pap smear if the patient cannot tolerate insertion of the speculum.
- If the exam is too challenging or frightening for the patient and you feel it is important to complete it, consider sedation.
- If the exam is for routine screening, consider coordinating it with a future procedure for which the patient will receive sedation or general anesthesia (e.g., MRI or dental work).
- Coercion and force should not be used.

31. What do you tell a parent who wants her mentally retarded daughter sterilized to prevent pregnancy?

State laws vary widely about this issue. In general, parents do not have the right to have cognitively impaired daughters sterilized against their will if they are deemed competent to object. The daughter does not have to demonstrate her competency to raise a child. All possible contraceptive methods should be tried and/or deemed unacceptable before the option of sterilization is considered. If no other means of contraception is medically feasible and sterilization is considered, consult state law and the hospital's ethics committee before proceeding.

BIBLIOGRAPHY

1. Bell DS, Jordan K, Robinson M: Thirteen-year follow-up of children and adolescents with chronic fatigue syndrome. Pediatrics 107:994–998, 2001.
2. Blum RW, Garrell D, Hodgman C, Slap GB: Transition from child-centered to adult health care systems for adolescents with chronic conditions. A position paper of the Society for Adolescent Medicine. J Adolesc Health 14:570–576, 1993.
3. Brown R: Adolescents with psychosomatic problems. Comprehen Ther 22:810–816, 1996.
4. Brown RT, Coupey SM (eds): Chronic and Disabling Disorders. Adolesc Med State Art Rev 5:197–366, 1994.
5. Edwards JP, Elkins TE: Just Between Us: A Social Sexual Guide for Parents and Professionals with Concerns for Persons with Developmental Disabilities. Pro-Ed, Austin, TX, 1988.
6. Gold D, Bowden R, Sixbey J, et al: Chronic fatigue: A prospective clinical and virologic study. JAMA 264:48–53, 1990.
7. Jordan KM, Landis DA, Downey JC, et al: Chronic fatigue syndrome in children and adolescents: A review. J Adolesc Health 22:4–18, 1998.
8. Krilov LR, Fisher M, Friedman SB, et al: Course and outcome of chronic fatigue in children and adolescents. Pediatrics 102:360–366, 1998.
9. Rangel L, Garralda E, Levin M, Roberts H: Personality in adolescents with chronic fatigue syndrome. Eur Child Adolesc Psychiatry 9:39–45, 2000.
10. Strasburger VC, Brown RT: Adolescent Medicine: A Practical Guide, 2nd ed. Philadelphia, Lippincott-Raven, 1998, pp 140–150.

6. NUTRITION

Lynda Peel, M.A., R.D., L.D.

1. What types of beverages are appropriate to replace sweat losses during a sports event or physical activity?

Water is excellent fluid replacement for recreational athletes who participate in physical activity that does not exceed 60–90 minutes. Water and almost any nonalcoholic fluid meet fluid replacement needs:

- Seltzer
- Juice
- Coffee or tea (decaffeinated)
- Herbal tea
- Lemonade
- Sports drinks
- Soups
- Milk
- Smoothies
- Watery foods (oranges, lettuce, tomatoes, cucumbers, watermelon) that are 85–95% water by weight

2. Can soft drinks be used to replace losses? What about diet soda?

Soft drinks are popular thirst quenchers, yet they offer zero nutritional value except for refined sugar-containing beverages, which offer 150 calories in a 10-oz serving. These may have some value in carbohydrate replacement, but natural sugars in juices can also replenish the carbohydrates as well as provide potassium (lost in sweat), vitamin C, and other nutrients.

Some people worry about aspartame in diet soft drinks. Aspartame is composed of two amino acids, aspartic acid and phenylalanine, that naturally occur in protein and exist in high amounts in the diet. Moderation is key for consuming sugar-free drinks. Some athletes fear that carbonation will decrease their performance. Studies indicate no deleterious effects of carbonation on athletic performance.

3. What types of sports drinks are appropriate?

Water is the fluid of choice for most physical activities lasting less than 60–90 minutes. Performance in marathons, hockey, long-distance running, or cross-country skiing (high-intensity endurance events) lasting more than 60–90 minutes can be enhanced by consuming beverages that contain a small amount of sugar (40–80 kcals/8 oz) and sodium (120–180 mg/8 oz). The sugar provides fuel; sodium enhances the body's ability to absorb water. There may be no physiologic need to replace sodium unless the athlete is exercising for more than 4 hours.

4. How should carbohydrates be replaced during high-endurance exercise?

Consuming carbohydrates during exercise provides muscles with added fuel, helps maintain normal blood sugar levels, and increases mental stamina, all of which contribute to increased endurance. Most sports drinks have half the carbohydrates of juices; in other words, one would have to drink 16 oz of a sports drink to get the same amount of carbohydrate in 8 oz of juice to replenish the glycogen burned during the event. If an athlete is snacking on bananas, dried fruits, pretzels, sports bars, or other high-carbohydrate snacks during exercise, water is appropriate as the fluid replacer. If a high-endurance athlete consumes a sports drink 20–45 minutes prior to the activity, the sugar content may trigger a hypoglycemic reaction.

35

5. Why is water important during exercise?

Water functions as a coolant during exercise: body temperature rises (even when it is cold outside), and the athlete sweats. The body cools down as the sweat evaporates from the skin, dissipating the heat to maintain a constant internal temperature of 98.6°F. A body temperature > 106°F damages the cells, whereas one of 107.6°F coagulates cell proteins, leading to cell death. Without adequate water, dehydration occurs. Dehydration can be dangerous: the body cannot cool down because the person cannot sweat. As much as 5% dehydration can cause a 20–30% decrease in endurance capacity.

6. What are symptoms of dehydration?

Early symptoms
- Thirst
- Chills
- Clammy skin

- Palpitations
- Nausea

Later symptoms
- Headache
- Cramps
- Shortness of breath

- Dizziness
- Dry mouth

Most serious level of dehydration
- Hallucinations
- Deafness
- Visual problems

- Swollen tongue
- Kidney failure

7. How can dehydration be prevented?

- Drink plenty of cool fluids before, during, and after the event (i.e., practice, exercise session, or competition).
- Drink 1–1½ cups of cool fluid 15 minutes before the event.
- Drink ½ cup of cool fluid every 10–15 minutes during the event.
- Weigh self before and after the event. For every pound lost (as sweat) drink 2 cups of fluid. Thirst alone is not an adequate guide to the amount of water that the body needs.
- Monitor the urine. Dark and scanty urine is concentrated with metabolic wastes and indicates the need for more fluids. If the urine is pale yellow, the body has returned to its normal water balance. Vitamins and other substances may discolor the urine; therefore, weighing oneself may be a better method of assessing fluid loss.
- Beware of diets that emphasize shedding "water weight." Such diets sap all reserves of water.
- Beware of techniques to drop weight quickly before competition (using a sauna, taking laxatives, and diuretics contribute to dehydration).

8. What tips should you give to athletes exercising in extreme temperatures?

Tips for exercising on hot, humid days
- Exercise (if at all possible) during the coolest time of the day—early morning or late evening. If exercise is scheduled for the middle of the day, build up tolerance to this activity over several days.
- Wear light clothing and equipment (e.g., mesh jerseys, lightweight shorts, cotton, low-cut socks) to allow sweat to evaporate.
- Weigh self, and drink plenty of fluids before, during, and after exercise.

Tips for exercising on cold days
- Wear several layers of loose clothing.
- Weigh self, and drink plenty of fluids before, during, and after exercise.

9. Do herbal supplements work? Are they safe?

Many dietary supplements and nutrition strategies have been promoted as "magic bullets" to improve athletic performance or reduce body fat. Herbal remedies are also known as botanicals, nutraceuticals, and phytomedicines. Some supplements may enhance exercise capacity, but most claims are based on anecdotal testimony or creative marketing rather than sound science.

The 1994 Dietary Supplement Health and Education Act (DSHEA) set minimal safety guidelines for dietary supplements: vitamins, minerals, herbs or botanicals, amino acids, and dietary substances. In reality, however, there is little government regulation of the production and sale of herbs. Supplements cannot make a medical claim unless they undergo a rigorous approval process according to the federal Food, Drug, and Cosmetic Act. A supplement may not always contain what is listed on the label, may contain ingredients not listed on the label, or may contain different purities or dosages than those listed. Lack of standardization leads to disparate amounts of active ingredients and possibly toxicity.

There is also a risk of drug-herb interactions. In 1998, Eisenberg and colleagues evaluated alternative medicine use trends in the United States and estimated that approximately 15 million adults were using herbal therapies. Furthermore, most of the adults were not routinely notifying their physicians of this use. In 1999, the American Society of Anesthesiologists issued a statement warning patients to discontinue herbal product usage 2–3 weeks before any surgical procedure.

10. Where can I get more information on herbal supplements?

- American Botanical Council
  P.O. Box 144345
  Austin, TX 78714-4345
  (512) 926-4900
  www.herbalgram.org
- National Center for Complementary and Alternative Medicine, NIH
  P.O. Box 8218
  Silver Spring, MD 20907-8218
  (888) 644-6226
  http://nccam.nih.gov/nccam
- Office of Dietary Supplements, National Institutes of Health
  31 Center Drive, Room 1B29
  Bethesda, MD 20892-2086
  (301) 435-2920
  http://odp.od.nih.gov/ods

11. Should physicians recommend that adolescents take supplements to compensate for poor eating habits?

Vitamins are metabolic catalysts that regulate biochemical processes. The recommended daily intakes (RDIs) reflect the minimal amount required daily plus a 30% safety margin to prevent vitamin deficiencies. Recommended amounts will be consumed if a variety of wholesome foods from all food groups are eaten. A supplement can correct a vitamin deficiency, but overall vitamin and mineral deficiencies are related to larger medical problems, such as anorexia, unhealthy weight reduction, malabsorption, poor eating habits, or an inadequate vegetarian diet.

12. Does taking extra vitamins enhance athletic performance?

Adequate vitamins help the body function properly. To date no scientific evidence indicates that extra vitamins enhance performance, increase strength and endurance, provide energy, or build muscles.

13. Does exercise increase the need for vitamins and minerals?

No. Exercise does not "burn" vitamins or minerals. Vitamin and mineral deficiencies are more likely to occur in an inactive person with a small appetite as opposed to a sports-active person eating lumberjack portions.

14. Which special populations of patients benefit from vitamin or mineral supplements?

Consider adding a vitamin supplement(s) to the diets of patients with the following clinical conditions:

- Calorie restrictions (diets < 1200–1500 calories/day): supplement with a multivitamin and calcium.
- Food allergies, such as fruits and wheat: supplement the nutrients absent from the diet.
- Lactose intolerance: supplement riboflavin and calcium.
- Pregnant women: additional vitamins and iron required with physician guidance.
- Contemplating pregnancy: start a "blue-ribbon" diet of folic acid, iron, and calcium to help reduce risks of birth defects.
- Total vegetarians: supplement with vitamin B_{12}, D, riboflavin and possibly protein, iron, and zinc.
- Fat malabsorption (e.g., cystic fibrosis): supplement fat-soluble vitamins (A, D, E, K).
- Sickle cell disease: supplement folic acid.
- Iron-deficiency anemia: supplement iron.
- Osteopenia or osteoporosis: supplement calcium.
- Adolescent females taking Depo-Provera: supplement calcium.

15. How should a physician choose a supplement for a particular patient?

First of all, think "food" first—a healthy eating plan works best. Choose a supplement with 100% of the RDIs. Multivitamins generally do not contain 100% of the RDI for calcium and magnesium because of their bulk. Choose a supplement with beta carotene, which acts as an antioxidant, rather than vitamin A. Take the supplement with a meal to optimize absorption. Store supplements in a cool, dry place, and do not use after the expiration date.

16. Which minerals are most likely to be deficient in an adolescent's diet?

As with vitamins, a wholesome eating plan provides the minerals needed with the possible exception of iron and calcium.

17. Who is at highest risk of developing iron deficiency?

Iron is a necessary component of hemoglobin and is therefore critical for optimal transport of oxygen from the lungs to the working muscles. People at the highest risk of developing an iron deficiency anemia include:

- Teenage athletes, particularly girls who do not consume adequate dietary iron
- Adolescents who do not eat red meat
- Girls with excessive iron loss through heavy or prolonged menses
- Marathon runners
- Endurance athletes with heavy sweat (iron) losses

18. What happens if an adolescent girl does not get enough iron?

She may report feeling tired or irritable, her work performance suffers, she has less resistance to infections, and healing may take longer after an injury.

19. How can adolescents increase their iron intake?

- Eat lean cuts of beef, lamb, pork, fish, and the dark meat of skinless chicken or turkey 3–4 times per week.
- Add vitamin C to the diet to enhance iron absorption.
- Select breads and cereals that are "iron-enriched" or "fortified" with iron.
- Use cast-iron skillets for cooking.
- Eliminate coffee and tea (caffeinated or decaffeinated) from the diet, or drink them at least 1 hour before a meal. These beverages interfere with iron absorption.
- Combine meat (animal sources of iron) with poorly absorbed vegetable sources of iron.

20. What are the RDIs for iron for male and female adolescents?

AGE (YR)	RDIS FOR MALES (MG)	RDIS FOR FEMALES (MG)
11–14	12	15
15–18	12	15
19–24	10	15

21. What is the typical daily iron intake of a female adolescent?
The average female adolescent consumes about 10 mg of iron/day.

22. How much calcium do adolescents need in their diets? Why is it important?
Adolescent males and females need at least 1200–1500 mg calcium/day. Calcium is needed for strong bone framework, strong and healthy teeth, and prevention of muscle cramps, high blood pressure, and osteoporosis.

23. What are good sources of calcium for adolescents?
Milk, cheese, yogurt, and ice cream are high in calcium and are available in low-fat versions. Vitamin D, potassium, and phosphorous, all found in milk, assist in the absorption of calcium.

24. How can patients with lactose intolerance get adequate calcium in their diets?
Alternate means of securing calcium include taking a lactaid tablet or drinking lactaid milk; possibility of tolerating yogurt, hard cheeses, or even small amounts of milk; eating green leafy vegetables such as spinach, turnip greens, and kale; and eating almonds, tofu, and perch.

25. What are the options for calcium supplementation?
The best supplemental sources of calcium are calcium carbonate, calcium citrate, and calcium phosphate. Calcium carbonate is cheapest and dissolves well but should be taken with meals for proper absorption. Calcium citrate and calcium phosphate are more easily absorbed than the carbonate salt and do not need to be taken with meals. Calcium citrate is recommended for people with kidney stones, but it is expensive. Food manufacturers fortify foods such as orange juice, cereals, and bread with calcium. Only 500–600 mg should be taken at one time. Fiber and iron supplements reduce calcium absorption and should be taken separately. Vitamin D aids in calcium absorption. Sources of vitamin D include sunlight and vitamin D-fortified products. Vitamin D RDI is 200 IU (5 μ) daily.

26. What are components of a healthy weight-loss plan?
• Reducing caloric density of meals (often by decreasing portion sizes)
• Increasing enjoyable physical activity, including regular aerobic and strength-building exercise
• Ensuring adequate sleep
All of the above may contribute to increased patient motivation and a positive mood.

27. How are caffeine intake and weight control related?
A common response to low perceived energy is to use caffeine. Patients on very-low-calorie-diet programs who drink several caffeinated beverages per day experience decreased sleep and loss of eating control. The use of caffeine and ephedra (popular in weight-management pills) also may exacerbate feelings of stress and lead to overeating as a method of coping. Foods often eaten during this time have a high sugar and fat content.

28. How can fat and sugar intake sabotage a weight loss plan?
In addition to being calorie-dense, a high-fat diet may cause shifts in the thyroid hormone profile, leading to a reduction in metabolic energy expenditure. A study by Rolls et al. showed

that a high-fat diet was associated with a reduction in energy expenditure. Intake of sugar may cause a subsequent drop in blood sugar that precipitates feelings of fatigue. A sugary snack can initially produce a brief surge of energy, but this is eventually followed by feelings of low energy and irritability.

29. Do most adolescents exercise?

According to the surgeon general's report on physical activity and fitness, activity levels decline as grade levels advance. Nearly 50% of people aged 12–21 years do not engage in regular vigorous activity. Nearly 25% engage in no vigorous activity, and 14% report no recent physical activity at all.

30. What health risks are associated with obesity in adolescents?

Increased incidence of hypertension, hyperlipidemia, type 2 diabetes, growth hormone dysregulation, and respiratory and orthopedic problems, not to mention self-esteem and socialization problems.

31. How can physicians assess and counsel patients about physical activity?

The surgeon general's report recommends 30 minutes of moderate activity on most days of the week for youth. An activity inventory can assist physicians in suggesting activities appropriate for the child's age, size, abilities, interests, and medical conditions. Discussion with the patient may focus on:
- Physical education (frequency and types of activities)
- Aerobic activities
- Sedentary activity (time spent with computers, video games, television, studying, talking on the phone)
- Recreational and other physical activities (e.g., hiking)

Strength training has gained popularity, and prepubescent children can achieve measurable gains with little risk of injury and no adverse effects on bone, joint, or muscle development. Adequate supervision, not lifting maximal weights, avoiding ballistic movements, and correct form and technique assist in the avoidance of injury.

32. What is the prevalence of obesity in children?

In the United States obesity is remarkably prevalent. Recent studies indicate that 22% of children between the ages of 6 and 17 years have a body mass index (BMI) greater than the 85th percentile, and 10.9% have a BMI greater than the 95th percentile. It appears that children in the upper BMI percentiles for age are now heavier than children in the same percentiles in previous studies.

33. Define obesity and overweight.

Obesity denotes excessive body fat, whereas **overweight** may refer to excessive fat or lean tissue relative to height. Using the standard conventional cut-offs, persons with BMI above the 85th percentile are considered "overweight" or "at risk for obesity;" persons whose BMI is greater than the 95th percentile are considered "obese."

34. What is BMI? How is it calculated?

BMI is the index of weight over height squared:
$$BMI = [wt\ (kg)] / [ht\ (m)]^2$$
This measurement reflects the amount of body fat compared with the amount of bone or muscle and is used in the absence of laboratory or radiographic determinations to determine whether a person is overweight.

35. List other methods of determining overweight.
- Underwater weighing
- Dual-energy x-ray absorptiometry

- Air displacement plethysmography (BOD-POD)
- Subcutaneous skinfold thickness
- Bioelectric impedance

36. Why is adolescence a crucial period for the development of obesity?

The older a child is when he or she or becomes overweight, the greater the chances that he or she will remain overweight into adulthood.

37. Discuss potential causes of obesity.

Biologic influences. Central to current thinking in obesity research is the idea that every-one is genetically programmed with homeostatic mechanisms to maintain a certain body weight or "set point." An obesity gene is a gene with alleles (natural variants) that cause monogenic obesity in families.

Family environment. Overweight parents are more likely to have overweight children than normal-weight parents. Environmental and genetic factors are unlikely to work independently. An interwoven network consisting of parent weight status, parent eating (food preferences, food selection, food availability, and dieting), child feeding practices (restriction, pressure to eat, and monitoring), child weight status, and child eating (food preferences, food selection, and regulation of energy intake) contributes to obesity.

Behavioral changes. Increased sedentary lifestyle due to increased reliance on technology and labor-saving devices and increased consumption of calorie-dense "fast foods" have contributed to an energy-saving lifestyle. Watching television or videotapes, playing video games, and using a computer contribute to time spent in sedentary activities.

Neuroendocrinology. Afferent neurologic and hormonal regulatory signals are generated at the liver, gut, and pancreas. Norepinephrine and serotonin, signaling satiety vs. hunger and thinness vs. fatness, are interpreted in various centers in the brain.

Energy expenditure and physical activity. Although the popular belief is that a reduced level of energy expenditure or physical activity leads to the potential for obesity, this hypothesis is difficult to prove and is still controversial. Many cultural, genetic, and hormonal factors drive energy intake and energy expenditure and contribute to the homeostatic regulation of body-energy stores.

38. What are some of the current guidelines for the prevention and treatment of over-weight in children?

American Academy of Pediatrics: The goal of treatment is to decrease morbidity and risk for morbidity rather than to achieve a cosmetically endorsed body habitus. The initial approach emphasizes a combination of exercise and a closely supervised dietary plan. A family-oriented approach is critical, and highly restrictive or fad "diets" are discouraged. Some children may be medically healthy at higher functional body fatness than is thought to be the ideal in Western culture.

American Dietetic Association: Goals include the promotion of a healthy lifestyle to achieve a desired body weight. A well-balanced diet, regular aerobic exercise, cognitive self-management, and frequent long-term monitoring by a pediatrician and dietitian are key elements. A family approach is promoted, including nutritional education about lifestyle behaviors, modification of the home/school environment, and motivation to change by modeling behaviors or contracting. A short-term, medically supervised, protein-sparing modified fast may be considered for pediatric patients with super obesity (> 140% of mean body weight for height).

American Heart Association: Goals include prevention of weight gain above what is appropriate for expected increases in height. Achievement of an ideal body weight for height is considered an unrealistic goal. Family lifestyle modification, endurance-type physical activity, and physician monitoring are encouraged.

39. What intensive therapies are available for pediatric obesity?

In general, only children and adolescents with a BMI > 95th percentile for age and sex who have demonstrable medical complications that may be remediable through weight reduction should be considered as candidates for intensive treatment regimens. Many of the intensive treatments for obesity are considered investigational when used in children. It may be advisable to obtain written informed consent from the parents for treatment in a specialized center with experience in pediatric treatments. All of the below procedures may present specific benefits and risks, and careful screening and selection of candidates are essential.

- **Dietary restriction**: protein-sparing modified fast.
- **Pharmacotherapy**: medications that reduce energy intake or absorption of nutrients or alter production of certain hormonal secretions.
- **Bariatric surgery**: roux-en-Y gastric bypass, which divides the stomach into a 15–30 ml pouch with additional jejunal alterations.
- **Lap-band procedure**: a silicone elastomer band is placed around the upper part of the stomach to create a small stomach pouch, which can hold only a small amount of food.

BIBLIOGRAPHY

1. Beck B, Shoemaker R: Osteoporosis: Understanding key risk factors and therapeutic options. Physician Sportsmed 28:69–84, 2000.
2. Clark N: Nancy Clark's Sports Nutrition Guidebook, 2nd ed. Brookline, MA, Human Kinetics, 1997.
3. Fereyt JP: Dieting and weight loss: The energy perspective. Nutr Rev 59:S25–S26, 2001.
4. Ganley T, Sherman C: Exercise and children's health. Physician Sportsmed 28:85–92, 2000.
5. Goran MI: Measurement issues related to studies of childhood obesity: Assessment of body composition, body fat distribution, physical activity and food intake. Pediatrics 101:505–518, 1998.
6. Skinner P, et al: Development of a medical nutrition therapy protocol for female collegiate athletes. Perspect Practice 101:914–917, 2001.

7. ADOLESCENT PREGNANCY AND PARENTING

Constance M. Wiemann, Ph.D., and Vaughn I. Rickert, Psy.D.

PREGNANCY AND BIRTH RATES

1. Why does the United States continue to have the highest teen birth rate in the industrialized world?

The teenage birth rate in the United States is almost twice as high as that in Great Britain, four times higher than in Germany, six times higher than in France, and 15 times greater than in Japan. Although American teenagers do not exhibit significantly different patterns of sexual activity compared with adolescents in many industrialized countries, they use contraception less consistently and effectively and receive significantly less formal education about responsible sexual behavior and contraception.

2. Why has the teenage birthrate declined in the United States?

During the past decade, teenage childbearing declined significantly. The greatest decreases were among African-Americans (23% decline) and non-Hispanic whites (16% decline). Girls aged 18 and 19 years continue to account for 62% of all teenage births. Greater access to and use of long-lasting contraception, increased use of condoms, and declines in the number of teens who are sexually active, the number of sexual partners, and the frequency of intercourse have been suggested as primary causes.

3. What are the major risk factors for teen pregnancy?
- Poverty
- Poor school performance or low educational attainment
- Low educational aspirations or absence of other life goals
- Perceived benefits of early parenthood
- Poor knowledge of contraception and sexuality
- Single-parent household
- Low self-esteem or depressive tendencies
- Older siblings or mothers who were teenage mothers
- Earlier age at first intercourse
- History of physical or sexual abuse
- Delinquent behavior

4. What is rapid repeat pregnancy? Why is it a problem for adolescent mothers?

Rapid repeat pregnancy is defined as a second pregnancy within 12–24 months of a previous pregnancy. Rapid repeat pregnancies are experienced by 25–50% of adolescent mothers and are associated with greater likelihood of poverty, school drop-out, child abuse, marital dissolution, depressive symptoms, and lower-birth-weight infants.

PREGNANCY PREVENTION

5. What do teens see as the best way to prevent pregnancy?
- Begin sex education in early elementary grades.
- Teach abstinence in grade school.
- Provide information about contraception and the realities of parenting in junior high and high school.

- Provide access to contraception.
- Discuss sexual feelings as well as mechanical aspects of sex.
- Educate about relationships.
- Do not preach abstinence but rather help guide decision making.
- Involve parents and other adults in helping adolescents understand sexuality and making decisions about sexual behavior.

6. Which contraceptive methods are most effective for preventing first and repeat pregnancy among adolescents?

Because of the user failure rate associated with oral contraceptives, depot medroxyprogesterone acetate is more effective than pills at preventing first pregnancies in sexually active adolescents over the first 6 months of use. Postpartum use of depot medroxyprogesterone acetate vs. oral contraceptives is associated with higher method continuation rates and lower incidence of repeat pregnancy at 12 months after delivery.

7. Does abstinence-only education work?

To date, abstinence-only education programs have not demonstrated that they reduce sexual initiation or activity. However, a number of components appear promising: parental involvement, solid theoretical grounding in health education, reinforcement of appropriate social norms, teaching/rehearsal of interpersonal skills necessary to remain abstinent, and use of written pledges to remain abstinent.

8. Do pregnancy prevention programs work? What are the most important components?

Sex education and abstinence-based programs generally have not been as effective as community-based life options pregnancy prevention programs in reducing pregnancy rates among teens. Effective programs should include the following characteristics:

- Focus on sexual behaviors that lead to pregnancy and clear messages about prevention
- Sensitivity to developmental and cultural diversity
- Theoretical soundness
- Sufficient duration (> 14 hours in length)
- Variety of teaching methods such as homework, role playing, didactic instruction, and skill-building exercises
- Discussion of societal and peer pressures related to sexual behavior
- Modeling and practice with regard to communication and assertiveness
- Skill building in areas beyond pregnancy (e.g., academic abilities and employment skills)
- Staff who believe in the program

PREGNANCY COMPLICATIONS AND OUTCOMES

9. What are the major complications of pregnancy among adolescents?

Medical complications	Adverse outcomes
• Inadequate weight gain	• Preterm delivery
• Pregnancy-induced hypertension	• Low–birth-weight infants
• Anemia	

10. How does continued growth during adolescence affect the course of pregnancy?

Although data are limited, evidence suggests that the pregnant adolescent who is still growing competes with her fetus for essential nutrients. Marked reductions in placental blood flow on Doppler ultrasound and reduced micronutrients in the fetus from the still-growing mothers have been observed. Competition between mother and offspring also may occur during lactation. Adolescents who breast-feed have significantly less milk volume compared with mature breast-feeding mothers.

11. Do adolescents lose bone mass at higher rates during pregnancy than adults?

Greater maternal bone loss during pregnancy has been associated with higher baseline bone measurement, nulliparity, and ongoing maternal growth. Thus, nulliparous adolescents who are still growing are likely to exhibit greater bone loss during their first pregnancy than fully grown multiparous women.

12. What are the major causes of poor obstetric outcomes to adolescents?

Poor nutrition and inadequate prenatal care.

13. What impact does pregnancy have on adolescent smoking behavior?

Many pregnant adolescents quit smoking cigarettes once they recognize they have conceived. Nevertheless, a significant number of adolescents continue to smoke throughout pregnancy. Risk factors for continued smoking during pregnancy include the belief that cigarettes prevent excessive weight gain, desire for a lower-birth-weight baby to avoid difficult delivery, tobacco use by partner, peers, or family members, prior history of physical or sexual assault, and depressive symptoms.

14. What do adolescent mothers report as benefits and barriers to breast-feeding?

BENEFITS	BARRIERS
Better infant nutrition	Less convenient
Convenience	Belief that formula is healthier for infant
Something only they can do for infant	Difficult to breast-feed and go to school or work or be with friends
Maternal–infant bonding	
Lower cost than bottle feeding	Dietary and substance use restrictions (e.g., proper diet, avoidance of alcohol)
Assistance with weight loss	
Encouragement by health care provider	Feelings of embarrassment if observed
	Lack of family support
	Concerns about pain associated with breast-feeding
	Belief that breast-feeding causes breasts to sag

SOCIOECONOMIC AND PSYCHOSOCIAL OUTCOMES

15. What are the major barriers to completing high school once an adolescent has a baby?

• Lack of adequate child care during school hours
• Lack of family or partner support
• Limited educational aspirations or perceived importance of education
• Having more than one child
• Poor school performance before pregnancy

16. Do all adolescent mothers fare poorly?

No. Adolescent mothers are surprisingly diverse, and some are highly resilient. Adolescent mothers who successfully prevent additional pregnancies, remain in school, and have high aspirations and strong community and family support systems have similar economic outcomes as older women. In addition, the birth of an infant propels many adolescents toward greater acceptance of adult roles, including discontinuation of substance abuse and delinquent behavior and a stronger desire to complete school and establish independent households.

17. What provisions of welfare reform are likely to have the greatest impact on adolescent mothers and their offspring?

• Abolishing cash benefits
• Limiting family benefits to no longer than 5 years over recipient's lifetime (limit may be shorter or longer in some states)

- Requiring recipients to work 20–30 hours per week after 2 years of Temporary Aid to Needy Families (TANF)
- Requiring minor mothers to live with a parent or legal guardian and to stay in school
- Requiring mothers to identify the fathers of their children and to cooperate with child support enforcement
- Family cap that gives no additional money for children born while mothers are on welfare (present in some states)

18. Are adolescent mothers more likely to abuse their children than older mothers?

Adolescent mothers appear to be at higher risk of child abuse, mainly because of low socioeconomic correlates of teenage childbearing (poverty, low educational attainment, limited resources) rather than age per se. In addition, adolescent mothers are more likely than older mothers to have been victims of child abuse.

19. Why are pregnant and parenting adolescents at high risk for physical or sexual violence?
- Victimization by multiple perpetrators, including parents, siblings, other teenagers, and one or more intimate partners
- Increased isolation and stress associated with pregnancy and early infant care
- Inexperience with romantic relationships, which may cause female adolescents to confuse jealousy, possessiveness, and violence with love

MALE PARTNERS

20. What barriers do fathers of infants born to adolescent mothers report as preventing their involvement with child-rearing?

Unemployment, perceived lack of parenting skills, inadequate role models, limited support in their role as parent, drug involvement (both use and dealing drugs), and resistance from both the adolescent mother and her parents.

BIBLIOGRAPHY

1. Aquilino ML, Bragadottir H: Adolescent pregnancy: Teen perspectives on prevention. Am J Matern Child Nurs 25:192–197, 2000.
2. Berne L, Huberman B: European Approaches to Adolescent Sexual Behavior and Responsibility. Washington, DC: Advocates for Youth, 1999.
3. DePaul J, Domenech I: Childhood history of abuse and child abuse potential in adolescent mothers: A longitudinal study. Child Abuse Negl 24:701–713, 2000.
4. Hacker KA, Amare Y, Strunk N, Horst I: Listening to youth: Teen perspectives on pregnancy prevention. J Adolesc Health 26:279–288, 2000.
5. Motil KJ, Kertz B, Thotath U, Chery M: Lactational performance of adolescent mothers shows preliminary difference from that of adult women. J Adolesc Health 20:442–446, 1997.
6. Nitz K: Adolescent pregnancy prevention: A review of interventions and programs. Clin Psychol Rev 19:457–471, 1999.
7. Scholl TO, Hediger ML, Schall JI, et al: Reduced micronutrient levels in the cord blood of growing teenage gravida. JAMA 274:26–27, 1995.
8. Sowers MF, Scholl T, Harris L, Jannausch M: Bone loss in adolescent and adult pregnant women. Obstet Gynecol 96:189–193, 2000.
9. Thomas MH: Abstinence-based programs for prevention of adolescent pregnancies. J Adolesc Health 26:5–17, 2000.
10. Ventura SJ, Mathews TJ, Curtin SC: Declines in Teenage Birth Rates, 1991–97: Nation and State Patterns. National Vital Statistics Reports, vol. 47, no. 12. Hyattsville, MD, National Center for Health Statistics, 1998.

8. ADOLESCENTS AND THE MEDIA

Victor C. Strasburger, M.D.

1. Do the media really influence teenagers?

Yes—in a variety of important and sometimes subtle ways. Children and teens spend more time in front of the television set than they do in formal classroom instruction (15,000 hours vs. 12,000 hours). By the time today's teenagers reach age 70, they will have spent 7–10 years of their lives watching television. Thus, simply from a time standpoint, the media are tremendously important, even if they had no other impact. Because it displaces other, more active pursuits, amount of television viewing per day is associated with child and adolescent obesity.

2. What are the major areas of concern?

Sex, drugs, and violence are the primary areas, but many other concerns exist. Many experts, for example, point to a significant association between the image of women in the media and eating disorders among teenage girls. Teenage girls may develop a distorted body image, particularly if they read women's magazines, in which models in advertisements are impossibly thin. Some studies show that up to 67% of fifth-grade girls have dieted at least once. The connection with obesity is well known, although still somewhat controversial. But the area that has been most thoroughly researched is the association between media violence and real-life aggression. There are more than 3500 studies in this area, and all but a handful show a significant effect.

3. Does media violence cause real-life violence?

Not necessarily. But media violence contributes significantly to real-life violence. Media violence contributes between 10% and 30% to violence in society. Although not the leading cause by any means, it is certainly a factor to be reckoned with.

4. How does media violence translate into real-life violence?

Many studies document that young people who witness violence are more likely to become violent themselves, whether due to role modeling, desensitization, normalization, or other factors. Witnessing real-life violence at home is clearly a major risk factor, but after that, there is no better place to "witness" violence than in the media. The U.S. has some of the most violent television shows, movies, and video games in the world. The average teenager witnesses 200,000 acts of violence by the time he or she graduates from high school. Viewing all of this violence may teach young people that (1) violence is an acceptable solution, even to complex problems; (2) violence is justifiable; and (3) the world is a violent place, and they had better protect themselves. Many excellent research studies document all of these effects.

5. How did the media contribute to the recent epidemic of schoolyard shootings?

Most experts believe that the cause of such shootings is multifactorial: disturbed teenagers, influence of violent media, teasing by peers, and access to guns. Although teenagers may give clues to their intentions, their plans remain undetected by friends or school officials until it is too late. Many of the teenaged shooters used and enjoyed violent media. One of the Columbine killers reprogrammed a video game so that it looked just like his neighborhood, complete with the houses of people whom he hated. Both of the Jonesboro shooters were avid players of video games. The 14-year-old boy responsible for the Paducah, Kentucky, schoolyard shooting had never fired a gun until the day of the shooting; yet his eight shots had eight hits, all to the head and upper torso, resulting in the deaths of three adolescents and the paralysis of one. In *Stop Teaching Our Kids to Kill*, Lt. Col. David Grossman and Gloria Degaetano hypothesize that exposure to violent video games helps teach disturbed teenagers how to shoot at targets and desensitizes them to killing. Of interest, the military uses similar video games to desensitize new recruits to killing.

6. How does rock music influence teens?

Rock music has always been an important badge of identity for teenagers. Unfortunately, as adult society has coopted mainstream rock music for its own commercial purposes, teens have been pushed into more extreme forms of music, such as gangsta rap, heavy metal, and hate metal. The good news is that teenagers rarely know the lyrics, even to their favorite songs. The bad news is that music videos have a far greater impact than lyrics, and many studies show that music videos are rife with violence, weapon-carrying, smoking, and drinking. Women in music videos are frequently portrayed as sex objects. Among the various genres of music, hip-hop, rap, and heavy metal videos tend to be the worst offenders.

7. What is the connection between sex in the media and sexual behavior in teens?

Unfortunately, far less is known about this subject. Compared with the 3500 studies of media violence, only seven studies have examined the impact of media on teens' actual sexual behavior. All seven found a significant contribution. At least four more studies are currently in progress. Again, numerous studies document that the media represent an extremely effective sex educator—perhaps the most effective currently, given the sad state of sex education in the U.S.—and that the media also contain an abundance of suggestive and unhealthy sexual content. The media may function as a "super peer," suggesting to teens that apparently everyone is having sex but them and that birth control is unnecessary. The latest content analysis of American television found that nearly 75% of primetime programs contain sexual content, but less than 10% responsibly portray the risks of sex and the need for birth control.

8. How may the media's portrayal of drug use influence teens?

On the one hand, we want teens to "just say no" to drugs. On the other hand, we allow tobacco manufacturers to spend $8 billion a year and alcohol manufacturers nearly $3 billion a year to get teens to "just say yes." In addition, one-fourth of all music videos contain either alcohol use or cigarette smoking. Cigarette smoking seems to be making a major comeback in popular Hollywood movies as well. According to the most recent study, which surveyed the 250 top-grossing movies from 1988 to 1997, 85% depicted characters using tobacco. Even G-rated movies are not immune to this pervasive depiction of tobacco: fully one-half contain scenes of smoking, including all 7 children's films released in 1996–1997. But the problem gets worse: 70% of school districts use the Drug Abuse Resistance Education (DARE) program for drug prevention efforts, despite complete absence of data that the program is actually effective. By contrast, social skills-building programs, which use media education as one component, can cut drug use to 25% of anticipated levels. Although the federal government expects to spend $200 million/year for the next 5 years on antidrug advertising, only illicit drugs will be targeted.

9. You present a rather bleak picture of the media so far. Are there any good aspects?

Certainly. Unfortunately, the positive aspects of media are overwhelmed by the 10,000 violent images, the 25,000 commercials, the 2,000 beer and wine ads, and the 15,000 sexual innuendoes that children and teens view every year. Of course, the media can be powerfully prosocial. They can teach teens racial tolerance, respect for their elders, respect for each other, the need for academic achievement, sexual responsibility and restraint, and even the need to avoid cigarettes, alcohol, and illicit drugs. Perhaps 5–10% of all media are prosocial, but the remainder are definitely problematic. Of interest, the entertainment industry is quick to point out how its finest products "ennoble" society. Films such as *Schindler's List* and *Boyz in the Hood* teach invaluable lessons to young people about the Holocaust and the tragedy of gang violence, respectively. Yet other products coming out of Hollywood—the ones with rampant violence, sex, or drug use—have no positive impact whatsoever.

10. What should concerned physicians and parents do about the impact of the media?

Dealing with the impact of media on young people requires a multifaceted approach, with contributions from parents, schools, physicians, the entertainment industry, and the federal government.

Parents need to be aware of how important the media can be in their children's lives. They need to take control of media, limiting total media time to no more than 1–2 hours per day and closely monitoring the media to which their children are exposed. Parents of teenagers obviously will exercise less control but still need to monitor what their teens are viewing and listening to and discuss the content with them. One way to achieve this goal, at least partially, is to keep TV sets and computers with Internet access *out* of teenagers' bedrooms.

Physicians need to be sensitized to the cultural lives of their patients and more cognizant of the current literature about media effects. Specifically, teens who are obese or have eating disorders and teens with aggressive behavior should be questioned about their media use. Physicians also need to advocate for effective sex education, drug education, and violence prevention programs in schools. Such programs need to incorporate media education into their materials.

The entertainment industry needs to be more aware of its public health responsibilities and less willing to sacrifice good standards to make profits. Collaboration with the public health community may well produce better, healthier programming. The ratings systems for the various media are deceptive and completely inadequate. A new universal ratings system, perhaps based on the Motion Picture Association of America (MPAA) system, needs to be devised to give parents more qualitative information about the content of movies, TV shows, and music lyrics.

The federal government needs to be far more proactive in protecting children and teens against potentially harmful influences. Specifically, greater restraints should be placed on the advertising and promotional activities of tobacco and alcohol manufacturers. Alcohol ads should be restricted to so-called tombstone ads, in which only the product is shown and discussed, not the "party animals" or "beach babes" that presumably accompany its use. The government also can mandate a universal ratings system for all media and fund far more media research. Finally, the last government report about the media was issued 18 years ago. There is an urgent need for a 2005 report that examines all modern media, including music videos, the Internet, and new video games.

BIBLIOGRAPHY

1. Grossman D, Degaetano G: Stop Teaching Our Kids to Kill. New York, Crown, 1999.
2. Singer DG, Singer JL: Handbook of Children and the Media. Thousand Oaks, CA, Sage, 2001.
3. Strasburger VC, Grossman D: How many more Columbines? What can pediatricians do about school and media violence? Pediatr Ann 30:87–94, 2001.
4. Strasburger VC, Wilson BJ: Children, Adolescents, and the Media: Medical and Psychological Impact. Thousand Oaks, CA, Sage, 2002.

9. LEGAL ISSUES IN CARING FOR ADOLESCENTS

Cynthia Holland-Hall, M.D., M.P.H., and Robert T. Brown, M.D.

1. What are the major legal issues involved in caring for adolescent patients?

Consent and confidentiality.

2. Define consent and informed consent.

Consent refers to the permission that the patient and/or parent gives to the clinician to provide medical care. **Informed consent** means that the patient has a good understanding of what the provision of care involves, alternatives to the proposed intervention, and its possible consequences as well as potential benefits.

3. Define confidentiality.

Confidentiality refers to the privileged nature of the relationship between clinician and patient, in which information provided during the health care encounter remains private. In a confidential relationship between clinician and patient, no information can be revealed to other parties, including parents, without the patient's permission.

4. Why is confidentiality an important concept in adolescent health care?

Under certain circumstances, adolescents are less likely to seek health care and/or to discuss health needs candidly with a provider if they believe that their parents will be informed. One study demonstrated that only 15% of adolescents would seek treatment for a sexually transmitted infection (STI) if parental notification is required, but 65% would seek care if confidentiality is assured.

5. Are consent and confidentiality related?

The ability to give consent and the right to have the nature of the health encounter kept confidential involve the adolescent's standing as a minor. Adolescents under 18 years of age (in most states) have not yet reached majority in the eyes of the law and therefore are not legally capable of entering into full, contractual relationships without parental/guardian involvement in most situations. However, certain exceptions to this generalization apply in the health care setting.

6. Define assent.

Assent refers to the agreement by a minor to allow a clinician to proceed with health care or to participate in a research study. Because minors often cannot legally consent to medical interventions, consent must be obtained from their parents or legal guardians. It is still appropriate, however, for the clinician to inform the minor patient of the potential risks and benefits of treatment and to take into consideration any serious objections that the patient has to treatment. Assent is not a legal concept, and the clinician obtaining assent should tailor the discussion to the patient's developmental level. Assent corroborates the consent given by the parent/guardian but is subservient to it.

7. What is an emancipated minor?

An emancipated minor is a person who by status of age is still a minor but because of special circumstances can legally assume the full responsibilities and privileges of an adult, including the right to consent to health care. Circumstances under which a minor may be emancipated vary from state to state but may include:

- Marriage
- Enlistment in the military
- Financial independence from parents
- Living independently from parents
- Parenthood or pregnancy
- Otherwise declared emancipated by a court of law

8. What is a mature minor?

A mature minor is a minor who by virtue of intellectual (cognitive) developmental status can provide informed consent and can be treated as an adult by the clinician. This status is relative; the clinician must consider the nature of the problem/procedure being considered vs. the ability of the minor to understand its implications and potential consequences. Therefore, an adolescent who is deemed a mature minor in one situation may not be considered adequately mature to consent to care in a more complicated situation. Responsible adults must be involved when the situation is deemed more serious and/or complicated than the adolescent can deal with in the estimation of the clinician.

9. What is the clinician's legal responsibility to the parents of a minor?

Legally, the adolescent patient is a minor until reaching the age of majority for medical issues in his or her state of residence. Technically, therefore, the clinician must involve the parents fully in the health care of adolescents with the exceptions of the emancipated minor or mature minor or when specific statutory rules take precedence. The physician's judgment is the deciding factor in the latter situations.

10. A parent says to you, "I pay for the roof over my daughter's head, and my medical insurance pays for this doctor's appointment. I therefore have a right to know everything that goes on during the visit." How do you respond?

The physician may respond to this attitude in a variety of ways. Each situation is different, but all must be handled with tact and respect for both patient and parent. Possibilities include:

- Validate the parents' feelings and let them know that you appreciate their concern for their child's well-being and share their concern.
- Discuss how normal development includes the adolescent's evolving ability to take responsibility for his or her own health and growing need for privacy.
- Explain that allowing the patient confidentiality makes it more likely that he or she will speak freely with you about health needs and that all health needs will be met.
- Describe the laws allowing minors to seek confidential health services in your state.
- Acknowledge that this policy may not seem "fair" on the surface, but that it was created with the child's best interest in mind.
- Ensure parents that you always encourage children to be open and honest with them about whatever is discussed during the visit.
- Inform parents that you will always inform them immediately if their child's life or health is in imminent danger.

11. Under what circumstances must a health care provider breach confidentiality in a physician-patient relationship and disclose to the parent something that the adolescent has revealed in confidence?

Parents must be notified if an adolescent reveals that he or she has suicidal ideations so that they can take an active role in their child's safety and pursue mental health intervention. Homicidal ideations must be disclosed to the authorities and/or the potential victim. If a patient under 18 years old reveals that he or she is being abused physically or sexually, parents and the proper authorities, such as child protective services, should be notified. To maintain good rapport and to build trust with the patient, the physician should discuss these special circumstances with patient and parents at the first visit.

12. What are the limitations to confidentiality other than what the provider chooses to tell the parent?

Providers must keep in mind that third-party payors may document provided services, such as Pap smears and STI testing, and that this information may be sent to the parents. In addition, certain STIs must be reported to the local health department, and sexual partners must be notified. Providers should inform patients who require absolute confidentiality to seek out family planning services and STI testing through organizations such as Planned Parenthood and other Title X federally funded programs that do not allow parents access to the adolescent's medical record.

13. In which specific situations may an adolescent consent to his or her own health care with the right to confidentiality?

Although the specific statutes vary from state to state, adolescents often may consent to their own care in the following situations:

- Testing and/or treatment of a sexually transmitted or otherwise communicable infectious disease, including HIV
- Prenatal care and delivery services
- Contraceptive services
- Evaluation and treatment for a substance abuse problem
- Evaluation and treatment for a mental health disorder
- Emergency care

Keep in mind, however, that the provider must still determine the cognitive maturity of the patient and his or her ability to understand the risks and benefits of medical interventions before proceeding with care. If the patient is cognitively immature, the provider may still choose to involve a parent. Several states set a minimal age of 12–16 years for a patient to consent to his or her own health care, even in the above situations, and some states allow the minor to consent to care but do not ensure confidentiality.

14. Are adolescents' rights to obtain contraception in a confidential manner secure in the United States?

Not entirely. Although no states have laws explicitly requiring parental consent for a minor to seek prescription contraceptives, many states have no laws addressing this issue. Clinical services supported by federal funds via the Title X Family Planning Program provide these services confidentially to anyone who needs them, regardless of age. In the past several years, however, some members of Congress have repeatedly attempted to require parental consent or notification when a minor accesses such services at a Title X-funded clinic. Several states have also made attempts to repeal minor consent statutes and require greater parental involvement. To date these provisions have not been enacted.

15. Can adolescents seek abortion services without their parents' knowledge?

Most states require either parental consent or parental notification before a minor can obtain abortion services. Mandatory 24-hour waiting periods after parental notification are common. In all but one state (Utah) with mandatory parental involvement, a minor may seek judicial bypass and often may be granted permission by a judge to undergo an abortion if she is deemed competent and/or the judge agrees that the abortion is in her best interest.

16. If an adolescent patient requests care to which the physician has a moral or ethical objection, is the physician legally obligated to provide that care?

No. Physicians are not legally obligated to provide services to which they are morally or ethically opposed. It may be appropriate, however, to refer the adolescent to another facility or provider who can better meet the adolescent's health care needs.

BIBLIOGRAPHY

1. American Academy of Pediatrics, Committee on Bioethics: Informed consent, parental permission, and assent in pediatric practice. Pediatrics 95:314–317, 1995.
2. American Academy of Pediatrics: Consent for medical services for children and adolescents. Pediatrics 93:290–291, 1993.
3. Society for Adolescent Medicine: Confidential Health Care for Adolescents. Blue Springs, MO, Society for Adolescent Medicine, 2000.
4. Council on Scientific Affairs, American Medical Association: Confidential health services for adolescents. JAMA 269:1420, 1993.
5. English A: Reproductive health services for adolescents. Critical legal issues. Obstetr Gynecol Clin North Am 27:195–211, 2000.
6. Lieberman D, Feierman J: Legal issues in the reproductive health care of adolescents. J Am Med Womens Assoc 54:109–114, 1999.
7. Wibbelsman CJ: Confidentiality in an age of managed care: Can it exist? Adolesc Med State Art Rev 8:427–432, 1997.

II. Physical Disorders Affecting Adolescents

10. ALLERGY AND ASTHMA

Roger A. Friedman, M.D.

ALLERGY

1. What conditions should be included in the differential diagnosis of rhinitis in adolescents?

Allergic rhinitis is the most common cause of noninfectious rhinitis, occurring in about 20% of adolescents. Nonallergic rhinitis (vasomotor or eosinophilic), anatomic obstruction (deviated septum, adenoidal hypertrophy, turbinate hypertrophy, nasal polyps), rhinitis medicamentosa, sinusitis, rhinitis of pregnancy, and illegal drug use may cause rhinitis.

2. What are the common environmental allergens and when do they cause problems?

Think of holidays!

Early spring–Easter: tree pollen

Spring/summer–Memorial Day: grass pollen

Late summer/early fall–Labor Day: ragweed pollen

Mid to late fall–Halloween: mold spores

Perennial allergens that may occur year-round include house dust mites, molds, animal dander, and foods.

3. Why are allergy skin tests still used?

Skin tests remain the most sensitive, specific, and cost-effective way to confirm the diagnosis of allergic disease. In addition, a large number of antigens can be tested and the results known immediately; thus, treatment options can be given and initiated in a timely manner.

4. How does a nasal smear help in the differential diagnosis of rhinitis?

Nasal secretions are stained by either Hansel's or Wright's stain to reveal eosinophils, neutrophils, and bacteria. The presence of > 10% eosinophils in the allergic patient confirms that the allergen is causing symptoms. Eosinophils in the absence of positive skin tests confirm the diagnosis of eosinophilic nonallergic rhinitis. Prominent neutrophilia with or without bacteria usually represents infection, possibly sinusitis.

5. What in vitro tests are available for allergy diagnosis and when should they be used?

The radioallergosorbent test (RAST), fluoro-allergosorbent test (FAST), and CAP RAST can help confirm the diagnosis of allergic rhinitis. They can be used instead of skin tests if the patient has severe skin disease or cannot stop antihistamines for 3–5 days. In vitro tests are preferred to confirm the diagnosis of latex allergy because of the lack of an approved standardized skin test. The CAP RAST may be helpful as a screening test and has the best sensitivity of the in vitro tests.

6. Describe the step-wise approach to the management of allergic rhinitis.

Identification of allergic antigens and avoidance are always the first steps of treatment. When they fail, pharmacotherapy and immunotherapy may be considered.

7. Which dust and mold avoidance measures are effective?

Decreasing dust mite concentrations involves decreasing indoor humidity to < 50%. Removing carpeting, especially from the bedroom and over concrete basement floors, can be extremely effective. Covering pillows, mattresses, and box springs with an allergen-proof encasing decreases dust mites, as does eliminating stuffed animals and chairs from the bedroom. Mold spores can be decreased by eliminating free-standing water, sealing house leaks, and using a dehumidifier. The use of an acaraside such as Acarosan, an allergy-control solution, can decrease mites, and the use of fungicides (Lysol) helps kill mold spores.

8. How can we decrease animal allergy?

The most effective way to decrease animal allergy is to eliminate all animals from the home. An outdoor pet leads to very few problems. When this is not possible, it is critical to keep the animal completely out of the bedroom. Bathing cats and dogs can also decrease dander. Decreasing the number of objects and carpets also may be helpful, because less animal dander will accumulate.

9. What is the first-line pharmacologic therapy for allergic rhinitis?

Traditionally, first-line therapy for allergic rhinitis is an antihistamine or antihistamine–decongestant combination. Many patients initiate therapy on their own by taking over-the-counter medicines. These agents, although effective, cause a great number of side effects, especially sleepiness, and may impair performance. The second-generation antihistamines, such as loratadine, fexofenadine, and cetirizine, have become the popular treatments because of their lack of such side effects.

10. Should the teenager with allergic rhinitis drive a car?

First-generation antihistamines may cause both sleepiness and performance impairment that affect the operation of motor vehicles. Driving performance can be affected even when the patient does not feel sleepy. The second-generation antihistamines are preferred for this reason.

11. When antihistamines are not sufficient treatment, what is next?

Nasal steroids are the most effective medications for allergic rhinitis. They can be used either as first-line therapy or when antihistamines are not adequate. Nasal steroids can be effective when used chronically to decrease symptoms and improve quality of life. They also can be effective even when used on an as-needed basis. Sodium cromolyn and azelastine are also effective additional therapy, but they are not as effective as nasal steroids.

12. What are the criteria to initiate immunotherapy for treatment of allergic rhinitis?

1. Symptoms are moderate to severe.
2. Avoidance measures and medications are ineffective or cause unacceptable side effects.
3. Symptoms are worsening in spite of treatment.
4. Symptoms are becoming more frequent.

Immunotherapy is effective in 80% of properly selected patients and is the best chance for a long time "cure."

13. How common is food allergy?

Food allergy occurs in 1–8% of the population. It is more common in infancy and becomes less common as the child grows. Cow's milk, egg, soy, wheat, corn, and peanut proteins are the most important food allergies in infancy. Peanuts, tree nuts, fish, and seafood become more common in older children and adults. Most food allergies are outgrown with the exception of nuts, peanuts, and seafood.

14. Why are teenagers and food allergies such a dangerous combination?

Food allergies can be a fatal disease, particularly for adolescents. In most young children with food allergies, diet can be limited by adults and dangerous foods avoided. With increased independence, teenagers may let down their guard and ingest offending foods. In addition, many allergic foods may be hidden in food products, and we may come across them more often as our diet expands.

ASTHMA

15. Why is the prevalence of asthma increasing?

Both allergies and asthma have increased tremendously over the past 40 years. Although the exact reason is uncertain, the latest theory is the clean hygiene hypothesis. Because children have become healthier and less exposed to severe illnesses, their immune system has remained in a TH_2 mode. This mode leads to the production of interleukin-4, interleukin-5, and interleukin-13, all of which tend to produce atopy. When children are exposed to serious diseases, such as tuberculosis, or frequent diseases, as in a daycare setting, there is a tendency for the immune system to switch to a TH_1 response, which produces gamma interferon and does not lead to the allergic diathesis.

16. How common is exercise-induced asthma?

Exercise-induced asthma (EIA) occurs in almost all people with asthma (80–90%). It is often the only manifestation of asthma. EIA may occur in 30–40% of severely allergic patients without any other evidence of asthma.

17. What can mimic asthma in teenagers?

The two most common masqueraders of asthma in adolescents are hyperventilation and vocal cord dysfunction. Many teenagers become short of breath with exercise and are diagnosed with EIA, when in fact they are hyperventilating. A careful history demonstrating rapid breathing, tingling in the hands and toes, and dizziness can usually cinch the diagnosis of hyperventilation. When bronchodilators fail to help improve asthma, a new diagnosis usually should be sought. Pulmonary function testing, both before and after exercise, can usually differentiate asthma from a hyperventilation syndrome.

18. What is vocal cord dysfunction?

Vocal cord dysfunction (VCD) is an involuntary adduction of the vocal cords that occludes the opening during breathing. VCD causes dyspnea and sometimes an upper airway wheeze. Chest auscultation often finds little obvious air entry into the lungs, and this finding can be confusing in an emergency setting when the patient presents with "asthma." Some patients are admitted to intensive care units or even intubated before the correct diagnosis is made. Psychological factors and esophageal reflux often play a role in VCD. Treatment can be successful with speech therapy, relaxation techniques, and treatment of any underlying psychologic problems.

19. How important are pulmonary function tests in diagnosing asthma?

Pulmonary function tests (PFTs) are extremely helpful in confirming the diagnosis of asthma and demonstrating airway reversibility. They are particularly important if the diagnosis is uncertain. A truncated, flattened inspiratory flow volume loop can help confirm the diagnosis of VCD as opposed to asthma, which is characterized by a concave expiratory loop (see figure, top of next page). Pulmonary functions are also helpful in following the patient with asthma and in determining severity on an objective basis.

20. Describe the proper characteristics, diagnosis, and treatment of mild persistent asthma.

Patients with mild persistent asthma need bronchodilators 2–6 times/week, wake up 2–4 times/month because of symptoms, and have an forced expiratory volume in one second (FEV_1) or peak flow of > 80% of predicted, with peak flow having < 20% variability. Chronic anti-inflammatory therapy is initiated either with inhaled nonsteroidal anti-inflammatory agents, such as cromolyn or nedocromil (Tilade); antileukotriene agents, such as montelukast or zafirlukast; or inhaled corticosteroids.

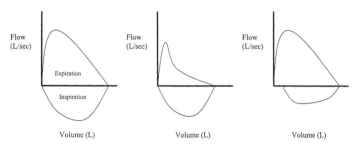

A normal flow-volume loop (*A*), the concave expiratory loop characteristic of asthma (*B*), and the flattened, truncated inspiratory loop seen in vocal cord dysfunction (*C*).

21. Define the proper diagnosis and management of moderate persistent asthma.

Moderate persistent asthma is defined as daily symptoms, waking up more than 5 times/month, peak flow or FEV_1 of 60–80% of predicted, and > 30% peak flow variability. Treatment for moderate or severe asthma should include inhaled corticosteroids as first-line therapy. The use of as-needed beta-agonists for occasional exacerbations or before exercise is indicated and, of course, avoidance of allergens.

22. What pharmacologic agent should be used for the treatment of persistent asthma?

Inhaled corticosteroid agents are the most effective treatment options for chronic persistent asthma and should be the initial therapy in all patients with moderate or severe persistent asthma. They are the one agent that most successfully reverses airway remodeling and decreases the death rate from asthma. In mild persistent asthma, leukotriene agents and cromolyn may be initiated as first-line therapy, but they should be supplanted by inhaled steroids when they are not rapidly effective.

23. What are the treatment options when corticosteroids are not completely effective?

When inhaled corticosteroids are not completely effective, there are three treatment options. The dose of inhaled corticosteroids can be increased, an antileukotriene agent can be added, or a long-acting beta agonist can be added. Studies have suggested that adding a long-acting beta agonist may be the most effective option. A new agent, Advair, combines an inhaled corticosteroid and salmeterol in an easy-to-use, disc-shaped inhaler and may be particularly appealing for compliance reasons.

24. What factors place teenagers at particular risk for death from asthma?

The death rate from asthma has increased greatly during the past 20 years, and adolescents are at risk. Most asthma deaths are preventable when appropriate chronic maintenance therapies are given. Unfortunately, adherence to maintenance drug regimens is often poor among adolescents. It is vitally important for physician educators to explain the necessity of drug therapy even when the patient feels good. New maintenance regimens that simplify therapy should be applied whenever possible.

25. When should you prescribe a peak-flow meter?

The peak-flow meter should be used with all patients who have persistent asthma. Because any level of asthma can progress to a severe exacerbation, monitoring of the disease is important, especially in patients who have labile asthma with a poor perception of their disease. Such patients are at risk for life-threatening asthma, and peak-flow monitoring can warn of worsening disease.

26. What is an asthma action plan?

An asthma action plan is a written document that allows patients to help manage their asthma. Self-management is a key concept for successful asthma care. The asthma action plan is a set of instructions from the doctor to the patient to initiate or change treatments based on symptoms and peak-flow meter recordings. Once normal peak flows are established, the patient uses symptoms and changes in peak flows to begin bronchodilator therapy, to increase inhaled corticosteroid therapy, or to begin oral steroids. The asthma action plan also tells patients when to call the doctor or go to an emergency department.

BIBLIOGRAPHY

1. Agertoft L, Pedersen S: Effects of long term treatment with inhaled budesonide on adult height in children with asthma. N Engl J Medicine 343:1064–1069, 2000.
2. Hay DB: Leukotrienes in asthma, old mediators up to new tricks. Trends Pharmacol Sci 16:304–309, 1995.
3. Kay AB: Allergy and allergic diseases: Part I. New Engl J Med 4:30–37, 2001.
4. Meltzer EO, Weil JM, Widlitz NM: Comparative outdoor study of the efficacy, onset and duration of action and safety of cetirizine, loratadine and placebo for seasonal allergic rhinitis. J Allergy Clin Immunol 97:617–626, 1996.
5. National Institutes of Health Expert Panel No. 2: Practical Guide to the Diagnosis and Management of Asthma. NIH publication no. 97-4053, 1997.
6. Skoner D: Management and treatment of pediatric asthma, an update. Allergy Asthma Proc 22:71–74.
7. Spergeo, JM, Beausoleil GO, Pawlowski NI: Resolution of childhood peanut allergy. Ann Allergy Asthma Immunol 85:473–476, 2000.
8. Sporik R, Hill DJ, Hosking CS: Specificity of allergen skin testing in predicting positive open food challenges to milk, egg, and peanut in children. J Allergy Clin Immunol 107:3–8, 2001.
9. Szefler SJ, et al for the Childhood Asthma Management Program Research Group: Long term effect of budesonide and nedocromil in children with asthma. N Engl J Med 343:1054–1063, 2000.
10. Szeinbach S, Barnes J, Sullivan TJ, et al: Precision and accuracy of commercial laboratories ability of classify positive and/or negative allergen specific IgE results. Ann Allergy Asthma Immunol 86:373–381, 2001.
11. Walker SM, Pajnog B, Lima, MT, et al: Grass pollen immunotherapy for seasonal rhinitis and asthma: A randomized controlled trial. J Allergy Clin Immunol 107:87–93, 2001.

11. CARDIOLOGY

Stephen C. Cook, M.D., and Curt J. Daniels, M.D.

1. What is the most common cause of syncope in children and adolescents?

Neurally mediated syncope, which is also known as vasovagal, vasodepressor, or neuro-cardiogenic syncope. The typical age of onset is 17 years for girls and 12 years for boys. Peak incidence occurs at ages 15–19 years for both males and females. These episodes tend to resolve over a period of 1–2 years. However, many adults have reported recurrences.

2. Which patients with syncope do not require additional cardiac evaluation?

Although it is unlikely that patients with vasovagal syncope have an underlying cardiac disturbance, it is important to rule out serious cardiac disease. The history is the most important tool for diagnosing vasovagal syncope. Important aspects obtained from the history should include events leading up to the episode, symptoms associated with the event, history of loss of consciousness, and status of the patient after the episode. Typically patients with vasovagal syncope describe standing for long periods, often in warm environments, before the syncopal event occurs. Overall hydration status also should be assessed. Most patients report inadequate oral intake before the event. Commonly associated symptoms include dizziness, a feeling of warmth, diaphoresis, nausea, and visual disturbance. Some patients report they "feel" as if they are about to pass out and will even attempt to adopt a supine position to prevent an attack. These historical points are classic for vasovagal syncope, and in patients with a normal physical exam and electrocardiogram (EKG), further testing is not indicated.

3. What clues suggest a potential cardiac cause of syncope?

Event history
- Event occurred during exertion or stress
- Palpitations, chest pain preceded syncope
- No premonitory warning symptoms, resulted in bodily injury
- Seizure-like activity, incontinence
- Event required cardiopulmonary resuscitation
- Event resulted in neurologic sequelae

Prior history
- Recent fatigue, exercise intolerance
- Known structural heart disease, arrhythmia

Family history
- Syncope
- Premature or unexplained sudden death
- Unexplained accidents (single motor vehicle accidents, drowning)
- Known arrhythmia, long QT syndrome, implanted cardiac device
- Early myocardial infarction
- Seizure disorder

Johnsrude CL: Current approach to pediatric syncope. Pediatr Cardiol 21:522–531, 2000.

4. What are the common causes of chest pain in adolescents?

Cardiac chest pain is rare in adolescents. Chest pain is more likely to present in girls than boys and is frequently due to chest wall pain. The most common noncardiac causes include:
- Musculoskeletal: costochondritis, muscle strain, myositis
- Pulmonary: asthma, pneumonia, pleuritis, bronchitis
- Gastrointestinal: esophagitis/gastritis (referred pain)
- Psychiatric

5. What historical features are suggestive of benign cardiac chest pain?
- **Timing**: fleeting pain, pain that lasts for hours, pain that occurs only at rest.
- **Location**: in one spot
- **Quality**: sharp

Again, the history is the essential tool in evaluating chest pain in adolescents. In the absence of features such as intermittent chest pain associated solely with exercise, pain that lasts for 5–10 minutes, and pain that is relieved by rest, a normal EKG and physical examination exclude the likelihood of cardiac chest pain.

6. What are the most common irregular rhythms detected in adolescents?

Sinus arrhythmia: a normal variant that occurs with variations in the respiratory cycle. Sinus arrhythmia is frequently detected in children because of their increased autonomic (vagal) sensitivity to respiratory variations. A bedside evaluation can confirm the diagnosis. The examiner should detect an increase in heart rate at the end of inspiration and a decrease in heart rate toward the end of expiration.

Premature atrial contractions: more common in very young patients but may be present in adolescents. Premature atrial contractions are insignificant and rarely cause hemodynamic compromise. They are frequently noted in adolescents who consume a significant amount of caffeine or use an over-the-counter remedy for cough and cold symptoms that contains a stimulant. Underlying cardiac defects are rarely associated with isolated premature atrial contractions.

Premature ventricular contractions: more common in adolescents than premature atrial contractions. An increase in frequency is noted with age. Premature ventricular contractions are considered benign in the following situations: when the contractions are isolated, uniform, and associated with a normal corrected QT interval on the EKG and when the cardiovascular examination is normal, the family history is negative for sudden cardiac death at a young age, and the contractions disappear with increased heart rate or exercise. If multiform premature ventricular contractions and ventricular tachycardia are present, a search for a cardiac cause should be sought.

7. Define supraventricular tachycardia (SVT).

This form of accessory connection-mediated tachycardia is due to antegrade conduction down the atrioventricular node and retrograde conduction up the accessory connection. During the tachycardia patients may report palpitations and the sensation of chest pain. These episodes start and stop abruptly and frequently last from minutes to hours. If an EKG is obtained during the event, the P waves may be difficult to discern or may even be retrograde. The QRS complex is characteristically narrow. The tachycardia may be terminated with vagal maneuvers. If vagal maneuvers fail, medical management should be attempted. Adenosine is usually a first-line agent because it prevents antegrade conduction at the level of the atrioventricular node.

8. How prevalent is sudden cardiac death in athletes?

The exact frequency of cardiac deaths in athletes is not known and is most likely underestimated. Estimations are based on reports from schools, institutions, and media. Such events are estimated to occur in about 1 in 200,000 high school athletes per academic year.

9. What are the most common causes of sudden cardiac death? How do they differ for adolescents and adults?

Please see figure, top of next page.

10. How should an athlete be evaluated before participation in sports?

Because the prevalence of sudden cardiac death in athletes is low, screening tools are unlikely to have a high specificity or sensitivity to detect an underlying cardiac cause. Currently

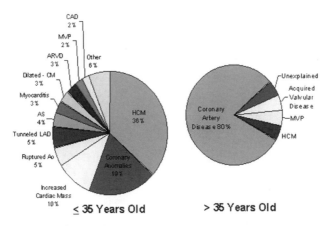

Comparison of the estimated prevalence of cardiovascular diseases responsible for sudden death in young (≤ 35 years) and older (> 35 years) trained athletes. *Left,* Causes of sudden cardiac death in young competitive athletes (median age: 17 years) based on systematic tracking of 185 athletes in the United States, primarily from 1985 to 1995. In an additional 2% of the series, no evidence of cardiovascular disease sufficient to explain death was evident at autopsy. "Possible hypertrophic cardiomyopathy" denotes hearts with some morphologic features consistent with (but diagnostic of) HCM. (Adapted from Maron BJ, et al: Sudden death in young competitive athletes: Clinical, demographic, and pathological profiles. JAMA 276:199-204, 1996.) *Right,* Causes of sudden death in older trained athletes. Data were assembled by collating findings from available published studies. (From Maron BJ, et al: Causes of sudden death in competitive athletes. J Am Coll Cardiol 7:204–214, 1986.)

available screening tools, such as the EKG or echocardiogram, are too costly to use for all United States high school and college athletes to identify such a small number of at-risk athletes. To make the problem more difficult, most athletes are asymptomatic before the event. There continues to be great difficulty in creating the ideal screening tool. To rectify these problems, the American Heart Association issued the following guidelines in 1996:

American Heart Association Recommendations for Cardiovascular Preparticipation Physical Evaluation.

A national standard is needed for preparticipation medical evaluations, including cardiovascular screening, because of heterogeneity in the design and content of preparticipation screening among states. Some form of cardiovascular preparticipation screening is justifiable and compelling for all high school and college athletes, based on ethical, legal and medical grounds.

Cardiovascular preparticipation screening, including a history and physical examination, should be mandatory for all athletes and should be performed before participation in organized high school (grades nine through twelve) and college sports.

A complete and careful personal and family history and physical examination designed to identify (or raise suspicion of) those cardiovascular lesions known to cause sudden death or disease progression in young athletes is the best available and most practical approach to screening populations of competitive sports participants, regardless of age.

The examination is to be performed by a health care worker (preferably a physician) who has the requisite training, medical skills and background to reliably obtain a detailed cardiovascular history, perform a physical examination and recognize heart disease.

For high school athletes, screening must occur every two years, with an interim history in intervening years.

From Maron BJ, et al: Cardiovascular preparticipation screening of competitive athletes. A statement for health professionals from the Sudden Death Committee (clinical cardiology) and Congenital Defects Committee (cardiovascular disease in the young), American Heart Association. Circulation 94:850–856, 1996, with permission.

American Heart Association Recommendations for Cardiovascular History and Physical Examination

Cardiovascular history

Inquire about and seek parental verification of:

Family history of premature death (sudden or otherwise)

Family history of heart disease in surviving relatives, or significant disability from cardiovascular disease in close relatives younger than 50 years, or specific knowledge of the occurrence of conditions (i.e., hypertrophic cardiomyopathy, long QT syndrome, Marfan syndrome, or clinically important arrhythmias)

Personal history of heart murmur

Personal history of systemic hypertension

Personal history of excessive fatigability

Personal history of syncope, or excessive/progressive shortness of breath (dyspnea) or chest pain/discomfort, particularly if present with exertion

Physical examination

Perform precordial auscultation in supine and standing positions to identify, in particular, heart murmurs consistent with dynamic left ventricular outflow obstructions.

Assess femoral artery pulses to exclude coarctation of the aorta.

Recognize physical stigmata of Marfan syndrome.

Assess brachial artery blood pressure in the sitting position.

From Maron BJ, et al: Cardiovascular preparticipation screening of competitive athletes. A statement for health professionals from the Sudden Death Committee (clinical cardiology) and Congenital Defects Committee (cardiovascular disease in the young), American Heart Association. Circulation 94:850–856, 1996, with permission.

11. What forms of heart disease are commonly diagnosed during adolescence?

Marfan syndrome. Marfan syndrome is a result of a mutation in the gene on chromosome 15 encoding for fibrillin protein. It is transmitted within families in an autosomal dominant fashion. This mutation results in abnormalities in connective tissue in many organ systems, including the heart. The mitral valve and the aortic root are the most dramatically affected by fibrillin mutation. Mitral valve prolapse is common, and occasionally mitral regurgitation also is present. Unless severe, mitral valve regurgitation is well tolerated. The greater concern is aortic root involvement. In fact, aortic root dilatation and dissection account for the morbidity and mortality associated with Marfan syndrome. The main risk factors for aortic dissection are the maximal aortic diameter, the rate of increase in the aortic diameter, and familial tendency to dissect. Therefore, referral to a cardiologist is prudent after diagnosis of Marfan syndrome. Aortic root dilatation can be followed echocardiographically with serial measurements of the aortic root. In the event of increasing aortic root size, treatment with beta blockers has been beneficial in decreasing the rate of progression. Surgery is an option in patients who progress despite medical management.

Mitral valve prolapse. This structural abnormality of the mitral valve results in prolapse of the leaflets into the left atrium. The exact cause is unknown; it appears to be multifactorial. The incidence and symptoms of mitral valve prolapse in children increase with age. Mitral valve prolapse commonly presents between the ages of 12 and 15 years. Most of these patients are asymptomatic. Symptomatic patients may report chest pain, dyspnea, fatigue, palpitations, and a variety of nonspecific neuropsychiatric complaints. The physical examination is significant for a mid-to-late systolic click. These physical findings in conjunction with the above history in a young, otherwise healthy person should suggest the diagnosis. The diagnostic evaluation should include an echocardiogram, which not only aids in making the diagnosis but also evaluates the degree of regurgitation, which in turn determines the need for endocarditis prophylaxis. Prolapse without regurgitation does not require prophylaxis.

Atrial septal defects. Atrial septal defects (ASDs) occur in 1 in 1500 live births and constitute 6–10% of congenital heart defects. The most common form of atrial septal defects is the secundum type, which is due to excessive resorption of the septum primum during cardiovascular development. Most patients are asymptomatic. They present most often for the evaluation of a "heart murmur." The murmur is not due to blood flow across the defect but rather to excessive blood flow through the pulmonary valve. This murmur is best appreciated in the left upper sternal border in the second intercostal space. Another cardiac finding is the fixed splitting of the second heart sound throughout the respiratory cycle. The diagnosis can be made with an echocardiogram. Treatment consists of surgical correction. Recently, transcatheter devices were approved for closure in the cardiac catheterization laboratory. Early detection and intervention can prevent the long-term complications associated with these defects. Complications include pulmonary hypertension, right ventricular enlargement, and ultimately right ventricular failure. Other complications include paradoxical embolization and atrial arrhythmias.

Bicuspid aortic valve. The congenitally bicuspid aortic valve is the most common congenital malformation, occurring in approximately 2% of the general population. Most patients are asymptomatic. The condition is detected by classic findings on cardiovascular examination: an ejection click and systolic ejection murmur. Patients with few or no symptoms related to their disease require prophylaxis for subacute bacterial endocarditis in addition to routine follow-up because the disease may progress. Patients who present with symptoms of chest pain and exertional dyspnea may have more severe disease and require additional evaluation. Historically, long-term complications include aortic stenosis, aortic insufficiency, aortic root dilatation, and an increased risk for aortic dissection. Treatment options include balloon valvuloplasty for aortic stenosis, and surgical aortic valve and root replacement.

12. How should young adults with congenital heart disease be followed?

As the adolescent becomes a young adult, he or she should continue to be followed by a family physician or internist. This transition should occur in an amicable and smooth fashion to prevent loss of follow-up. Resources for young adults with congenital heart disease should include a family physician or internist in conjunction with a cardiologist knowledgeable about their condition. The current recommendations from the 32nd Bethesda Conference, "Care of the Adult with Congenital Heart Disease," state that follow-up every 3–5 years for lower-risk patients is sufficient. Low-risk lesions were defined as isolated congenital aortic and mitral valve disease, isolated patent foramen ovale or small atrial septal defect, and isolated small ventricular septal defect. Also included was a previously ligated or occluded ductus arteriosus, repaired secundum or sinus venosus ASD without residua, and a repaired ventricular septal defect without residua. Examples of higher-risk lesions include valved or nonvalved conduits, cyanotic congenital heart disease, double-outlet ventricle, Eisenmenger syndrome, and single ventricle. Such patients require much closer follow-up at intervals of 12–24 months. Higher-risk patients need follow-up to monitor cardiovascular problems that may lead to hemodynamic instability. Settings specific to this category of patients include:

- Significant intracardiac shunting
- Greater than "mild" pulmonary vascular disease
- Greater than "moderate" left ventricular or "mild" right ventricular dysfunction or failure
- Systemic right ventricle
- Single-ventricle physiology
- Greater than "mild" obstructive intracardiac valvular or vascular disease, including patients with peripheral pulmonary artery stenosis or aortic coarctation and excluding patients with isolated aortic valve and many patients with isolated mitral valve disease
- Significant congenital coronary arterial abnormalities
- Pregnancy in the setting of significant congenital heart disease
- New onset of tachyarrhythmias that require institution of antiarrhythmic medication or ablation therapy or bradyarrhythmias that include atrioventricular block or symptomatic sinus node dysfunction, in any of the patients listed above, repaired or unrepaired

BIBLIOGRAPHY

1. Aburawi EH, O'Sullivan J, Hasan A: Marfan's syndrome: A review. Hosp Med 62(3):153–157, 2001.
2. Allen HD, Gutgesell HP, Clark EB, Driscoll DJ (eds): Moss and Adams' Heart Disease in Infants, Children, and Adolescents, Including the Fetus and Young Adult, 6th ed. Philadelphia, Lippincott Williams & Wilkins, 2001.
3. 32nd Bethesda Conference: Care of the adult with congenital heart disease. J Am Coll Cardiol 37: 1161–1198, 2000.
4. Case CL: Diagnosis and treatment of pediatric arrhythmias. Pediatr Clin North Am 46(2):347–354, 1999.
5. Daniels CJ, Franklin WH: Common cardiac diseases in adolescents. Pediatr Clin North Am 44(6):1591–1601, 1997.
6. Driscoll DJ: Left-to-right shunt lesions. Pediatr Clin North Am 46:355–368, 1999.
7. Gutgesell HP, et al: Common cardiovascular problems in the young. Part I: Murmurs, chest pain, syncope and irregular rhythms. Am Fam Physician 56:1825–1830, 1997.
8. Jeresaty RM: Mitral valve prolapse: Definition and implications in athletes. J Am Coll Cardiol 7:231–236, 1986.
9. Johnsrude CL: Current approach to pediatric syncope. Pediatr Cardiol 21:522–531, 2000.
10. Lyznicki JM, Nielsen NH, Schneider JF: Cardiovascular screening of student athletes. Am Fam Physician 62:765–774, 2000.
11. Maron BJ: Heart disease and other causes of sudden death in young athletes. Curr Probl Cardiol 23:477–529, 1998.
12. Ohara N, et al: Mitral valve prolapse in childhood: The incidence and clinical presentations in different age groups. Acta Paediatr Jpn 33:467–475, 1991.

12. DERMATOLOGY

Mark Allen Bechtel, M.D.

1. What causes acne?
Acne results from physiologic and pathologic changes in the pilosebacious unit. The incidence of acne peaks during the period of increased sebum production during adolescence. Androgen production is a prerequisite for the development of acne. Stress, increased sweating, mechanical trauma, and genetic factors may play a role. Diet has not been shown in clinical studies to be a significant factor.

2. Is acne common among adolescents?
Yes. The prevalence of acne in adolescents 15–17 years of age approaches 85%. Girls usually note the onset of acne between 12 and 13 years of age and boys between 13 and 14 years of age.

3. What are the major objectives of managing adolescent acne?
1. Correct the abnormal follicular keratinization.
2. Decrease sebaceous gland activity.
3. Decrease the bacterial population in the follicles.
4. Promote an anti-inflammatory effect.

4. Are topical retinoids helpful in the treatment of acne?
Topical retinoids are essential in the treatment of comedonal acne. Open and closed comedones in the T-zone area are the earliest manifestation of adolescent acne. Topical retinoids are comedolytic and promote desquamation by decreasing cellular adhesion and altering differentiation of epithelial cells. Topical tretinoin (Retin-A) was the first topical retinoid used for acne. Tretinoin should be initiated at lower strengths that are less irritating and gradually increased in strength. Recently Retin-A has been developed with a 0.1% microsponge formulation (Retin-A Micro). Adapalene (Differin) is a naphthoic acid derivative that is less irritating and has both comedolytic and anti-inflammatory activities. Tazarotene (Tazorac) is a new retinoid used for acne and psoriasis.

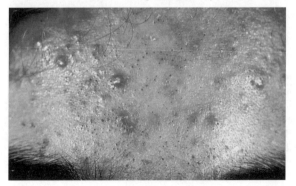

Comedonal and pustular acne.

5. Does bacterial resistance to antibiotics occur in the treatment of acne?
Propionibacterium acnes is an anaerobe that contributes to the pathogenesis of acne. Antibiotic resistance to *P. acnes* has significantly increased over the past several years.

Resistance to topical and oral erythromycin, clindamycin, and tetracycline is especially common, and these agents should be avoided as monotherapy. Combining benzoyl peroxide with topical erythromycin (Benzamycin) or topical clindamycin (Benzaclin) significantly reduces resistant bacteria. Including benzoyl peroxide washes or gels in various topical regimens is helpful in reducing resistance. Minocycline demonstrates the lowest incidence of resistance among oral antibiotics.

6. Discuss the important aspects of acne treatment in patients with darkly pigmented skin.

Darkly pigmented skin has a propensity to develop marked postinflammatory hyperpigmentation. Comedonal acne tends to be more inflammatory. Pomades used to improve the manageability of hair and scalp dryness are common contributing causes of acne in African-Americans. Papules and comedones are often noted on the forehead and temples. Early and aggressive treatment of acne in darkly pigmented skin is important to prevent postinflammatory hyperpigmentation. Topical retinoids and azelaic acid (Azelex) are helpful in reducing postinflammatory hyperpigmentation. Noncomedogenic pomades for the scalp hair included TCB Easy Comb, Soft N' Sheen, Stay Soft-Fro, Afro Soft, and Carefree Curl.

7. When should oral isotretinoin (Accutane) be considered in the treatment of acne?

Oral isotretinoin should be reserved for patients who have severe nodulocystic acne with scarring. Patients should demonstrate resistance to conventional systemic antibiotics and topical therapies before Accutane is considered.

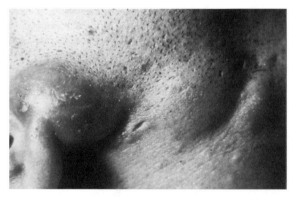

Cystic acne lesions.

8. What are important side effects of oral isotretinoin therapy?

Mucocutaneous side effects, including cheilitis, epistaxis, xerosis, and dry eyes, are common. Muscle soreness and bone tenderness may occur. Calcification of the ligamentous insertion on vertebrae and other joints has been noted. Pseudotumor cerebri has been reported in rare cases, especially with concomitant tetracycline or minocycline use. Cholesterol, triglycerides, and liver functions need to be monitored because they may become elevated. Teratogenicity remains the major concern. Women of child-bearing potential must be counseled, be reliable, and understand pregnancy prevention. They must practice strict effective contraception; two methods are preferred unless total abstinence is chosen.

9. Does oral isotretinoin cause depression and suicide?

Suicide and depression have been reported in patients on isotretinoin therapy. However, a direct relationship among suicide, depression, and oral isotretinoin therapy is not clearly documented by epidemiologic data. The total number of suicides on isotretinoin therapy is below the expected population number based on age. The biologic plausibility of an isotretinoin/suicide link has not been established. Physicians, however, should be vigilant and warn patients on isotretinoin therapy about possible depression, mood swings, and suicidal behavior.

10. Are oral contraceptives helpful in the treatment of acne?

Estrogens in combination with a progestin can be used to treat acne. Unfortunately, some progestins have intrinsic androgenic activity, which may exacerbate acne. Second-generation progestins, including ethynodiol diacetate, norethindrone, and levonorgestrel, have low androgenic activity. The third-generation progestins, including desogestrel and norgestimate, have the lowest intrinsic androgenic activity. Only the oral contraceptive containing ethinyl estradiol and norgestimate (Ortho Tri-Cyclen) has been approved by the Food and Drug Administration (FDA) for treatment of acne, although many are effective.

Oral Contraceptives to Treat Acne

TRADE NAME	ETHINYL ESTRADIOL (μg)	PROGESTIN (MG)
Desogen	35	Desogestrel 150
Ortho-Cept	35	Desogestrel 150
Ortho-Cyclen	35	Norgestimate 250
Ortho Tri-Cyclen	35	Norgestimate 180, 215, 250
Ortho-Novum 777	35	Norethindrone 500, 750, 1000
Ovcon-35	35	Norethindrone 400
Demulen	35, 50	Ethynodiol diacetate 1000
Triphasil	35, 50	Levonorgestrel 50, 75, 125

11. What is the current treatment for tinea capitis?

Griseofulvin microsized, 20 mg/kg/day for 8 weeks, is still the first-line therapy for tinea capitis. Griseofulvin should be taken with a fatty meal. Recent data support the efficacy and safety of the new antifungals terbinafine, itraconazole, and fluconazole in the treatment of tinea capitis, but they are not FDA-approved for this disorder. Selenium sulfide lotion or ketoconazole shampoo, 2–3 times weekly, should be used by the patient and siblings.

12. Is cervical lymphadenopathy an important finding in tinea capitis?

In a recent study, all pediatric patients with cervical lymphadenopathy and scalp alopecia had positive fungal cultures. A high percentage of patients with scaling of the scalp and adenopathy also had positive fungal cultures of the scalp.

13. Does griseofulvin help tinea versicolor (pityriasis versicolor)?

No. Tinea versicolor is due to the lipophilic yeast organism, *Malassezia furfur*. Griseofulvin does not treat tinea versicolor or other yeast infections; it is effective only against dermatophytes. Oral ketoconazole in a dose of 3–5 mg kg/day to a maximum of 200 mg/day may be administered daily for 5–7 days. Physicians should be aware of the risk for hepatotoxicity and avoid use in younger children. In adult-sized adolescents, ketoconazole can be given as a single dose of 400 mg. Patients are encouraged to stimulate a heavy sweat 1–2 hours later. The drug is excreted in high concentrations in sweat, and excretion facilitates eradication of the fungus. Itraconazole, 200 mg daily for 5 days, has been reported to be effective in adult-sized adolescents with tinea versicolor. The risk for hepatotoxicity is still present.

14. List the possible topical therapies for tinea versicolor (pityriasis versicolor).

- Zinc pyrithione shampoo daily for 7 days
- Selenium sulfide shampoo daily for 7 days and weekly for 1 month
- Topical imidazole creams (Nizoral, Lotrimin) daily for 2 weeks
- Ketoconazole shampoo daily for 5 minutes for 3 days
- Terbinafine spray (Lamisil) twice daily for 1 week

15. What are the important infectious cutaneous disorders in wrestlers?

Tinea gladiatorum is a fungal infection that is common on the neck and shoulders. Large outbreaks may cause exclusion from competition. Important viral infections transmitted by wrestlers include herpes simplex, molluscum contagiosum, and verrucae vulgaris. Scabies, lice, and impetigo are also of concern. Wrestlers with exposed active infections should be excluded from competition.

16. What are the important cutaneous manifestations of pediatric acquired immunodeficiency syndrome (AIDS)?

Manifestations in younger children usually start by 3–6 months with persistent oral candidiasis and generalized lymphadenopathy. Cutaneous findings in adolescent patients often represent severe and atypical forms of common skin disorders. Cutaneous infections caused by *Staphylococcus aureus* are frequent. Oral pseudomembranous candidal infections are common and may be associated with candidal esophagitis. Chronic candidal paronychia and severe atypical dermatophyte infections may occur. Cutaneous lesions of sporotrichosis, histoplasmosis, and cryptococcosis have been reported. Viral infections with molluscum contagiosum, herpes simplex, varicella-zoster, and human papilloma virus may be severe and recalcitrant to therapy. Seborrheic dermatitis and psoriasis may flare. Drug eruptions caused by trimethoprim-sulfamethoxazole are especially common. Kaposi's sarcoma occurs much less frequently in adolescents than in adults.

17. How is molluscum contagiosum treated?

Molluscum contagiosum is common, affecting 10% of children. Infections eventually undergo spontaneous resolution. The choice of treatment must be individualized for every patient and practitioner. Discomfort is the most important limiting factor for young people. Treatments include the following:
- Gentle manipulation
- EMLA (eutectic mixture of local anesthetics) plus curettage
- Cryotherapy (gentle)
- Cantharidin (apply for 4 hours and wash off. Do not use on face; it causes blisters and possibly scarring.)
- Salicylic acid preparation
- Topical tretinoin (Retin-A)
- Imiquimod (Aldara)
- Watchful waiting (active nonintervention)

18. What are the possible treatment options for common warts?

The choice of treatment should be individualized for every patient and practitioner. Special consideration should be made for discomfort, risks of scarring, and costs. Options include the following:

• Active nonintervention	• Tape occlusion on fingers and toes
• Salicylic acid preparations	• Curettage and electrosurgery (may scar)
• Cryotherapy	• Laser
• Cantharidin	• Imiquimod (Aldara)
• Cimetidine	• Formalin–glutaraldehyde (for plantar warts)

19. What factors have been identified in the pathogenesis of atopic dermatitis?

Atopic dermatitis is a manifestation of a complex interrelationship of genetic, immunologic, and environmental factors. Infectious agents, super antigens, pattern of local cytokine expression, differentiation of helper T cells, skin-directed responses, and IgE are important components.

20. Should patients with atopic dermatitis avoid bathing?

Drying of the skin by poor bathing and moisturizing practices is a major exacerbating factor in atopic dermatitis. Bathing dries the skin through evaporation of water from wet skin and damages the epidermal barrier. Daily bathing followed by applications of a moisturizer within 3 minutes after a bath hydrates the skin and keeps it soft.

21. List important management principles of atopic dermatitis.

1. Avoid irritants. Limit exposure to wool, rough fabrics, tobacco smoke, pet danders, and dust mites.

2. Reduce pruritus. It is critical to break the itch-scratch cycle. Oral antihistamines should be used as needed. Nonsedating antihistamines are helpful during school attendance. Sedating antihistamines may be used at night.

3. Hydrate the skin. Dryness of skin exacerbates pruritus. Apply moisturizers within 3 minutes after each bath.

4. Reduce inflammation of the skin. Topical steroids are excellent for reducing inflammation. Tacrolimus ointment has excellent anti-inflammatory properties.

5. Reduce infection. Colonization of the skin with *S. aureus* is common in patients with atopic dermatitis. Treatment of active infection helps decrease pruritus and promotes healing. Dicloxacillin and cephalosporins are most helpful.

22. How does topical tacrolimus work? Is it safe in children?

Tacrolimus ointment is a nonsteroidal topical immune modulator specific for the treatment of atopic dermatitis in children over the age of 2 years. Tacrolimus blocks the early phase of T-cell activation and inhibits the phosphatase activity of calcineurin. It is safe and effective for long-term treatment in children. Transient burning and itching of the skin are the most common side effects.

23. What are the early warning signs of malignant melanoma?

Cutaneous melanoma is uniquely visible, and early detection is the key to possible cure. An ABCD guideline helps the clinician and patient suspect the diagnosis of melanoma:

A = **A**symmetry
B = **B**order irregularity
C = **C**olor (varied or dark)
D = **D**iameter greater than the size of a pencil eraser

The possibility of melanoma should be considered when a patient reports a new pigmented lesion or a change in a preexisting mole. Any change in size, color, shape, or surface should be evaluated carefully. Varying shades of black, brown, blue, red, and white within the individual nevus are significant. Melanomas often have irregular or scalloped borders.

24. Are tanning beds safe?

Many tanning salons promote themselves as "safe" because they use ultraviolet A (UVA) light sources. However, UVA light sources have been suspected to promote malignant melanoma and may damage the immune system. Many tanning lamps also emit significant amounts of ultraviolet B rays. Studies indicate that tanning beds can induce skin and eye burns, alter the immune system, cause photo aging, and promote nonmelanoma skin cancers. Many adolescents take medications such as tetracycline, which are photosensitizing. Herpes labialis can be exacerbated by tanning beds. Adolescents who are fair-skinned and burn easily without tanning are at greater risk. Patients with collagen vascular diseases should avoid tanning beds.

25. What are important measures to take for sun protection?

1. Limit the amount of time in midday sun. The sun's ultraviolet rays are strongest between 10 AM and 4 PM.

2. Always use a sunscreen. A sunscreen with a sun protective factor of at least 15 is important and should block ultraviolet A and B rays. An excellent sunscreen component is Parsol. Sunscreens should be applied liberally before exposure and should be reapplied every 2 hours with sweating or swimming.

3. Wear a wide-brimmed hat and tightly woven protective clothing.
4. Wear sunglasses that block ultraviolet radiation to reduce the risk of cataracts.

26. Can sunless-tanning products provide a safe protective tan?

Sunless-tanning products, such as self-tanning creams, bronzers, and extenders, are not harmful but do not provide any sunscreen protection. They may be a safer alternative to the use of tanning beds before the prom. Sunless tanning pills often contain canthaxanthin, which can form crystal deposits in the eye and be harmful.

27. What can help axillary hyperhidrosis or sweaty palms?

Drysol solution (20% aluminum chloride hexahydrate in anhydrous ethyl alcohol) applied at bedtime to the axillae or palms can help reduce sweating. Xerac AC solution is less irritating and can be used in milder cases.

28. Can any topical medication help decrease excessive facial hair?

Vaniqa, a cream containing eflornithine hydrochloride, inhibits the enzyme ornithine decarboxylase found in hair follicles; it thus inhibits cell division and retards the rate of hair growth. Vaniqa does not permanently remove hair and is not a depilatory but slows hair growth and is cosmetically helpful.

BIBLIOGRAPHY

1. Hubbard TW: The predictive value of symptoms of diagnosing childhood tinea capitis. Arch Pediatr Adolesc Med 153:1150–1153, 1999.
2. Hurwitz S: Clinical Pediatric Dermatology, 2nd ed. Philadelphia, W.B. Saunders, 1993.
3. Leung DY, Soter NA: Cellular and immunologic mechanisms in atopic dermatitis. J Am Acad Dermatol 44:S1–S10, 2001.
4. Schaner LA, Hansen RC (eds): Pediatric Dermatology, 2nd ed. New York, Churchill Liningstone, 1995.
5. Thomas L, Trachand P, Berard F: Semiological value of ABCDE criteria in diagnosis of cutaneous pigmented tumors. Dermatology 197:11–17, 1998.
6. Toffe SJ, Hanifin JM: Current management and therapy of atopic dermatitis. J Am Acad Dermatol. 4:513–516, 2001.

13. ENDOCRINOLOGY

John A. Germak, M.D.

SHORT STATURE

1. What are three main determinants of the regulation of growth in children and adolescents?

Growth represents a complex series of events regulated by **genetic, endocrinologic**, and **environmental** factors. Recently described genes important for growth include the ontogenetic pituitary genes (*Pit-1* and *Prop-1*) and genes for growth hormone-releasing hormone (GHRH), growth hormone (GH), and the growth hormone receptor. Environmental factors include nutrition, normal body metabolism, lack of disease, and a healthy psychosocial milieu. The important endocrine factors include growth hormone, thyroid hormone, sex steroids, and growth factors, particularly insulin-like growth factor I (IGF-1).

2. Should short stature be considered a disease?

Short stature is defined by statistical criteria and assessed by plotting an accurately measured height on a standard growth chart, yielding a growth curve for measurements over time. By definition, 3% of the general population plots below the third percentile for height and therefore is considered to have short stature. Although the majority have no identifiable abnormality, pathologic causes of short stature do exist. In general, if the growth in height is parallel to the normal curve, growth velocity is normal and a pathologic cause of short stature is unlikely.

3. When is an evaluation for short stature indicated?

An evaluation of short stature should be considered in any child whose growth velocity is below normal. Although the normal rate of growth depends on the age of the child and is highest in the first year after birth, it should generally be consistent (5–6 cm per year) between 4 years of age and puberty. The most practical means of making this determination is to plot an accurately measured height on a standard growth chart. A linear growth curve that is less than parallel or shows downward crossing of percentiles should prompt a screening evaluation. However, even without longitudinal measurements, if the height is profoundly affected (more than 3 standard deviations below the mean), an evaluation should be strongly considered.

4. How is short stature classified?

Given the above consideration, there are two major categories of short stature: (1) normal variant short stature and (2) pathologic short stature or insufficient growth. Normal variant short stature can be subdivided into familial short stature and constitutional delay of growth and puberty, colloquially referred to as the "late bloomer." The causes of pathologic short stature include chronic systemic disease; chromosomal disorders (e.g., Down syndrome, Turner syndrome); other genetic disorders (e.g., osteochondrodystrophies, Prader-Willi syndrome); malnutrition (relative or absolute); endocrine disorders (e.g., growth hormone deficiency, hypothyroidism, Cushing syndrome); and psychosocial growth retardation. The vast majority of cases of short stature fall into the normal variant category.

5. What are the differences between familial short stature and constitutional growth delay?

In both conditions the growth curve is parallel to the normal curve, at least after about 2 years of age. Although constitutional delay is a diagnosis of exclusion, it can initially be distinguished from familial short stature by delayed bone age and eventually a delay in puberty. Unlike familial short stature, the "late bloomer" eventually catches up with the normal growth curve after puberty begins. There may or may not be a family history of a similar growth pattern in children with constitutional growth delay. However, there is always a family history of short adults in familial short stature, in which the bone age is equivalent to the chronologic age. Items helpful in determining a family history of delayed puberty and growth are age at menarche in female relatives and, for boys, whether the father or a male relative continued to grow beyond high school graduation (i.e., after age 17 or 18). In either condition of normal-variant short stature, monitoring growth is important to ensure continued normal growth velocity. However, although a delayed bone age is a hallmark of constitutional delay, most pathologic causes of short stature also have some degree of delayed skeletal maturation.

6. What is a bone age x-ray? How is it helpful in the evaluation of growth disorders?

Bone age is usually determined by a radiograph of the left hand and wrist that is compared with a standard atlas of x-rays for boys and girls of different ages. The hand/wrist x-ray is adequate for this determination in adolescents. A delay in bone age relative to chronologic age indicates growth potential beyond the currently plotted height percentile. For example, although a patient with constitutional growth delay may plot at or below the fifth percentile, he or she will usually catch up to the normal growth curve. The same is true in children treated for growth hormone deficiency who have a delayed bone age at diagnosis. On the other hand, children with precocious puberty have an advanced bone age due to the effect of premature secretion of sex steroids that accelerate skeletal maturation. Although patients with precocious puberty may plot at the upper percentiles in early childhood, they eventually may end up with short stature because of early epiphyseal closure if the progression of puberty is not interrupted. As a follow-up measure, bone age generally is not needed more often than annually except in the longitudinal evaluation of precocious puberty, in which the rate of skeletal maturation can exceed the increase in chronologic age.

7. What is idiopathic short stature?

This term is reserved for adolescents who, after careful evaluation, have no explanation for short stature. Parents and family members are generally of normal height, and there is no family history of constitutional growth delay. Growth velocity is usually below normal, and bone age may or may not be delayed. The physical examination and laboratory tests are within normal limits. The height percentiles of these children are below the calculated midparental target heights, which can be determined by the following formula:

For girls: $$\frac{[\text{Father's ht (in)} - 5\text{ in}] + \text{mother's ht (in)} \pm 3\text{ inches}}{2}$$

For boys: $$\frac{[\text{Mother's ht (in)} + 5\text{ in}] + \text{father's ht (in)} \pm 3\text{ inches}}{2}$$

Plotting the height for bone age can also give a rough estimate of ultimate height potential. A few reports indicate that patients with idiopathic short stature have a relative deficiency of the growth hormone receptor, but this finding is by no means definitive. The response to growth hormone therapy has been variable and usually minimal, making it difficult to recommend this therapy for most patients with idiopathic short stature. On the other hand, beneficial effects of growth hormone therapy have been observed in patients with Turner syndrome and chronic renal insufficiency. In both of these conditions, growth hormone secretion has been shown, for the most part, to be normal by standard testing.

8. In addition to age, what else contributes to variations in growth velocity?

Both a seasonal variation and a more frequent or saltatory variation in growth rate over the year are seen in prepubertal children. Height tends to increase maximally in spring until autumn and to slow down in the winter months. The inverse is true for weight. In addition, several periods of accelerated growth are followed by relative lack of growth over the year.

Children with congenital growth hormone deficiency often grow normally for the first 1.5–2 years of age for reasons that are not entirely understood. However, patients with growth hormone deficiency due to a genetic mutation in the development of the GH–IGF-1 axis are often small from birth.

9. What historical information is important in evaluating short stature?

Birth history, previous measurements, family heights and history, psychosocial history, medications, and review of systems are important factors in evaluating short stature. Whether the child was premature or small for gestational age at birth is important. Breech presentations, significant hypoglycemia, and prolonged neonatal jaundice have been associated with pituitary deficiency. The system review may uncover symptoms of hypothyroidism, malabsorption, chronic disease, or diabetes insipidus, visual impairment, and increased intracranial pressure associated with a tumor in the area of the hypothalamus. Concurrent medication for attention-deficit hyperactivity disorder (ADHD), such as methylphenidate (Ritalin), can suppress appetite and thereby inhibit growth. Bizarre behavior can be a manifestation of psychosocial growth failure. Previous growth records help determine whether the current measurement represents a decrease in percentiles or is consistent with the previous growth pattern.

10. What parts of the physical examination are helpful?

Dysmorphic features on physical examination are consistent with a genetic cause of short stature. Measurements of body dimensions screen for a skeletal abnormality, such as one of the skeletal dysplasias. In achondroplasia, the arm span is significantly shorter (> 5 cm) than stature, and the upper-to-lower body segment ratio is increased. The body segment ratio is normally well above 1.0 in infancy but becomes equal to unity by 7–10 years of age. On the other hand, the body segment ratio is decreased in spinal abnormalities, such as spondyloepiphyseal dysplasia or severe scoliosis, or as a result of spinal irradiation therapy. The relation of weight to height, plotted on the appropriate curve, is important for identification of nutritional deficiency as a cause of short stature. Pubertal staging is important. Even without classical stigmata, Turner syndrome should be considered in any girl with short stature, especially when pubic hair is present without concurrent breast development. In boys, short penile length since infancy may be a sign of hypopituitarism and growth hormone deficiency.

11. In addition to a bone age, what initial laboratory tests should be considered in evaluating short stature?

If growth velocity is abnormally low, a general laboratory screen should be considered, taking into account the various causes of poor growth. The screen includes a complete blood count, paying particular attention to anemia of chronic disease. In addition, a sedimentation rate can screen for occult inflammatory bowel disease. Assessment of blood urea nitrogen, creatinine, and electrolytes and urinalysis are important to look for renal disease, acidosis, or diabetes insipidus. Measuring calcium, phosphorus, and alkaline phosphatase screens for rickets or pseudohypoparathyroidism. In girls, a chromosomal karyotype should be considered to look for Turner syndrome. From an endocrine standpoint, levels of thyoxine (T_4) and thyroid-stimulating hormone (TSH) should be measured to rule out hypothyroidism, even when no signs other than short stature are present. IGF-1 (somatomedin C) is an insulin-like growth factor directly regulated by growth hormone. IGFBP-3, its binding protein, is also regulated by growth hormone. These peptides show no significant diurnal variation. Both are low to varying degrees in growth hormone deficiency (GHD), and therefore are used as a screening test for GHD. One caveat is that both of these factors also may be low because of malnutrition. Another test to consider in evaluating short stature is serum antiendomysial antibodies to look for celiac disease.

12. When should a provocative growth hormone stimulation test be considered?

If all screening tests are normal except for a low IGF1 and/or IGFBP-3 and malnutrition is not the explanation, a provocative growth hormone stimulation test is the next step. Because growth hormone is secreted mainly during slow-wave sleep, it is difficult to assess by a random blood sample in the office or clinic. Various secretagogues have been used to determine normal pituitary reserve of growth hormone, including intravenous arginine and glucagon, and oral levo-dopa and clonidine. These agents seem to work by stimulating growth hormone-releasing hormone (GHRH) or inhibiting somatostatin. In addition, insulin-induced hypoglycemia has been used as a stimulus for release of both growth hormone and adrenocorticotropic hormone (ACTH)/cortisol and has the advantage of analyzing the response of both hormones.

13. What are the currently approved indications for growth hormone therapy?

The Food and Drug Administration (FDA) has approved growth hormone therapy for children with growth hormone deficiency, short stature associated with Turner syndrome and chronic renal insufficiency, and Prader-Willi syndrome and for adults with bona fide growth hormone deficiency. The most recent indication approved by the FDA is use in small-for-gestational age infants who have shown no catch-up growth by 2 years of age. As the supply of growth hormone derived from recombinant DNA technology is virtually unlimited, newer indications are always under consideration.

14. What are the potential side effects of growth hormone therapy?

At the appropriate dose, side effects are extremely rare. Two possibilities, however, deserve mention. Slipped capital femoral epiphysis is seen on rare occasions, especially in children with an increased body mass index. Pseudotumor cerebri is rare and unpredictable. If benign increased intracranial pressure should develop, cessation of growth hormone usually leads to resolution, and resumption of therapy is often possible without recurrence. Although historically leukemia was mentioned as occurring with increased frequency, this side effect was noted only in Japan and on subsequent analysis found not to be a problem. However, leukemia should be considered in patients with genetic risk factors, such as disorders characterized by chromosomal fragility (e.g., Fanconi syndrome.)

PUBERTY

15. What mechanism controls the onset of puberty?

The mechanism controlling the onset of puberty is unknown. What has been established is that the limiting factor regulating development of puberty is the mature physiologic and pulsatile secretion of luteinizing hormone-releasing hormone (LHRH), also known as gonadotropin-releasing hormone (GnRH), from the hypothalamus. Although the critical regulatory component of GnRH release at the onset of puberty is not known, contributing factors include nutrition (critical body weight), skeletal age, insulin-like growth factors, and sex hormones (e.g., earlier onset of puberty is seen in patients with poorly controlled congenital adrenal hyperplasia).

16. When is the development of puberty considered precocious?

Precocious puberty is defined by statistical criteria. Currently any sign of puberty before 8 years of age in girls or 9–9.5 years of age in boys is considered precocious. Recently interest in lowering the threshold age for diagnosis in girls has been renewed because of data suggesting that pubertal onset is occurring earlier. Recent data show that in African-American girls onset of normal puberty may occur as early as 7 years of age. True precocious puberty is most common in girls and usually idiopathic, whereas in boys it is often associated with pathology such as a brain tumor.

17. What is premature adrenarche?

A common presentation of precocious puberty in both sexes is premature adrenarche, isolated premature development of pubic and/or axillary hair with or without adult-like body odor. Although it is a diagnosis of exclusion, this entity is not uncommon, occurs more often in children with exogenous obesity, and is considered a variation of normal. Its biochemical hallmark is selective, mild-to-moderate elevation in serum dehydroepiandrosterone sulfate (DHEAS) in relation to Tanner stage. Bone age is usually normal or mildly advanced and consistent with height age, and linear growth is not significantly accelerated.

18. How is a delay or lack of puberty classified?

Delayed puberty is usually defined as lack of initiation of secondary sexual characteristics in boys by 14 years and in girls by 13 years of age. Failure of pubertal development can be classified into three main categories: (1) hypergonadotropic hypogonadism or primary gonadal failure, (2) hypogonadotropic hypogonadism or central hypothalamic/pituitary failure, and (3) deferred or delayed function. Examples of the first category include Turner syndrome, Klinefelter syndrome, or acquired gonadal failure after chemotherapy or radiation therapy for malignancy. Serum concentrations of luteinizing hormone (LH) and/or follicle-stimulating hormone (FSH) generally are elevated when measured at the usual age of puberty. Hypogonadotropic hypogonadism can be either congenital (e.g., Kallmann syndrome, which is associated with anosmia; Prader-Willi syndrome) or acquired secondary to central nervous system tumors, radiation therapy, or surgery. Although constitutional delay of puberty, usually associated with growth delay, is an example of hypogonadotropic hypogonadism, it is more accurately placed in the category of delayed or deferred function. The same can be said for pubertal delay associated with exercise (athletes, ballet dancers), anorexia nervosa, or chronic illness.

19. Describe a reasonable approach to the evaluation of delayed pubertal development.

In patients meeting the definition of delayed puberty, evaluation should begin with a comprehensive medical history and physical examination. Because constitutional delay is the most common cause of delayed sexual development, a careful family history is important to help determine the extent of evaluation. Constitutional delay, acquired gonadal failure, and various syndromes, such as Turner or Klinefelter syndrome, may be suspected at this stage of evaluation. Absence of the sense of smell provides evidence for Kallmann syndrome. A bone age x-ray is delayed significantly and corresponds to the height age in constitutional delay. Serum FSH and/or LH are abnormally increased in primary gonadal failure, whereas values are low or characteristic of prepubertal levels in hypogonadotropic hypogonadism. A serum estradiol in girls and serum testosterone in boys should be obtained. A serum prolactin is sometimes helpful, especially in the presence of secondary amenorrhea in girls, to look for a prolactin-secreting adenoma. Other hormones, such as thyroid hormone and TSH, should be obtained as clinically indicated. A serum DHEAS may help determine the presence of adrenarche. An LHRH stimulation test is not useful before 11–12 years of age in girls and 13 years of age in boys, because it is impossible to distinguish results from a normal prepubertal pattern. A karyotype should be considered as clinically indicated, especially to look for Turner or Klinefelter syndrome. Other tests, such as brain imaging, should be considered if clinically indicated.

20. Describe a reasonable approach to treatment of delayed pubertal development.

If constitutional delay is the likely diagnosis, treatment of delayed puberty is based on psychological factors, because tincture of time generally solves the problem. However, when significant delayed development causes undue psychological stress, treatment can be considered if the skeletal age is at least 2 years behind the chronologic age and no physical signs of puberty are present. For boys, a short course of depot testosterone in the form of testosterone enanthate or cypionate at a dose of 50 mg intramuscularly every 4 weeks for 5 or 6 doses often "jump-starts" endogenous puberty. Care must be taken to avoid prolonged treatment, which may lead to an unanticipated and undesirable continued acceleration of skeletal maturation that curtails ultimate height potential. In boys who are unable to progress through puberty because of hypergonadotropic or hypogonadotropic hypogonadism, testosterone therapy can be initiated as in patients with constitutional delay. However, the dose of testosterone should gradually be increased to simulate normal pubertal progression, generally increasing by 25 mg to 50 mg every 6 months. The adult male testosterone replacement dose is equivalent to 100 mg weekly and usually is administered as 300 or 200 mg every 3 weeks or every 2 weeks, respectively. Adults can then be treated with other testosterone preparations, such as topical patches or gels, but these options are not recommended for adolescents because of the difficulty in titrating a dose that is appropriate for Tanner stage.

21. Are girls treated for constitutional delay of growth?

For selection bias and other reasons, girls are treated less often than boys for constitutional delay of puberty. However, treatment is needed for girls with Turner syndrome and other causes of hypogonadism. Although various approaches are available, one option is to begin with daily low-dose estrogen for 6–12 months, either in the form of Premarin, 0.3 mg, or ethinyl estradiol, 0.02 mg. After this period or when breakthrough menstruation occurs, cyclic hormonal replacement therapy can be instituted with estrogen administered on days 1–21 and progesterone on days 10–21 of the cycle. No medication is given on day 22 through day 28 to allow menstruation, after which the medication cycle is repeated. The doses of estrogen and progesterone can be increased as puberty progresses and, after a certain time, hormonal replacement with oral contraceptive therapy may be considered. In both sexes, care must be taken in patients with short stature so that doses of sex hormones are increased gradually in order not to compromise adult height potential.

OBESITY AND POLYCYSTIC OVARY SYNDROME

22. When should an endocrine problem be considered in the evaluation of obesity?

The vast majority (> 90%) of children referred for obesity do not have an endocrinologic problem. However, depending on the family constellation, long-standing obesity can lead to insulin resistance and type 2 diabetes. Therefore, obesity is not usually caused by an endocrinopathy but can result in one over time. Two endocrinologic diagnoses that can cause obesity (albeit relatively mild) in children and adolescents are hypothyroidism and Cushing syndrome. In both conditions, statural growth velocity is impaired in contrast to the normal-to-accelerated height velocity seen in exogenous obesity. Therefore, overweight children who have a normal height generally do not require endocrine tests. However, for patients with significant obesity and patients with acanthosis nigricans, a simultaneous fasting serum glucose and insulin or C-peptide level should be considered. Although this test rarely uncovers diabetes in children without symptoms of hyperglycemia, inappropriate elevation in serum insulin as a sign of insulin resistance is not uncommon. A serum glucose ≥ 126 mg% (fasting) or ≥ 200 mg% (nonfasting) is significant and consistent with early diabetes. Even if normal, the results may be helpful for therapeutic purposes, including anticipatory guidance, weight management, and dietary counseling. For patients with profound obesity, measurement of serum transaminases to check for hepatic steatosis and, if symptoms exist, evaluation for sleep apnea may be indicated.

23. What about the overweight patient with short stature or decreased linear growth velocity?

Measurement of T_4 and TSH is indicated in this situation. Depending on signs and symptoms of endogenous Cushing syndrome, a fasting serum ACTH, cortisol, electrolytes, and a 24-hour urine free cortisol (standardized to urine creatinine) may be indicated. Although growth hormone deficiency does not usually result in frank generalized obesity, an overweight child may suffer from growth hormone deficiency, and the standard evaluation for short stature should be considered. Although other syndromes, such as Prader-Willi or Laurence-Moon-Biedl syndrome, may be associated with obesity, the clinical history and physical examination should lead to these diagnoses.

24. What is polycystic ovary syndrome?

Polycystic ovary syndrome (PCOS) is a term used loosely to describe a heterogeneous, incompletely understood family of disorders characterized by elevated intraovarian concentrations of androgens and the clinical manifestations of hyperandrogenism. The primary form of the disease is also called functional ovarian hyperandrogenism or Stein-Leventhal syndrome.

25. Describe the clinical features of PCOS.

Signs and symptoms of PCOS include evidence of virilization (e.g., acne, hirsutism, alopecia), which may be mild. Menstrual irregularities are common and may range from amenorrhea or oligomenorrhea to frequent, heavy menses. Anovulation underlies most of these irregularities. Obesity, acanthosis nigricans, and insulin resistance frequently occur. Onset of symptoms is typically peripubertal, and a family history of similar clinical features is often present.

26. What are potential long-term sequelae of PCOS?

Women with PCOS have an elevated risk of developing diabetes mellitus and endometrial cancer later in life. Because many affected women are anovulatory, fertility is impaired.

27. What other conditions should be considered in an adolescent with clinical evidence of hyperandrogenism?

Although **Cushing disease** can present with findings similar to those of PCOS, they are usually more severe and associated with hypertension, striae, and central adiposity. Cushing disease usually is not associated with acanthosis nigricans. Screening for latent **congenital adrenal hyperplasia** (e.g., mild 21-hydroxylase deficiency) can be considered, although it is often associated with more marked evidence of virilization and usually is not associated with obesity and acanthosis nigricans. A striking elevation in serum testosterone is consistent with an **adrenal or ovarian tumor**. The use of **androgenic drugs** also should be considered.

28. What laboratory features are suggestive of PCOS?

A mild elevation in plasma testosterone, particularly free testosterone, is consistent with PCOS. Androstenedione may be increased as well. Levels are not suppressed during a dexamethasone suppression test, although this test is not routinely indicated. Sex hormone-binding globulin levels may be low. Elevation of the LH-to-FSH ratio and elevated insulin levels are consistent with PCOS but not specific for the disorder. Pelvic ultrasound may show excessive stroma and a polycystic follicular appearance of the ovaries, but these findings are neither sensitive nor specific for PCOS.

29. How is PCOS treated?

Treatment of PCOS should be individualized, based on clinical findings. Combination oral contraceptive pills suppress ovarian androgen hypersecretion, thereby improving acne and slowing the progression of hirsutism as well as regulating the menstrual cycle. Alternatively, a cyclic progestin may be given to induce periodic menses in an oligomenorrheic or amenorrheic adolescent. Both regimens decrease the risk of endometrial cancer due to unopposed estrogen. Adolescents with severe hirsutism may benefit from an androgen blocker such as spironolactone. Other cosmetic measures, such as waxing, electrolysis, and laser treatment, may be used alone or in conjunction with spironolactone. The use of metformin in PCOS is currently under evaluation and may be considered in patients with concurrent insulin resistance. Referral to a specialist in endocrinology, adolescent medicine, or gynecology should be considered. Women desiring pregnancy should be referred to a reproductive endocrinologist to discuss pharmacologic means of inducing ovulation.

THYROID DISEASE

30. How does hypothyroidism present in children and adolescents?

Hypothyroidism in older children presents in a variety of ways. Often, but not always, it may present with a goiter incidentally noted on physical examination. The majority of such patients have autoimmune (Hashimoto) thyroiditis. The thyroid gland is usually mildly to moderately enlarged, nontender, firm, and symmetrical; at times it has a pebbly or bosselated surface on palpation. There are usually no discrete nodules, although multinodular goiter occasionally occurs in autoimmune thyroiditis. Symptoms of hypothyroidism (e.g., infrequent bowel movements, cold intolerance) usually are not present unless the T_4 level is low. An elevated TSH, despite a normal T_4, is consistent with compensated hypothyroidism. Relatively asymptomatic long-standing hypothyroidism also may occur, usually in the context of significant linear growth failure. Although autoimmune thyroiditis is the likely etiology, a goiter is not present in most cases (lymphocytic infiltration has "scarred down" to the point of a small gland). The bone age is significantly delayed, often more than the height age.

31. What if the thyroid gland is not symmetrical?

In an adolescent with an asymmetrical goiter, nodular goiter, or isolated nodule, thyroid cancer should be suspected. In that case, a thyroid ultrasound is helpful as an initial diagnostic step in addition to measurement of thyroid antibodies, T_4, TSH, and serum thyroglobulin. Such patients should be referred to a pediatric endocrinologist and, depending on results of the ultrasound, probably will proceed to a diagnostic fine-needle aspiration and/or surgical exploration.

32. What are the usual laboratory findings in patients with a simple goiter?

Laboratory tests can reveal a normal T_4 and TSH, a normal T_4 and elevated TSH, or a low T_4 and high TSH. Although a serum TSH can be used to screen for primary hypothyroidism, in which case TSH is elevated, the TSH level is usually in the normal range (but with a low T_4) in hypothalamic or tertiary hypothyroidism and, therefore, is not helpful in the diagnosis of this condition. Thyroid peroxidase and antithyroglobulin antibodies are elevated in ≥ 50% of patients with autoimmune thyroid disease. Measurement of the resin T_3 uptake (rT3U), a test that indirectly assesses the binding capacity for thyroid hormone, is rarely helpful or diagnostic. TSH is an adequate screening test for hypothyroidism in most cases.

33. What is the recommended treatment for hypothyroidism?

Treatment with L-thyroxine should be instituted in patients with abnormally elevated TSH with or without a low T_4. In the adolescent with acquired hypothyroidism, synthetic L-thyroxine at the appropriate dosage (1–3 µg/kg body weight/day) is sufficient for treatment. There is generally no need to consider treatment with triiodothyronine (Cytomel) because the enzymatic conversion of T_4 to T_3 is augmented in the hypothyroid state. Caution must be used in prescribing generic preparations of L-thyroxine, which historically have had problems with biologic potency. There is no place for the use of desiccated thyroid hormone, derived from animal thyroid tissue. These preparations have unknown amounts of T_4, T_3, and other metabolites, making titration of the appropriate dosage difficult. In the child with long-standing hypothyroidism and growth failure, catch-up growth occurs with L-thyroxine replacement, but ultimate height potential can be jeopardized because during treatment the bone age often advances more rapidly than chronologic age. Consideration can be given in this context to starting at a lower replacement dose of L-thyroxine that is gradually increased over time. The patient and parents should be counseled that temporary mild hair loss and a decrease in school performance may occur during treatment. The decrease in school performance is due to the child's "waking up," noticing the outside world, and becoming more easily distracted. Serum T_4 and TSH should be monitored periodically. After initiation of therapy or a dose adjustment, these tests should be obtained within 6–8 weeks to ensure adequacy of dosage. When the results are normal, serum T_4 and TSH can be monitored every 6 months in the older growing child and annually after puberty is completed.

34. Describe the usual presentation of hyperthyroidism in children and adolescents.

Although less common than hypothyroidism, hyperthyroidism is seen not infrequently in older children and adolescents. Symptoms and signs of hyperthyroidism (heat intolerance, weight loss, polyuria, fatigue, sleeplessness, irritability, tremor, tachycardia, systolic hypertension, goiter) are usually apparent. Some patients complain of muscle weakness and cramps. The thyroid gland is symmetrically enlarged, not as firm as in Hashimoto thyroiditis, and smooth to palpation; it may be slightly tender. There is often an audible bruit over one or both thyroid lobes. Exophthalmos is frequently seen, and, if present, increases the likelihood of autoimmune hyperthyroidism or Graves' disease.

35. What are the typical laboratory findings in hyperthyroidism?

Laboratory tests reveal an elevated T_4 and T_3 and a suppressed or undetectable TSH. Thyroid antibodies are usually positive, but an elevated TSH receptor antibody (TSI) confirms the diagnosis of Graves' disease, although this parameter is not elevated in every patient. An I^{123} thyroid uptake scan shows high 6- and 24-hour uptake and a symmetrical goiter. However, this test is not always indicated if other clinical findings are obvious. Often the serum T_3 is elevated out of proportion to T_4 in Graves' disease or in the unusual condition of an autonomous hyperfunctioning thyroid nodule.

36. What are the different treatment methods for hyperthyroidism?

Three treatment options are available: antithyroid medicinal therapy, radioactive iodine (RAI) therapy, or surgery. Usually antithyroid medicinal therapy is begun with either propylthiouracil (PTU) or methimazole (Tapazole). PTU has the advantage of inhibiting conversion of T_4 to T_3. Methimazole has the advantage of a longer half-life and potential twice-daily dosing (compared with 3 times daily). RAI therapy is often reserved as a second-line treatment in older children (> 12 years old) after medicinal therapy has been unsuccessful or if rare side effects (e.g., bone marrow suppression, hepatopathy) develop during PTU or Tapazole therapy. However, RAI is considered more frequently as a first-line treatment in older pediatric patients. Beta-adrenergic blockers, such as propranolol or atenolol, often improve significant tachycardia and systolic hypertension. Symptoms of hyperthyroidism may not begin to improve for 1 or 3 weeks after initiation of therapy. Initially, patients need to be seen frequently for follow-up.

HYPOGLYCEMIA

37. Is hypoglycemia a frequent concern and real entity in adolescents?

Bona fide hypoglycemia is a rare condition that is often overly suspected in older pediatric patients in contrast to neonates or young infants, in whom close and frequent glucose monitoring, in conjunction with unambiguous signs and symptoms, confirms the diagnosis. In adolescents, most of the symptoms attributed to hypoglycemia, such as dizziness, headache, and weakness, are not due to hypoglycemia. The existence of reactive or postprandial hypoglycemia as a distinct entity is questionable. In adult studies, more than 70% of patients with temporal symptoms consistent with reactive hypoglycemia were found to have normal blood glucose levels at the time of symptoms. Most of the remainder had mildly low glucose levels. A relative decrease in blood glucose after the postprandial peak and the attendant adrenergic response may be one explanation. The omission of breakfast by adolescent patients has been associated with this problem. In any case, most symptoms resolve with the institution of dietary changes, such as adequate calories, regular meals and snacks, and avoidance of concentrated sugars. An oral glucose tolerance test (OGTT) to evaluate for hypoglycemia is rarely necessary. If done, it should be at least 5 hours in duration, obtaining both glucose and insulin levels and observing for behavioral changes at each time point. Dietary preparation, including high complex carbohydrates for 3 days before the OGTT, is important to avoid the apparent flat glucose response seen in some patients with poor nutritional habits.

38. How is hypoglycemia defined?

Although a blood glucose < 60 mg/dl is considered abnormal in most laboratories, a diagnosis of hypoglycemia should be considered if the blood glucose is < 50 mg/dl and is made definitively if blood glucose is < 40 mg/dl or plasma glucose is < 46 mg/dl. Clinical signs and symptoms vary significantly among patients. Causes of hypoglycemia vary according to the age of the patient. There are three major etiologic categories: (1) abnormalities in hormone secretion, (2) abnormalities in the production or utilization of metabolic fuels, and (3) other causes. Abnormalities in hormone secretion include hormone overproduction, as seen in hyperinsulinism, and underproduction, as seen in hypopituitarism (ACTH, growth hormone) and adrenal insufficiency (Addison disease, congenital adrenal hyperplasia). Adrenal insufficiency is characterized by a lack of secretion of hormones to counterregulate insulin and to stimulate endogenous glucose production. Abnormalities in the production or utilization of metabolic fuels include the rare inborn errors of metabolism of amino and fatty acids or glycogen storage and delayed development of normal metabolic mechanisms, as seen in premature or small-for-gestational age infants or idiopathic ketotic hypoglycemia. Other causes include hypoglycemia due to drugs (exogenous insulin, sulfonylurea, or alcohol).

39. How is hypoglycemia evaluated?

If hypoglycemia is documented or strongly suspected in any patient, referral to pediatric endocrinology is indicated. If hypoglycemia was not documented but symptoms are compatible with the diagnosis, a diagnostic fast under close observation in the hospital setting is sometimes needed. Frequent monitoring of blood glucose is conducted, and the critical blood sample is obtained if hypoglycemia should develop. Although any child beyond 2 years of age is expected to tolerate at least 24 hours of fasting without hypoglycemia, normal adolescents should be capable of withstanding 36–48 hours of fasting without becoming hypoglycemic. With any evaluation for hypoglycemia it is important to obtain the necessary diagnostic blood/urine tests at the time of hypoglycemia. The so-called critical blood sample should include blood glucose, electrolytes, serum insulin, cortisol, growth hormone, and beta-hydroxybutyrate. Other tests to consider, especially in the presence of hepatomegaly, are uric acid, liver transaminases, and blood lactate. A urinalysis including ketones and a urine metabolic screen and organic acids also should be obtained, especially in younger children.

40. Why is the measurement of ketones important in evaluating hypoglycemia?

Hypoglycemia without ketones is seen in hyperinsulinism (endogenous or exogenous), carnitine deficiency, and other metabolic errors such as medium chain acyl-CoA dehydrogenase (MCAD) deficiency. This finding emphasizes the need to assess for urinary and serum ketones (beta-hydroxybutyrate) at the time of hypoglycemia. Surreptitious delivery of insulin to a patient without diabetes, either self-administered by a psychologically depressed adolescent or given in the form of child abuse, is associated with no significant ketone production and is assessed by simultaneous measurement of serum insulin, C-peptide, and glucose at the time of hypoglycemia. An elevated insulin and low C-peptide confirms exogenous insulin administration, whereas simultaneous elevation of insulin and C-peptide is consistent with either endogenous hyperinsulinism or sulfonylurea ingestion. Given the latter condition, a careful medical history for family members with type 2 diabetes on oral therapy is important to suggest the possibility of sulfonylurea-induced hypoglycemia. As part of the diagnostic evaluation, one must indicate a specific drug screen for sulfonylurea, because it is not routinely included.

41. How is the family history important in the evaluation of hypoglycemia?

In older children and adolescents, a family history of multiple endocrine neoplasia type I (MEN I) is important because this autosomal dominant condition, although sporadic in some cases, may run in families. MEN I consists of three levels of endocrine tumors: pituitary adenomas (e.g., prolactinoma, somatotropinoma, corticotropinoma), hyperparathyroidism, and insulinoma or gastrinoma (Zollinger-Ellison syndrome). Hypoglycemia in the infant of an adolescent mother with diabetes is secondary to poor control of maternal diabetes. This form of temporary neonatal hypoglycemia is due to pancreatic islet beta cell hyperplasia and resultant hyperinsulinism in the fetus and infant from continuous exposure to maternal hyperglycemia.

DIABETES MELLITUS

42. Describe the common presentation of diabetes mellitus in older children and adolescents.

Although type 2 diabetes is becoming more prevalent in the pediatric population, the majority of diabetic patients (90%) have autoimmune type 1 diabetes and present with symptoms of insulin deficiency and hyperglycemia. Symptoms include a 3- to 6-week history of polyuria, nocturia, polydipsia, and often weight loss or lack of weight gain. Polyphagia also may occur, although it is less apparent because patients usually are more interested in drinking than in eating. About 30–40% of pediatric patients present with varying degrees of diabetic ketoacidosis (DKA). DKA may be slow to develop, appearing several days or weeks after initial symptoms, or relatively precipitous in some patients. New-onset diabetes is confirmed at the bedside or in the office with a capillary blood glucose and urinalysis for glucose and ketones. Although the peak incidence for onset of diabetes remains during adolescence, over the past few years the onset of diabetes in children less than 4 years of age has increased significantly.

43. Describe the recommended evaluation and treatment of new-onset diabetes.

Although there may be less urgency for adolescents suspected of having new-onset type 2 diabetes, such patients are frequently difficult to differentiate from patients with type 1 diabetes and may present with significant ketosis and/or ketoacidosis requiring hospitalization and insulin therapy. Therefore, a physician with adequate experience in childhood and adolescent diabetes should be contacted for any child with significant symptoms or lab results. Insulin is often the initial therapeutic modality in pediatric type 2 as well as type 1 diabetes. However, older patients with type 2 diabetes, depending on the degree of metabolic decompensation, may be treated initially with oral agents, as in the case of hyperglycemia without ketosis. In any case, a thorough review, including diabetes and dietary education, is essential.

After stabilization, patients with newly diagnosed diabetes should be seen on average every 3 months by a specialist and other members of a diabetes management team for evaluation of insulin dose, diet, home glucose monitoring, hemoglobin A_{1C}, height and weight, and potential complications. In addition, regular telephone or facsimile contacts between the patient and diabetes clinic for review of blood glucose patterns and insulin adjustment and regular communication between the diabetes team and primary care physician about the evaluation and treatment plan are crucial.

44. What are the main components and principles of therapy for pediatric and adolescent diabetes?

The main components of diabetes therapy are insulin, diet, exercise, and emotional and psychological support. The guiding principles of therapy are elimination of symptoms of hyperglycemia, prevention of DKA, avoidance of hypoglycemia, maintenance of normal growth and puberty, detection of associated disease (e.g., autoimmune thyroiditis), detection and prevention of emotional disorders, and prevention of chronic vascular and neurologic complications. Any hospitalization for DKA after initial diagnosis should be viewed as a failure of therapy and of the diabetes therapeutic team.

45. Ideally, who should be included in the diabetes therapeutic team?

The diabetes therapeutic team should include the following members: diabetes nurse educator; social worker with access to psychological/psychiatric consultants; dietitian; physician;

and patient and parents. The patient and parent (or guardian) are the most important team members, and this approach encourages the patient to take more ownership in the day-to-day management of diabetes. Each professional on the team should be well versed in the nuances and management issues of diabetes in children and adolescents. The multicenter Diabetes Control and Complications Trial (DCCT) demonstrated clearly that the multidisciplinary approach of a diabetes team is an integral part of successful management.

46. What is the DCCT?

The DCCT is the first multicenter, large scale, clinical study to demonstrate that improved metabolic control decreases the risk of microvascular complications of type 1 diabetes. It was conducted at 29 national centers and involved 1,441 patients between the ages of 13 and 39 years; 195 patients were between 13 and 17 years of age. The duration of diabetes was between 1 and 15 years, and patients included in the study could have no major complications of diabetes. Patients were randomized into intensive and conventional treatment groups. Conventional treatment consisted of absence of symptoms of hyperglycemia, 1–2 daily insulin doses, one or two home blood glucose measurements (or four urine glucose measurements) per day, and standard medical contact. The intensively treated patients had much closer surveillance and higher expectations. They received 3–4 insulin doses per day or used a continuous subcutaneous insulin infusion (CSII) pump; blood glucose was tested at least 4–5 times per day; preprandial blood glucose was maintained at 70–120 mg/dl and postprandial glucose at < 180 mg/dl; and frequent contact was maintained with the therapeutic team, including weekly phone calls and monthly visits. The goal of the intensive treatment group was achievement of a normal hemoglobin A_{1C} (< 6.05%).

47. What were the results of the DCCT?

The intensive treatment group achieved a mean hemoglobin A_{1C} of 7.12% compared to the conventional group mean of 9.02%. The subset of adolescent patients in the intensively treated group achieved a hemoglobin A_{1C} of 8.06% compared with 9.76% in the conventional treatment group. Among both adolescents and adults, the intensively managed patients had the following reduced risks of complications compared with the conventional group: retinopathy, 76%; nephropathy, 54%; and neuropathy, 60%. One of the more important findings was that the reduction in complication risk represented a continuum of benefit from a reduction in hemoglobin A_{1C}. For example, in most patients a two percentage point reduction in hemoglobin A_{1C} reduced the risk of retinopathy by 50%. Despite the importance of an intensified insulin approach, the investigators were cautious not to attribute the results to intensive insulin therapy alone. Other components of enhanced management, such as the multidisciplinary team, frequency of contacts and visits, and frequent adjustments in therapy, were deemed equally important in achieving the improved glycosylated hemoglobin results. Adverse events were somewhat higher in the intensive group and included hypoglycemia, weight gain, and cutaneous infections in pump patients.

48. What were the recommendations of the DCCT?

Recommendations were to embrace the DCCT results as significant evidence that diabetic metabolic control does matter. A multidisciplinary team and frequent visits, including quarterly measurements of hemoglobin A_{1C}, should be the standard of care. Behavioral scientists were valuable during the trial and should be included in diabetes management. In addition, more steps should be adopted in an attempt to avoid hypoglycemia while still achieving improved metabolic control. Finally, legislation or other means should be enacted to reimburse more completely nonphysician team members.

49. In addition to the DCCT recommendations, what other strategies can be used to improve diabetes metabolic control?

Newer, fast-acting, and earlier-peaking insulins, such as Lys-Pro (Humalog), allow better control of postprandial blood glucose, which is now recognized as an important variable in the development of chronic complications of diabetes. Multiple daily insulin injections, 3 or 4 times/day with a combination of long-acting and short-acting insulin, or use of the CSII pump can lead to improved control in many patients. Of course, attention to diet and exercise is of continuing importance in type 1 and type 2 diabetes.

50. What are the complications of type 1 diabetes in children and adolescents?

The potential complications of diabetes in the pediatric age group can be divided into acute, intermediate, and chronic. The acute complications are DKA, hypoglycemia, and inappropriate weight loss or gain. Potential intermediate complications include growth failure, delayed puberty, impaired cognition (from recurrent hypoglycemia, especially in young children), failure of glucose counterregulation or hypoglycemia unawareness, hyperlipidemia, and emotional or psychiatric disturbances. Chronic or long-term complications are the most familiar and include microvascular retinopathy, nephropathy, neuropathy, and, at a later age, macrovascular disease.

51. What are the therapeutic objectives and tools for managing diabetes in adolescent patients?

Therapeutic objectives include normalization of blood glucose levels while at the same time avoiding hypoglycemia. The goals include a fasting glucose between 80 and 120 mg/dl, postprandial glucose between 80 and 140 mg/dl, and 3 AM blood glucose levels > 70 mg/dl to avoid overnight hypoglycemia. One advantage of the CSII pump is a reduced propensity for overnight hypoglycemia because the steady background basal infusion of insulin does not have an unwanted peak activity in the early morning hours, as can be seen after an evening dose of intermediate-acting neutral protamine Hagedorn (NPH) or Lente insulin. Other goals, as mentioned, are postponement or avoidance of chronic complications and detection and treatment of associated disease, such as hypothyroidism. To this end, glycosylated hemoglobin should be measured at quarterly clinic visits and thyroid antibodies and functions (T_4, TSH) every 1–2 years or more often as clinically indicated. Between 30% and 40% of children with type 1 diabetes develop positive thyroid antibodies; although most remain euthyroid, some develop hypothyroidism and, in rare cases, hyperthyroidism. Once puberty begins, annual screening should be done for proteinuria by assaying urine microalbumin relative to creatinine excretion, as surveillance for early diabetic nephropathy. Although microvascular complications generally do not appear before puberty even in poorly controlled patients, the clock for onset of complications can be accelerated once puberty begins in the presence of chronically poor metabolic control. As part of prevention of macrovascular complications, fasting plasma lipids should be periodically evaluated. Although mild hyperlipidemia is part and parcel of poor diabetic control, annual measurements of total, low-density lipoprotein (LDL), and high-density lipoprotein (HDL) cholesterol can alert the physician to abnormally elevated levels and also can be used to convince patients and families of the need for improved metabolic control.

52. What is glycosylated hemoglobin? How is it useful?

Glycosylated or glycated hemoglobin refers to the passive binding of glucose to the hemoglobin protein by an Amadori rearrangement of the Schiff base (glucose-protein unit) into the glycated protein product. The reaction depends on the ambient glucose concentration and is generally irreversible so that more glycosylation of protein can accumulate over time but glucose is not released from the protein after binding has taken place. Because the life span of any one red blood cell, including its hemoglobin content, is approximately 100 days, the glycosylated hemoglobin represents an average value, at one point in time, for red cells of different ages in the 100-day life cycle. Therefore, it reflects an integrated concentration of ambient blood glucose for the previous 3 months. The hemoglobin A_{1C} is the glycosylated A_1 component of the hemoglobin molecule and the gold standard used by clinical labs. It can be assayed every 3 months to assess changes in average blood glucose for that period. In conjunction with daily home blood glucose monitoring, it is useful for assessing the degree of metabolic control. The DCCT used hemoglobin A_{1C} as one of the main variables in predicting risk for development of microvascular complications. Given the DCCT results, a reasonable goal is to maintain hemoglobin A_{1C} below 8% and as close to normal ($\leq$ 6%) as possible. Hemoglobn A_{1C} can also be helpful in deciphering whether home glucose measurements are accurate or fabricated (as may be seen on occasion in adolescent patients).

53. Discuss the peculiarities of type 1 diabetes in adolescent patients.

Sex hormones of puberty and the attendant rise in growth hormone secretion induce a degree of insulin resistance. The average insulin dose per body weight increases from < 1 to > 1 unit/kg/day during puberty in most patients. Adolescent patients with diabetes have the usual issues of adolescence, including searching for independence in function and decision-making and balancing peer relationships. The transition from childhood to adolescence, therefore, may be associated with deviation from the recommended treatment plan and often is manifested by lack of adherence to home blood glucose testing and occasionally by omission of insulin doses. The number-one cause of recurrent DKA in adolescents with type 1 diabetes is omission of insulin. In addition, in some adolescent patients with long-standing diabetes, a blunted epinephrine response to nocturnal hypoglycemia and hypoglycemia unawareness have been observed. These factors can make adjustments in insulin dose, diet, and exercise potentially difficult.

54. What are the psychological comorbidities in adolescent diabetes?

A number of studies have shown potentially significant psychological problems in pediatric and adolescent patients with diabetes. A study by Kovacs et al. in 1997 of 92 children between 8 and 13 years of age reported that 48% of participants had a major depressive, conduct, or anxiety disorder identified by 10 years after diagnosis of diabetes. Another study by Blanz et al. in 1993 of 93 patients between the ages of 17 and 19 years showed that 33% were identified with a psychological disorder compared with 9.7% of nondiabetic controls. Examples included somatic, sleep, compulsive, and depressive disorders. The study by Rydall et al. in 1997 of 91 female patients with diabetes reported that 29% manifested some degree of disordered eating behavior and were at greater risk for the development of diabetic retinopathy. Overall psychological and physical health of adolescents with diabetes appears to revolve around four main areas: knowledge about diabetes, adherence to the medical plan, stress, and family dynamics. Given these complex and dynamic issues, a multidisciplinary approach to diabetes care in children and adolescents should include the participation of behavioral scientists, such as social workers, psychologists, and, at times, psychiatrists.

55. How has the nature or type of pediatric diabetes changed over the past decade?

About 10 years ago, type 1 diabetes accounted for > 98% of childhood and adolescent diabetes; the remaining cases consisted mostly of classic type 2 diabetes, with a few cases of maturity-onset diabetes of youth (MODY). Over the past 10–15 years, the prevalence of type 2 diabetes has increased dramatically in the pediatric age group—in some studies as much as tenfold. For example, one report showed that the incidence of type 2 diabetes in Cincinnati increased from 0.7 per 100,000 pediatric population per year in 1982 to 7.2/100,000 in 1994. The same trend has been seen in many U.S. metropolitan areas. The end result is that now as many as 10–15% of childhood/adolescent cases may be type 2 diabetes. A definite ethnic predilection has emereged: type 2 diabetes is more likely to occur in African-American, Hispanic, and Native American adolescents. In addition to ethnicity, the predominant risk factors are a family history of type 2 diabetes in first- or second-degree relatives, adolescent age, obesity, and insulin resistance as manifested by acanthosis nigricans or associated polycystic ovarian syndrome.

56. What factors explain the increasing prevalence of pediatric type 2 diabetes?

The reason for the increase in type 2 diabetes is not clear, but the trend is associated with a more sedentary lifestyle and a high-calorie diet that for many children consists of fast foods high in fat and simple carbohydrates. This combination leads to obesity at a young age and the propensity for insulin resistance and type 2 diabetes. There are also two seemingly opposing developmental theories that involve the perinatal environment and early neonatal period. One is the thrifty gene hypothesis, espoused by Barker, that stems from epidemiologic studies showing that infants born small for gestational age (SGA) are more likely to develop insulin resistance and type 2 diabetes as adults. Of note, some SGA infants have been shown to have paradoxical hyperinsulinism after birth, including some with attendant hypoglycemia. The other theory derives from epidemiologic studies showing that infants of diabetic mothers have a greater incidence of later type 2 diabetes. The purported pathogenesis involves pancreatic islet beta-cell hyperplasia and increased insulin secretion that may have a permanent effect on later islet cell function. In addition, numerous studies have shown increased insulin resistance during puberty in nondiabetic children and an even greater degree of insulin resistance in African-American and Hispanic adolescents.

57. Describe the typical clinical presentation of pediatric type 2 diabetes.

The major hallmarks of pediatric type 2 diabetes are obesity (> 85th percentile body mass index), acanthosis nigricans (insulin resistance), family history, and peripubertal age. Symptoms of hyperglycemia are often present, but other clinical signs, such as polycystic ovarian dysfunction, may predominate. Of particular interest is that up to 25% of pediatric patients present with varying degrees of DKA at diagnosis, requiring intravenous fluids and insulin. This finding contrasts with the presentation in adults, who generally do not have DKA. The reason for this difference is not clear but obviously indicates severe insulin deficiency at presentation in some pediatric patients.

58. What is the recommended treatment for adolescent patients with type 2 diabetes?

For patients who present with DKA or have significant ketosis, insulin is the recommended initial therapy. Diabetes education, therefore, is similar to that given to patients with type 1 diabetes. The insulin dose should be adjusted to achieve euglycemia. However, diet and exercise are extremely important to avoid the tendency for increasing weight gain, which is more prominent in type 2 diabetes. Once blood glucose and insulin dose are stabilized, an insulin-sensitizing agent can be carefully added to the treatment regimen. The only FDA-approved oral agent for patients younger than 18 years old is metformin (Glucophage). Metformin increases insulin sensitivity and decreases hepatic glucose production. Potential untoward effects are the same as those reported in adults: hepatic and renal toxicity and lactic acidosis. Gastrointestinal symptoms, such as nausea and diarrhea, can occur but fortunately are transitory in most patients. In some patients who are successful in following a recommended diet and controlling their weight, the insulin dose can be gradually reduced over time while metformin is continued. Occasionally, both insulin and oral agents can be discontinued in highly motivated patients who achieve significant weight loss through diet and exercise.

59. What are the long-term complications of pediatric type 2 diabetes? Are they different from the long-term complications of type 1 diabetes?

Long-term microvascular complications, including retinopathy, nephropathy, and neuropathy, occur in both type 1 and type 2 diabetes. However, type 2 diabetes may be relatively silent in adolescents before diagnosis, even though microvascular damage may already be taking place. Onset of microvascular complications in patients who maintain poor metabolic control, therefore, may occur earlier than otherwise expected. In addition, given the obesity and often-attendant hypertension in such patients, macrovascular complications may occur earlier and be more severe than in patients with type 1 diabetes. Furthermore, relative or absolute hypertension may place the kidneys at even more risk for development of nephropathy.

60. Given the often insidious nature and associated findings of type 2 diabetes in adolescents, what are the recommendations for diagnostic screening?

The American Diabetes Association recommends obtaining a fasting serum/plasma glucose every 2 years beginning at the age of 10 in patients with a body mass index above the 85th percentile for age and any two of the following criteria:

- Family history of type 2 diabetes in first- or second-degree relative
- Member of a high-risk ethnic group (African American, Hispanic, Native American, or Asian Pacific Islander)
- Clinical signs of insulin resistance (e.g., acanthosis nigricans, PCOD)

A fasting serum glucose $\geq$ 126 mg/dl or random serum glucose $\geq$ 200 mg/dl is consistent with diabetes, and therapy is recommended. However, it is hoped that anticipatory and preventive treatment will have been initiated before diagnosis in any patient at risk for type 2 diabetes.

61. What are the risk factors for DKA in children and adolescents?

DKA is the presenting finding in 30–40% of pediatric patients at diagnosis of type 1 diabetes. Outside of newly diagnosed diabetes, the most common cause of recurrent DKA in children and adolescents is omission of insulin doses. Infection is a much less frequent precipitating event for DKA in pediatric patients. Studies have shown that when insulin administration is assured, repeated hospitalizations for DKA decline dramatically. Patients generally have significant psychological or psychiatric illness or come from a profoundly dysfunctional home environment. In such cases, psychological intervention for the patient and family is critical, although often not well received, and involvement of governmental child protection agencies may be necessary. Although relatively infrequent, an emerging risk factor for DKA is the continuous subcutaneous insulin infusion (CSII) pump. Because insulin pumps use very short-acting insulin and pump patients do not receive long- or intermediate-acting insulin, any interruption in subcutaneous insulin infusion can result in significant ketosis and eventual acidosis. Therefore, patients using the CSII pump need to be counseled thoroughly about this potential complication.

62. Describe the typical presenting signs of DKA.

One should assume a minimum of 10% dehydration in moderate or severe DKA in children, even though some patients do not manifest signs commensurate with the degree of dehydration on physical exam. For example, although dry mucus membranes, tachycardia, and sunken eyes are common in severe DKA, skin tenting is not a usual finding. Patients have a prodromal history of polyuria and polydipsia, and many have had frequent vomiting as ketoacidosis progresses. Kussmaul respirations are common in moderate-to-severe DKA. In rare cases, however, when blood pH is profoundly decreased, the respiratory drive may be suppressed until the pH begins to increase, thereby resulting in a paradoxical change in respiratory pattern. DKA is generally a hypothermic illness due to ketoacidosis-induced peripheral vasodilation and heat loss. Therefore, significant infection can be present in the face of a normal or minimally elevated body temperature. Patients frequently have significant abdominal pain related to ketoacidosis and attendant ileus that often mimics an acute abdomen. However, the abdominal pain is usually diffuse rather than localized and resolves with treatment if due to DKA. The sensorium can be affected to varying degrees because of the hyperosmolar state and severe acidosis. Although rare, patients have been reported to have cerebral edema and cerebral thrombotic events at the time of clinical presentation of severe DKA.

63. Discuss the diagnostic dilemmas in DKA.

Certain laboratory tests and clinical findings may be confusing during the initial evaluation of a patient with DKA. For example, the serum sodium (Na^+) concentration is artifactually decreased in an inverse relationship with the serum glucose due to osmotically driven dilution of Na^+ in the intravascular space. A rough calculation for corrected serum Na^+ is an increase of 1.6 mmol/L Na^+ for every 100 mg/dl glucose > 150 mg/dl. Similarly, despite total body potassium depletion, the serum potassium (K^+) concentration may initially be normal or mildly elevated because of the extracellular localization of K^+ in acidosis and insulin deficiency. Serum amylase can be elevated predominantly from salivary gland secretion; therefore, measurement of serum lipase is also necessary in the assessment for acute pancreatitis. Leukocytosis with a mild left shift is common in DKA because of a stress-induced leukemoid reaction. Therefore, an elevated white cell count is not diagnostic of infection in patients with DKA. Likewise, because DKA is usually associated with mildly low body temperature, a normal temperature at presentation does not rule out significant infection.

64. What is the recommended intravenous (IV) fluid therapy for DKA?

Although the numerous treatment protocols arrive at the same endpoint, certain basic tenets of therapy for DKA are widely accepted. Intravascular volume depletion should be initially corrected with isotonic (0.9%) normal saline, usually administered as a bolus of 10–20 ml/kg body weight over 1 hour. After this initial correction of intravascular volume (which is not included in subsequent calculations), replacement fluid therapy is based on the calculated deficit and ongoing fluid maintenance needs. Although some protocols recommend replacing up to half of the fluid deficit in the first 8–12 hours, a more practical approach includes even replacement of the deficit and maintenance needs over the first 24 hours of therapy. If significant hypernatremia is present, fluid replacement can be calculated over 36–48 hours. Given the usual state of dehydration in DKA, calculating total fluid replacement at 2.5 times maintenance requirements over 24 hours is another accepted method, as long as it does not exceed 4 L/24 hours/m^2 body surface area. To replace significant electrolyte deficit and to decrease the risk for cerebral edema, total osmolarity of IV fluids should be isotonic and consist of adequate NaCl and K^+ replacement (usually 40 mmol K^+/L). If potassium phosphate is used it usually administered as 20 mmol/L in combination with 20 mmol/L of potassium chloride (KCl). Dextrose is added to IV fluids when blood glucose is $\leq$ 300 mg/dl. The patient usually must take nothing by mouth (NPO status) until ketoacidosis is corrected to avoid overhydration and a resultant increased risk for brain swelling. In addition to hourly blood glucose determinations, serum electrolytes and blood pH should be monitored every 2–4 hours. Finally, because DKA is associated with total body depletion of phosphate, calcium, and magnesium, these elements also should be monitored and replaced as clinically indicated.

65. What is the recommended method for insulin administration in diabetic ketoacidosis?

Continuous intravenous insulin administration is the preferred method of delivery for DKA for a number of reasons. Although frequent (hourly) intramuscular injections of regular insulin have been used in DKA and may suffice temporarily under dire circumstances, this method is inadequate because decreased tissue perfusion from significant dehydration prevents sufficient insulin delivery and distribution. Furthermore, because the intravenous half-life of insulin is $\leq$ 15 minutes, IV administration enables more frequent adjustments for titration of insulin and fluid therapy. The usual starting dose of IV insulin is 0.1 unit/kg body weight/hour. Capillary blood glucose is measured at least hourly, and the blood glucose should not decrease more than 80–100 mg/dl/hour. When the decrement in blood glucose is greater or when blood glucose approaches 300 mg/dl, dextrose is added or increased in the IV fluids. An eventual target blood glucose during IV insulin therapy for DKA should be between 150 and 250 mg/dl to avoid impending hypoglycemia and at the same time to bring the blood glucose concentration toward or below the renal glucose threshold to lessen osmotic diuresis. If the patient is still acidotic while blood glucose continues to drop, it is best to increase the amount of dextrose in the IV solution (e.g., from 5% to 10% dextrose) rather than lower the rate of insulin infusion. This strategy avoids persistence or exacerbation of ketoacidosis due to inadequate insulin. Conversion from intravenous to subcutaneous insulin should not be done until ketosis and acidosis have been corrected.

66. Discuss the major controversies involved in the treatment of DKA.

Although significant phosphate depletion in DKA results in a reduction in erythrocyte 2,3-diphosphoglycerate and an attendant left shift in the oxyhemoglobin saturation curve, the use of phosphate in IV replacement fluids has not been shown to have a significant effect on the clinical course of DKA. The one practical benefit of using phosphate is a decrease in the total amount of chloride administered during therapy. This strategy reduces the likelihood of developing a nonanion gap hyperchloremic acidosis that, although transitory, can prolong the metabolic acidosis.

The more traditional controversy has been with the use of sodium bicarbonate. Because DKA is primarily a state of ketoacidosis due to insulin deficiency, insulin and fluid administration will correct the acidosis. Sodium bicarbonate theoretically can augment central nervous system (CNS) acidosis because the end products of the Hendersen-Hasselbach reaction are water and carbon dioxide (CO_2). CO_2 readily diffuses across the blood-brain barrier, but sodium bicarbonate does not, thereby potentially increasing CNS acidosis while correcting peripheral acidosis. This effect presents a theoretical risk for development of cerebral edema. However, sodium bicarbonate occasionally may be needed in states of profound acidosis associated with cardiovascular instability. If needed, it generally should not be administered as an acute IV bolus.

67. Discuss the potential complications of DKA and their management in pediatric and adolescent patients.

Although myocardial infarction and stroke can complicate DKA in adults, they are not usually seen in pediatric patients. The acute complications in adolescents include hypoglycemia, hypokalemia, hyper- or hyponatremia, hypocalcemia, and hyperchloremia.

The most significant and devastating complication, however, is cerebral edema. For reasons that are not clear, cerebral edema can occur in children but not usually in adults with DKA. This finding suggests a developmental predilection in pediatric patients. Although younger infants and children are at highest risk for cerebral edema, it may develop in adolescent patients and is estimated to occur in 0.3–3% of children with DKA. Morbidity and mortality from cerebral edema are substantial. The mortality rate is 40–90%, and cerebral edema accounts for 50–60% of diabetes-related deaths in the pediatric age group. Although the cause remains unknown, risk factors for cerebral edema include new-onset diabetes with DKA, younger age, less than isotonic fluid replacement with injudicious overhydration, severity of acidosis, hypoglycemia, and use of sodium bicarbonate. Furthermore, brain imaging studies in asymptomatic pediatric patients with DKA are consistent with subclinical brain swelling. Most often cerebral edema develops several hours into therapy for DKA, but it also has been reported at clinical presentation.

Symptoms and signs include development or recurrence of headache and vomiting, changes in sensorium, and other signs of increased intracranial pressure, such as bradycardia and hypertension. Decorticate/decerebrate posturing indicates impending brain herniation. Laboratory results consistent with the syndrome of inappropriate secretion of antidiuretic hormone (SIADH) also may be a sign of impending cerebral edema.

The only treatment that has been shown to be effective is immediate administration of intravenous mannitol to reduce brain swelling osmotically. Mannitol must be given within the first several minutes of clinical signs to avoid major neurologic sequelae. Other measures to reduce intracranial pressure also should be instituted.

BILBIOGRAPHY

1. Aceto T, Dempsher DP, Garibaldi L, et al: Short stature and slow growth in the young. In Becker KL (ed): Principles and Practice in Endocrinology and Metabolism. Philadelphia, Lippincott Williams & Wilkins, 2001, pp 1784–1808.
2. Alemzadeh R, Lifshitz F: Childhood obesity. In Lifshitz F (ed): Pediatric Endocrinology, 3rd ed. New York, Marcel Dekker, 1996, pp 753–774.
3. Arslanian S: Type 2 diabetes in children: Clinical aspects and risk factors. Horm Res 57(Suppl 1):19–28, 2002.
4. Diabetes Control and Complications Trial (DCCT)/Epidemiology of Diabetes Interventions and Complications (EDIC) Research Group: Beneficial effects of intensive therapy of diabetes during adolescence: Outcomes after the conclusion of the diabetes control and complications trial. J Pediatr 139:804–812, 2001.

5. Drash AL: Management of the child with diabetes mellitus: Clinical course, therapeutic strategies and monitoring techniques. In Lifshitz F (ed): Pediatric Endocrinology, 3rd ed. New York, Marcel Dekker, 1996, pp 617–629.

6. Eastman RC, Siebert CW, Harris M, Gorden P: Implications of the diabetes control and complications trial. J Clin Endocrinol Metab. 77:1105–1107, 1993.

7. Foley TP Jr: Disorders of the thyroid in children. In Sperling MA (ed): Pediatric Endocrinology. Philadelphia, W.B. Saunders, 1996, pp 171–194.

8. Lee PA: Pubertal neuroendocrine maturation: Early differentiation and stages of development. Adolesc Pediatr Gynecol 1:3, 1998.

9. Rosenbloom AL: Psychosocial aspects of diabetes mellitus. In Lifshitz F (ed): Pediatric Endocrinology, 3rd ed. New York, Marcel Dekker, 1996, pp 653–664.

10. Rosenfield RL: The ovary and female sexual maturation. In Sperling MA (ed): Pediatric Endocrinology. Philadelphia, W.B. Saunders, 1996, pp 329–385.

11. Tanner JM: Issues and advances in adolescent growth and development. J Adolesc Health Care 8:470, 1987.

12. Walvoord, EC, Waguespack SG, Pescovitz OH: Precocious and delayed puberty. In Becker KL (ed): Principles and Practice in Endocrinology and Metabolism. Philadelphia, Lippincott Williams & Wilkins, 2001, pp 893–908.

13. Warren MP: Clinical review 77: Evaluation of secondary amenorrhea. J Clin Endocrinol Metab 81:437–442, 1996.

14. GENETIC SYNDROMES AFFECTING ADOLESCENTS

Joan F. Atkin, M.D.

1. Is Turner syndrome a common sex chromosomal abnormality?

Turner syndrome, 45,X, is the most common chromosomal abnormality at the time of *conception* (1–2% of all conceptions). However, most of these pregnancies (about 99%) end in miscarriage, making the incidence at *birth* approximately 1 in 5000, which is not very common. For comparison, Klinefelter syndrome, 47,XXY, has a birth incidence of 1 in 1000.

2. Why do so many pregnancies end in miscarriage?

The fetus has lymphatic dysplasia resulting in lymphatic obstructive sequence with severe edema, hydrops, cystic hygromas, ascites, and interference with normal fetal development.

3. Why do some fetuses survive?

In some cases, lymphatic dysplasia does not develop. This occurs more often in those who have a mosaic karyotype or an X chromosome structural abnormality. In other cases, a connection between the lymphatic and venous system develops, allowing for release of the obstructive effects. In these cases, there may have been cystic hygromas that resolve, leaving residual features such as increased nuchal skin or webbed neck.

4. How many persons with Turner syndrome have a karyotype other than 45,X?

A wide range of karyotypic abnormalities is seen in Turner syndrome. About 50% of Turner patients have a 45,X karyotype. About 25% have a mosaic karyotype such as 45,X/46,XX; 45,X/46,XY; or 45,X/46,XX/47,XXX. Approximately 25% have a structural change to one of X chromosomes such as an isochromosome of Xq or deletions of part of the X chromosome.

5. Is Turner syndrome associated with advanced maternal age?

No. The average age of mothers of girls with Turner syndrome is the same as the background population. About 80% of girls with a 45,X karyotype are missing the paternal X chromosome. There is no increased risk for future pregnancies.

6. What are the most consistent clinical findings in Turner syndrome?

The most consistent findings are **infertility**, resulting from gonadal dysgenesis, and **short stature**. Virtually all patients with a 45,X karyotype will have short stature, as will 95% of those with mosaicism or a structural X chromosome abnormality. Some girls are small from birth, but most tend to fall off the growth curve by 3 years of age. Untreated girls have an average adult height of 4 feet, 7 inches. Gonadal dysgenesis is present in greater than 90%.

7. What are other common clinical findings in Turner syndrome?

- Congenital lymphedema with puffiness of hands and feet
- Broad chest with widely spaced hypoplastic or inverted nipples
- Unusual shape and rotation of ears
- Facial features consisting of narrow maxilla, small mandible, and inner canthal folds
- Webbed neck with low posterior hair line and appearance of short neck
- Extremity abnormalities, most commonly cubitus valgus and short 4th and 5th metacarpals

- Narrow, hyperconvex nails
- Pigmented nevi
- Renal anomalies such as horseshoe kidney or duplication of collecting system
- Congenital heart disease, primarily left sided such as bicuspid aortic valve, coarctation of the aorta, aortic stenosis, hypoplastic left heart, and dissecting aortic aneurysm

8. Are there cognitive problems associated with Turner syndrome?

Girls with Turner syndrome have normal intelligence, and many go on to have professional careers. However, there are some areas of difficulty in learning such as visual-motor coordination, spatial-temporal processing, and mathematics. Because girls with Turner syndrome have only one X chromosome, they have the same risk for X-linked conditions as males.

9. What medical conditions are associated with Turner syndrome?

A variety of medical conditions including thyroid disease, diabetes, inflammatory bowel disease, and hypertension are seen more often in patients with Turner syndrome than in the general population.

10. At what age is Turner syndrome usually diagnosed?

With the increased use and accuracy of prenatal ultrasound, most cases of Turner syndrome associated with cystic hygroma or edema can be picked up **prenatally**. These findings or other anatomic defects (e.g., congenital heart disease or structural renal anomalies) are an indication for amniocentesis and fetal chromosomal analysis. Also, an elevated maternal serum alpha-fetoprotein (AFP) is associated with Turner syndrome. In **newborns**, Turner syndrome is diagnosed based on common clinical findings such as edema of the hands and feet, cystic hygroma, or short, webbed neck. In **infancy**, the diagnosis may be made during evaluation for congenital heart disease. Any time that a girl falls off the growth curve, evaluation for Turner syndrome should be considered. A common time for diagnosis is in **adolescence**, prompted by either a lack of development of secondary sexual characteristics or primary amenorrhea, which results from ovarian dysgenesis. On rare occasions, an individual is diagnosed in **adulthood** after evaluation for infertility.

11. Is treatment available?

Unless they maintain normal growth (as may be seen in mosaicism), girls are often treated with growth hormone by a pediatric endocrinologist. This treatment usually brings girls to an adult height of about 5 feet, which is 5 inches taller than otherwise expected and within the normal range. Estrogen or progesterone replacement therapy is started peripubertally to obtain normal female secondary sexual characteristics and menses and to prevent osteopenia. This treatment is continued throughout life. Pregnancy is obtained by donor eggs fertilized in vitro and implanted into the woman's uterus. The pregnancy is maintained with hormonal supplementation. Many times, a sister or other female relative is able to donate the eggs. It is important to follow these pregnancies carefully because women with Turner syndrome are at increased risk for hypertension and dissecting aortic aneurysm.

12. What is Klinefelter syndrome?

Klinefelter syndrome is a sex chromosome abnormality caused by an extra X chromosome in a male. Most affected individuals (about 80%) have a 47,XXY karyotype. Examples of other Klinefelter karyotypes include 48,XXYY, 48,XXXY, and mosaic 46,XY/47,XXY. All have at least one Y chromosome and two X chromosomes. The syndrome occurs in approximately 1 in 500 male newborns.

13. What are the common clinical characteristics of Klinefelter syndrome?

- Hypogonadism with small testes, decreased testosterone, and infertility
- Decreased facial and pubic hair

- Gynecomastia
- Disproportionately long limbs
- Learning and behavior problems with lower IQ than expected (usually still in the normal range)
- Feminine distribution of adipose tissue

Boys with Klinefelter syndrome do *not* have an increased incidence of birth defects or a dysmorphic appearance.

14. When is Klinefelter syndrome diagnosed?

Persons with Klinefelter syndrome often appear normal and may never be diagnosed. However, the incidence of Klinefelter syndrome increases with advanced maternal age, and many patients are diagnosed **prenatally** by amniocentesis, an option offered in advanced maternal age. As a **preschooler**, a boy may come to the attention of physicians because of speech delays or behavioral problems. In **elementary school**, he may present with learning or behavioral problems. A common time for presentation is **adolescence**, when poor development of masculine secondary sexual characteristics or lack of testicular growth becomes evident. It is important always to include a genitalia exam as part of a routine physical examination. Some patients present in **adulthood** as part of an evaluation for infertility. Chromosome analysis should always be considered in males with learning or behavioral problems, infertility, or small testes.

15. What treatments are available?

Testosterone therapy is an integral part of treatment and is usually begun prepubertally, around 11–12 years of age. Besides helping with virilization, many parents report that it helps with behavior. It will *not* treat infertility or small testicular size but definitely helps with libido, penile size, and erectile dysfunction. Parents should be encouraged to meet with an endocrinologist well before puberty to discuss therapy. Most individuals are given an intramuscular dose of testosterone every 3 weeks, but other treatment modalities are now available. Psychological and educational therapies are very helpful in those with emotional, behavioral, or learning problems. Surgery is available for gynecomastia when necessary.

16. How can the infertility be treated?

The vast majority of men with Klinefelter syndrome are infertile and should be handled the same as any other male with infertility. Artificial insemination with donor sperm and adoption should be discussed. Rarely, some men with Klinefelter syndrome are fertile, particularly those with the mosaic karyotype.

17. Are there other health-related issues?

Breast cancer, which is extremely rare in most males, is more common in males with Klinefelter syndrome (about 20 times the background incidence in males). **Osteoporosis** is also more commonly seen and is helped with testosterone therapy. There is also an increased incidence of **autoimmune disorders** such as diabetes, lupus, rheumatoid arthritis, and thyroid disease.

18. Is fragile X syndrome a chromosomal or a single gene disorder?

Fragile X syndrome is a single gene disorder inherited in an X-linked fashion; it is an X-linked dominant disorder. Many people had thought of it as a chromosomal disorder because there is a visible fragile site on the X chromosome in some cells. This is the site of the gene mutation at Xq27.3.

19. Is fragile X syndrome the only form of X-linked mental retardation?

There are approximately 130 described different X-linked mental retardation (MR) syndromes, with close to 200 gene loci on the X chromosome associated with MR. X-linked mental retardation conditions account for the excess of males with mental retardation over fe-males (about 30% excess). Fragile X is the most common X-linked MR syndrome and one of the most common causes for inherited mental retardation.

20. How common is fragile X syndrome?

About 1 in 4500 males and 1 in 9000 females are affected. Approximately 1 in 400 fe-males and 1 in 1000 males are premutation carriers. All ethnic groups are affected.

21. What is a premutation carrier?

The fragile X gene (*FMR1*) is associated with a trinucleotide repeat sequence (CGG). In the normal population, there are about 30 repeats. In those affected with fragile X syndrome, there are greater than 230 repeats (up to 4000). These individuals are said to have the full mu-tation, resulting in the lack of gene transcription and absence of the gene product. A **premu-tation carrier** has 50–200 repeats and exhibits transmission instability dependent on the gender of the carrier and the size of the repeat. Premutation carriers do produce the gene prod-uct and therefore are clinically normal. They can be male or female. The repeat sequence can expand in size when passed on from the mother. A woman with a premutation (who is clini-cally unaffected) can produce a child with the full mutation (who is affected).

22. Does this mean that a man can be an unaffected carrier? Does that ever happen in X-linked conditions?

A man can be a premutation carrier. He carries the premutation, not the full mutation. This premutation is passed on to all of his daughters and none of his sons. The repeat size does not expand from him to his daughters but can expand from his daughters to their chil-dren. He can have affected grandchildren through his daughters. He can also have an affected brother with the full mutation. This is not usually seen in X-linked inheritance, which is why these pedigrees can look very unusual for an X-linked condition. With most X-linked condi-tions, females who have the mutation are unaffected carriers, and men who have the gene mu-tation are all affected.

23. Do the premutation carriers have any clinical symptoms?

The only consistent documented finding is premature ovarian failure (POF). Based on studies, 21% of premutation females have POF compared to 1% of the general population. The reason for this is unknown. The POF seen in premutation females is not seen in full mu-tation affected females.

24. Other than mental retardation, what other symptoms can be seen in an affected person?

Typically, patients with fragile X syndrome have unusual facial features including long narrow facies, large ears, and prominent nose and jaw. Males have large testicles (macro-or-chidism) generally seen after puberty. Typical behavior patterns include hyperactivity, autistic features, and repetitive speech pattern. Affected females seem to have problems with shyness, anxiety, and social adaptation. Many have evidence of connective tissue problems including mitral valve prolapse, hyperextensible joints, and high arched palate. Other medical problems include seizures, frequent otitis media, and visual abnormalities. As a general rule, males tend to function in moderate range of MR, females in the mild range.

25. How is an individual tested for fragile X?

DNA testing is available for fragile X through most large commercial laboratories and many private and research labs. This testing is much more reliable than the "old" testing, which consisted of cytogenetic testing for the X chromosome fragile site. The DNA testing can give the number of repeats, which will allow for diagnosis of premutation-unaffected car-riers as well as full mutation affected individuals.

26. Who should be tested?

This is a difficult question. Many people believe that there should be large population screening since this is a common cause of mental retardation and excellent testing is available for both affected and premutation carriers. Certainly all those with the characteristic findings should be tested. Any family with more than one person with MR and no other explanation should be tested. If an individual is tested for fragile X, routine chromosomes should be done as well. In large surveys, when individuals with MR were tested for fragile X, there were as many chromosomal abnormalities picked up as fragile X.

27. Is treatment available?

There is no specific treatment to replace the *FMR1* protein. However, there are effective interventions to treat the symptoms. As with most conditions involving cognitive impairment, early intervention programs, therapies, and special education programs are quite helpful. Attention deficit–hyperactivity disorder (ADHD) and seizures can be treated with medication. Hearing, vision, and cardiac problems should be evaluated by appropriate specialists. Genetic counseling is extremely valuable in this genetically difficult condition.

28. How common is neurofibromatosis type 1 (NF-1)?

NF-1 is a common inherited condition affecting 1 in 4000 people. It affects both sexes and has no particular racial, ethnic, or geographic distribution.

29. How is NF-1 inherited?

NF-1 is inherited in an autosomal dominant fashion; the affected individual has a 50% chance of passing on the gene, and therefore the condition, to each of his or her offspring. In about half of those affected, the condition arises from a new mutation, which means that neither parent is affected.

30. Why is there is such a high mutation rate?

The NF-1 gene is extremely large, resulting in a greater chance for mutation. The gene is located on chromosome 17 in band q11.2. The NF-1 gene codes for a protein, neurofibromin, which may act as a tumor suppressor.

31. Is there a DNA test for NF-1?

Because the gene for NF-1 is very large, there are many different mutations in many places along the gene that can lead to malfunction. Most families have fairly unique mutations. To sequence the entire gene is tedious, time-consuming, and expensive. This testing is not commercially available. A test known as the protein truncation assay that is not specific for any one mutation is available commercially and is positive in two thirds of people with NF-1. There can be false-negative results, so this test is not recommended in isolated cases to confirm the diagnosis. No laboratory test allows for clinical outcome predictions. DNA linkage studies can be done in families with multiple affected members for purposes of prenatal and presymptomatic testing.

32. What are common signs of NF-1?

1. **Neurofibromas**, the tumors that give NF its name, are benign tumors that grow on nerves usually just under the skin, but also may be in deeper tissue. Nodule-like surface growths are called dermal or cutaneous neurofibromas. Plexiform neurofibromas are complex, large, entangled growths that are usually present from birth. Most other neurofibromas develop later, often around puberty.

2. **Café-au-lait spots**, named for their color of coffee with milk, are the most common finding in NF-1. They may be present at birth or develop at any age; they usually increase in size and number with age, especially at puberty and with pregnancy. They are flat and vary in size and shape but are often round or ovoid.

3. **Axillary freckling** or freckling in an area not exposed to the sun such as the inguinal region is common.

4. **Lisch nodules** are iris nevi visible only with slit lamp exam and should not to be confused with iris freckling. These are not present at birth but begin to appear in childhood and are present in almost all individuals with NF-1 by the age of 20. They cause no problems to vision but are helpful as a diagnostic aid.

33. How is the diagnosis of NF-1 made?

A National Institutes of Health (NIH) Consensus Development Conference listed seven major features of NF-1, two of which need to be present to make the diagnosis.

1. Six or more café-au-lait spots at least 5 mm in diameter in children and 15 mm in diameter in adults

2. Two or more neurofibromas of any type or one plexiform neurofibroma

3. Axillary or inguinal freckling

4. Two or more Lisch nodules

5. Distinctive osseous lesions such as sphenoid dysplasia or thinning of long bones with or without pseudarthrosis

6. Optic glioma

7. A first-degree relative with NF-1 (based on above criteria)

34. Is NF-1 a serious debilitating disease?

Although there can be serious complications with NF-1, the vast majority of affected persons lead normal, healthy lives. Manifestations of NF-1 are variable; some patients have only café-au-lait spots and a few neurofibromas, whereas others have major disfigurement and serious complications. There is no test to predict who will have the more serious complications.

35. What complications may be seen in NF-1?

1. **Disfigurement**, while uncommon, can be quite challenging. Cosmetic problems can result from multiple raised dermal neurofibromas on the face or other exposed areas of the body. Removal is usually unsuccessful. Plexiform neurofibromas can be quite disfiguring, especially those behind the eye, and very difficult to resect surgically. A variety of bony defects can result in macrocephaly, scoliosis, pseudarthrosis, absence of the orbital wall, and asymmetry.

2. **Central nervous system (CNS) problems** are usually rare except for learning disabilities and ADHD, which may be seen in 50% of individuals. Less common findings include mental retardation and seizures. CNS tumors are more common than in the general population.

3. **Tumors**, both malignant and benign, are seen in NF-1. The most common benign tumors are the neurofibromas. Optic pathway gliomas are seen in 15%. Sometimes, these do not need to be surgically removed. Dumbbell neurofibromas of the spine can be very difficult to remove. Other CNS or nerve cell tumors (seen rarely) include malignant schwannomas, astrocytomas, neurilemomas and meningiomas. In addition to these nerve cell tumors, juvenile chronic myeloid leukemia is seen more often than in the general population.

4. **Hypertension** can be seen due to renal artery stenosis (from pressure of a neurofibroma) or due to a pheochromocytoma, which is another tumor seen more commonly in NF-1.

36. Are there other findings to look for in NF-1?

Other findings include:

1. **Unidentified bright objects (UBOs)**. UBOs are seen on MRI in the basal ganglia, thalamus, cerebellum, and brain stem regions. These are common and distinctive lesions although their significance is unknown. UBOs have not yet been shown to be specific for NF-1 and are therefore not used as a diagnostic criterion. Often, they disappear with age.

2. **Pubertal disturbances**. Both precocious and delayed puberty have been reported, but the incidence is low. Short stature (although not dramatic) is also seen. If there are signs of

precocious puberty, the individual should be evaluated for an optic glioma or hypothalamic lesion.

   3. **Pruritus**. Itching is a major complaint in about 10% of affected individuals. Some respond to routine methods of treatment, but many are not helped by medications, lotions, or baths. This is particularly problematic and more common in the patient with actively growing or multiple neurofibromas.

37. Are there specific management recommendations for persons with NF-1?

Persons with NF-1 should have regular (at least yearly) examinations either by their primary care physician or by a physician who specializes in NF-1. Areas of concentration should include:

- Careful history and neurologic exam
- Blood pressure measurement
- Developmental assessment with careful attention to learning disabilities and ADHD
- Scoliosis evaluation
- Annual exam by an ophthalmologist familiar with NF

BIBLIOGRAPHY

1. Bock R: Understanding Klinefelter Syndrome: A Guide for XXY Males and Their Families. Bethesda, MD, National Institutes of Health, 1993, NIH publication 93-3202.
2. Gutmann DH, Aylsworth A, Carey J, Marks, J, et al: The diagnostic evaluation and multidisciplinary management of neurofibromatosis 1 and neurofibromatosis 2. JAMA 278:51–57, 1997.
3. Policy statement of American Academy of Pediatrics Committee on Genetics: Health supervision for children with fragile X syndrome. Pediatrics 98:297–300, 1996.
4. Policy Statement of American Academy of Pediatrics Committee on Genetics: Health Supervision for Children with Neurofibromatosis. Pediatrics 96:368–372, 1995.
5. Policy Statement of American Academy of Pediatrics Committee on Genetics: Health Supervision for Children with Turner Syndrome. Pediatrics 96:1166–1173, 1995.
6. Rosenfeld R: Turner Syndrome: A Guide for Physicians. Houston, Turner Syndrome Society, 1992.
7. Smyth CM, Bremner WJ: Klinefelter syndrome. Arch Intern Med 158:1309, 1998.
8. Warren S, Sherman S: The fragile-X syndrome. In Scriver C, Beaudet A, Sly W, Valle D (eds): The Metabolic and Molecular Bases of Inherited Disease, 8th ed. New York, McGraw Hill, 2001, pp 1257–1289.

15. GASTROENTEROLOGY

Wallace V. Crandall, M.D.

ABDOMINAL PAIN

1. What are the most common causes of acute abdominal pain in adolescents?

Viral gastroenteritis is the most common cause of acute abdominal pain in all ages outside the neonatal period. Other common considerations in adolescents include:

- Appendicitis
- Urinary tract infection
- Trauma
- Pelvic inflammatory disease
- Pneumonia
- Mittelschmerz
- Gallstones

2. How does this list differ from the causes of chronic abdominal pain?

Chronic abdominal pain occurs in 10–15% or more of all adolescents. Most adolescents with chronic abdominal pain (defined as pain of more than 3 months' duration) suffer from a form of "functional" abdominal pain. This term refers to conditions in which structural or biochemical abnormalities or inflammatory processes cannot be identified.

3. List other causes of chronic abdominal pain.

- Inflammatory bowel disease (IBD)
- Gastritis/peptic ulcer disease (with or without *Helicobacter pylori* infection)
- Gastroesophageal reflux disease
- Constipation
- Gallstones
- Renal stones
- Hepatitis
- Lactose intolerance
- Ureteropelvic junction obstruction
- Gynecologic disease
- Psychiatric disease

4. How are the different types of functional abdominal pain classified?

They are classified according to the (pediatric) Rome II criteria under the umbrella of functional gastrointestinal (GI) disorders:

1. **Functional dyspepsia**: epigastric pain or discomfort, often associated with nausea, bloating, belching, and vomiting but not associated with a change in bowel habits.

2. **Irritable bowel syndrome** (IBS): pain relieved with defecation and/or associated with a change in bowel habits.

3. **Functional abdominal pain**: pain that is often periumbilical but not related to physiologic events and for which no pathologic cause can be found.

4. **Abdominal migraine**: chronic abdominal pain often associated with some combination of headache, photophobia, family history of migraine, and/or an aura.

5. **Aerophagia**: air swallowing, abdominal distention, and belching or flatus.

Depression and anxiety are common cofactors in adolescents with chronic abdominal pain.

5. Describe the pathophysiology of functional GI disorders.

The pathophysiology of functional GI disorders is an area of ongoing research. Currently, at least three factors are thought to cause or influence symptoms: intestinal dysmotility, visceral hypersensitivity (increased awareness and decreased pain threshold to visceral stimuli), and coping skills/early pain experiences. Other factors, such as cultural values, social support, secondary gain, and pain expectations, further modify the symptoms as well as an individual's response to symptoms.

6. What treatments are available for functional GI disorders?

Symptoms improve in a subset of patients after a knowledgeable explanation of the condition and reassurance that they will not progress to a more serious disease. Dietary manipulation includes increased dietary fiber (particularly in constipation-predominant IBS); limited intake of lactose, fruit juice, and soda on a trial basis; avoidance of foods that repeatedly exacerbate symptoms; and eating smaller portions of food. Exercise and maintenance of normal activities should be encouraged. If symptoms are associated with anxiety or depression, counseling that includes stress reduction may result in improvement.

If diet and lifestyle changes do not make the symptoms tolerable, medications are often used. Antispasmodic medications such as hyoscyamine sulfate (Levsin) and dicyclomine (Bentyl) result in symptomatic improvement in some people but often are of limited utility. A trial of a H_2 receptor antagonist should be considered in patients with dyspepsia. In more severe cases, tricyclic antidepressants at low doses may be useful for the management of chronic pain.

7. If chronic abdominal pain is so common in adolescents, when should I worry about it?

The following red flags should prompt further evaluation, although many patients with these features eventually are diagnosed with a functional GI disorder:
- Pain localized away from the umbilicus
- Pain radiating to the shoulder or back
- Pain awakening them from sleep
- Vomiting (especially hematemesis or bilious emesis)
- Diarrhea (particularly if blood or mucus is present)
- Fevers
- Unintentional weight loss
- Rashes
- Arthritis
- Sudden and/or discrete episodes of pain
- Family history of diseases that may explain symptoms

INFLAMMATORY BOWEL DISEASE

8. Compare the symptoms of irritable bowel syndrome (IBS) and inflammatory bowel disease (IBD).

	IBS	IBD
Abdominal pain	+	+
Diarrhea	+ (intermittent)	+
Rectal bleeding	−	+
Involuntary weight loss	± (depression)	+
Poor linear growth	−	+
Decreased Hb/albumin, increased ESR	−	+
Fever, rash, joint pains	−	+
Nausea, vomiting	+	+
Perianal disease	−	+
Abdominal tenderness/mass	−	+

Hb = hemoglobin, ESR = erythrocyte sedimentation rate.

9. Describe the work-up to rule out IBD.

The first step is a complete history (including family history) and physical exam. Particular attention is paid to the following findings:

- Pallor
- Body habitus (i.e., short stature and/or a decreased weight-to-height ratio)
- Iritis
- Arthritis
- Digital clubbing
- Mouth lesions
- Abdominal tenderness or masses
- Perianal fissures or skin tags
- Stool occult blood

There is no single diagnostic test for Crohn's disease or ulcerative colitis. If IBD is suspected, blood work should include a complete blood count (to evaluate for anemia or thrombocytosis), albumin (to assess for a protein-losing enteropathy), and an erythrocyte sedimentation rate (normal in 10% of people with Crohn's disease, 50% with ulcerative colitis). Stool studies to rule out infectious colitis also should be obtained. Many physicians obtain liver enzymes and a bilirubin panel to evaluate for associated liver diseases such as autoimmune hepatitis or sclerosing cholangitis. Consider ordering these lab tests before referral.

10. If clinical suspicion remains high, how does the evaluation proceed?

Complete colonoscopy with ileoscopy and biopsy may be performed to look for both microscopic and gross evidence of an inflammatory disorder. Some physicians also perform an upper endoscopy, because approximately one-third of patients with Crohn's disease have upper GI tract findings. An upper GI series with small bowel follow-through is usually obtained to evaluate the remainder of the small bowel, particularly the terminal ileum.

11. What therapies may be used to treat IBD?

Therapy for IBD should be viewed as a two-step plan: induction of remission and maintenance therapy. In mild disease, induction of remission may be attempted with a 5-aminosalicylic acid (ASA) preparation (e.g., Pentasa, Dipentum, Asacol) alone or in combination with an antibiotic such as metronidazole (in patients with Crohn's disease). Moderate-to-severe disease is usually treated with oral steroids at initial diagnosis, often in combination with a 5-ASA. Some centers restrict diet to an elemental or polymeric formula, often given by nasogastric tube infusion. Successful induction of remission is determined by a combination of history, physical examination, and selected lab tests (e.g., hemoglobin, albumin, sedimentation rate). After remission is achieved, it is critical to try to maintain the remission as long as possible. Common maintenance medications include 5-ASA drugs and 6-mercaptopurine (a purine analog that inhibits DNA synthesis).

If the above medications are unsuccessful, other medications used for induction of remission or maintenance therapy include infliximab (anti-tumor necrosis factor antibody), methotrexate, mycophenolate, and cyclosporine.

GASTROESOPHAGEAL REFLUX DISEASE AND GASTRITIS

12. Are gastroesophageal reflux (GER) and gastroesophageal reflux disease (GERD) the same thing?

GER is the passage of stomach contents into the esophagus, usually after the ingestion of food. This normal process occurs as often as up to 4–6% of the day. GERD refers to reflux that causes symptoms or complications.

13. What symptoms suggest GERD?

- Recurrent vomiting
- Epigastric or chest pain
- Heartburn, regurgitation
- Hematemesis
- Acid brash (an acidic taste in the mouth)
- Dysphagia
- Nausea
- Halitosis
- Asthma refractory to typical management
- Dental erosions

14. What complications can result from untreated GERD?
- Esophagitis
- Strictures
- Anemia
- Hypoproteinemia
- Barrett's esophagus (intestinal metaplasia, a premalignant condition)

15. How do I evaluate a person with suspected GERD?
A variety of tests may be obtained, depending on the clinical situation. However, in the absence of complications, an empirical trial of an acid blocker (H_2 receptor antagonist [H_2RA] or proton pump inhibitor [PPI]) may be attempted first.

If testing is deemed necessary, an upper GI series may be obtained to look for evidence of mucosal inflammation, hiatal hernia, stricture, or an anatomic abnormality that may predispose to reflux or vomiting. However, an upper GI series is neither sensitive nor specific for the diagnosis of GERD. Esophagogastroduodenoscopy allows better direct visualization of the mucosa and also evaluates for the microscopic presence of esophagitis or Barrett's esophagus with esophageal biopsies. Esophageal pH monitoring allows quantitation of the time that the esophagus is exposed to acid. This test can be useful in carefully selected situations (i.e., to assess for a temporal relationship between symptoms and episodes of GERD or to assess the adequacy of acid blockade) but usually is not needed or indicated in the evaluation of GERD.

16. Does GERD require surgical management?
GERD usually can be managed with medications (H_2RAs and/or PPIs). Occasionally, adolescents require PPIs twice daily as well as a nighttime dose of an H_2RA to control nighttime acid breakthrough. In rare cases, acid suppression sufficient to induce mucosal healing cannot be adequately achieved. In such circumstances, surgery may be indicated. The cost and benefit of antireflux surgery vs. life-long acid suppression in a young person with severe GERD is a point of debate.

Prokinetic medications are also sometimes prescribed for GERD. Although they appear to be helpful in some patients, none of the currently available prokinetics has proven efficacy in the treatment of GERD.

Lifestyle modifications, such as elevating the head of the bed and avoidance of smoking, alcohol, high-fat foods, and caffeine (chocolate), also should be encouraged.

17. What other diseases mimic GERD?
The list is extensive but depends in part on what specific symptoms the patient experiences. Functional dyspepsia presents with many of the same symptoms as GERD, including epigastric discomfort and nausea. Recurrent vomiting may be caused by any number of conditions, ranging from migraine headaches and stress to intracranial lesions. Dysphagia may represent achalasia, dysmotility, or stricture. Epigastric pain may result from any number of conditions, including peptic-ulcer disease with or without *Helicobacter pylori* infection.

18. What is *H. pylori*?
H. pylori is a gram-negative spiral bacterium that colonizes the stomach and frequently is implicated in duodenal ulcer, gastric ulcer, and gastritis.

19. Which populations are most likely to be infected?
Poor socioeconomic status is the greatest risk factor. In developed countries, up to 50% of children living in poor socioeconomic conditions are infected compared with less than 10% of children overall.

20. Describe the evaluation for *H. pylori* infection.
Several tests are available. Serology allows for the detection of antibody to *H. pylori* but does not distinguish between past and current (active) infection in treated patients. C13 breath

testing for *H. plyori* (urease-positive organisms) is relatively sensitive for current infection. However, patients must discontinue PPI therapy for 2 weeks before testing. A stool test for *H. pylori* antigen also has been developed and is becoming more commonly available. Endoscopic biopsy is currently considered the gold standard and, in contrast to the other tests, allows the determination of associated mucosal pathology.

21. If *H. pylori* is present, it is probably the cause of the patient's symptoms, right?

If only life were so simple. *H. pylori* gastritis without ulcer is asymptomatic in most young people. Furthermore, eradication of *H. pylori* in people with abdominal pain but no ulcer often does not lead to resolution of symptoms.

22. If the patient has no ulcer, should I treat *H. pylori* infection?

For:

H. pylori has been associated with the development of gastric cancer and is classified as a group 1 carcinogen by the International Agency for Research on Cancer. Several studies have shown an association between gastric cancer and *H. pylori*, with odds ratios ranging from 2 to 16.

Against:

Other studies have shown that some areas with high rates of *H. pylori* infection have relatively low rates of gastric cancer and that some areas with variable rates of gastric cancer have similar rates of infection with *H. pylori*. Furthermore, other factors, such as blood type A, increased dietary intake of smoked or salted foods, and decreased vitamin C consumption, also may be associated with an increased risk of gastric cancer. It is not known whether eradication of *H. pylori* will lead to a significant reduction in the cases of gastric cancer in the presence of other risk factors.

Note: The above discussion refers to gastric adenocarcinoma. Gastric B-cell lymphomas, known as mucosa-associated lymphoid tissue (MALT) lymphomas, are known to be associated with *H. pylori* infection. Treatment of *H. pylori* leads to regression of MALT lymphoma in adults.

23. What is the bottom line?

Certainly, patients with ulceration and *H. pylori* should be treated. Although there is currently insufficient evidence to suggest population screening and treatment for *H. pylori* in an attempt to prevent gastric cancer, most experts recommend treatment for an individual patient with *H. pylori* infection in an attempt to resolve the symptoms for which the evaluation was initially started. However, the patient should understand that treatment may not necessarily lead to resolution of symptoms. It is also important to note that empirical treatment for *H. pylori* generally is not recommended.

24. What are the current treatment recommendations for *H. pylori*?

Several combinations of acid blockers and antibiotics are efficacious. These treatment plans usually include either ranitidine or a PPI and two different antibiotics (clarithromycin, amoxicillin, metronidazole, or tetracycline). Some drug manufacturers prepackage the antibiotics and acid blockers together for ease of use.

OTHER GASTROINTESTINAL CONDITIONS

25. What are the symptoms of lactose intolerance?

Lactose intolerance and IBS present with similar symptoms. Patients with lactose intolerance often have abdominal discomfort, bloating, flatulence, and loose stools. Although frequently occurring within 3–4 hours of ingesting lactose, symptoms may be delayed, making the connection to lactose intake more difficult in some patients. Symptoms are also dose-dependent; some patients have only minimal symptoms with ordinary quantities of milk or milk products.

26. Are some people born with lactose intolerance?

Congenital lactase deficiency is extremely rare. Lactase activity after the first few years of life depends on a genetic polymorphism. "Lactose absorbers" tend to have persistently high levels of lactase activity, whereas "lactose malabsorbers" lose 90–95% of lactase activity. Lactose absorbers are more commonly of northern or central European descent, whereas malabsorbers are often of Asian, African, or Native American heritage. Although lactose intolerance may develop by 3 years of age in some populations, it usually presents in adolescence.

27. How is lactose intolerance diagnosed?

If lactose intolerance is suspected on clinical grounds, a simple first step is a 2-week trial of a lactose-free diet. Lactose breath hydrogen testing is readily available when the results of a lactose-free diet are equivocal. It is also possible to measure the lactase activity of an intestinal biopsy specimen, but this step generally is not indicated.

28. Does a positive diagnosis mean that lactose-intolerant adolescents can never have ice cream again?

The symptoms of lactose intolerance generally can be managed by avoiding foods that contain large quantities of lactose. Many lactase-deficient people are able to tolerate small quantities of lactose without experiencing significant symptoms. Furthermore, milk containing predigested lactose and capsules containing beta-galactosidases (which digest milk sugar) are available.

29. A patient has right upper quadrant pain and elevated liver function tests. What do those tests actually tell you about liver function?

Liver function tests can be a confusing term for two reasons. First, it may refer to any number of different tests. Second, most liver function tests give no indication of how the liver is actually functioning.

Aspartate aminotransferase (AST) and alanine aminotransferase (ALT) are elevated in response to hepatocellular injury but do not indicate whether synthetic activity has been affected. Elevations of conjugated bilirubin, alkaline phosphatase, or gamma-glutamyltransferase (GGT) indicate impaired bile flow but, again, are not indicative of synthetic function. Commonly obtained tests that give some indication of synthetic activity include serum albumin, prothrombin time (PT), partial thromboplastin time (PTT), and individual clotting factors.

30. What work-up needs to be initiated before referring the patient to a gastroenterologist?

Tests for synthetic function, including albumin levels, PT, and PTT, should be obtained to ensure that the patient does not need to be seen emergently. Infectious causes such as hepatitis A, B, and C as well as Epstein-Barr virus also should be excluded.

31. What other diagnoses need to be excluded?

Depending on the patient's symptoms and which enzyme levels are elevated, other possibilities may include:
- Steatosis/steatohepatitis (alcoholic and nonalcoholic fatty liver)
- Alpha$_1$ antitrypsin deficiency
- Autoimmune hepatitis
- Wilson's disease
- Thrombosis (Budd-Chiari syndrome, portal vein thrombosis)
- Sclerosing cholangitis
- IBD
- Celiac disease
- Cystic fibrosis
- Gallstones
- Drugs

Of course, treatment depends on the underlying diagnosis.

32. A patient presents with scleral icterus after a recent cold but no other symptoms. His hepatic transaminases are normal. Does he have Gilbert's syndrome?

Gilbert's syndrome is a hereditary, mild, chronic, intermittent elevation in the serum unconjugated bilirubin concentration due to a decrease in hepatic bilirubin uridine diphosphate glucuronosyltransferase (BUGT) activity. Gilbert's syndrome is the major potential diagnosis in this patient.

33. How is Gilbert's syndrome diagnosed?

Specific testing usually is not necessary. The diagnosis can be made if the patient has a mild, fluctuating, unconjugated hyperbilirubinemia (1–4 mg/dl); normal levels of AST, ALT, alkaline phosphatase, and GGT; and no evidence of hemolysis. Fasting can sometimes induce the elevation of unconjugated bilirubin.

34. What treatment should be offered?

The patient should be reassured about the diagnosis. Because Gilbert's syndrome is not associated with a significant increase in morbidity or mortality, no specific treatment is required.

BIBLIOGRAPHY

1. Camilleri M: Management of the irritable bowel syndrome. Gastroenterology 120:652–668, 2001.
2. Drumm B, Koletzko S, Oderda G: *Helicobacter pylori* infection in children: A consensus statement. J Pediatr Gastro Nutr 30:207–213, 2000.
3. Gold BD, Colletti RB, Abbott M, et al: *Helicobacter pylori* infection in children: Recommendations for diagnosis and treatment. J Pediatr Gastroenterol Nutr 31:490–497, 2000.
4. Horwitz BJ, Fisher RS: The irritable bowel syndrome. N Engl J Med 344:1846–1850, 2001.
5. Rasquin-Weber A, Hyman PE, Cucchiara S, et al: Childhood functional gastrointestinal disorders. Gut 45(Suppl II):II60–II68, 1999.
6. Sands BE: Therapy of inflammatory bowel disease. Gastroenterology 118:S68–S82, 2000.
7. Shanahan F: Inflammatory bowel disease: Immunodiagnostics, immunotherapeutics, and ecotherapeutics. Gastroenterology 120:622–635, 2001.
8. Suchy FJ, Sokol RJ, Balistreri WF (eds): Liver Disease in Children, 2nd ed. Philadelphia, Lippincott Williams & Wilkins, 2001.
9. Uemura N, Okamoto S, Yamamoto S, et al: *Helicobacter pylori* infection and the development of gastric cancer. N Engl J Med 345:784–789, 2001.
10. Walker WA, Durie PR, Hamilton JR, et al (eds): Pediatric Gastrointestinal Disease, 3rd ed. Philadelphia, B.C. Decker, 2000.

16. HEMATOLOGY AND ONCOLOGY

Jeffrey D. Hord, M.D.

ANEMIA

1. What is the major cause of anemia during adolescence?

The major cause of anemia during adolescence is iron deficiency. Anemia is defined as a level of hemoglobin or hematocrit less than the fifth percentile for age and gender. Iron deficiency occurs in both sexes and is the result of increased iron requirements during rapid growth, increased iron losses in females during menses, and inadequate iron intake due to poor dietary habits.

2. Why are adolescent athletes who are involved in lengthy, intense physical activities at greater than average risk for iron deficiency?

During endurance events intravascular hemolysis occurs as older, more fragile red cells break down in capillaries. Gastrointestinal hemorrhage occurs in highly trained long-distance runners as the intestines become ischemic because of diminished splanchnic blood flow during prolonged maximal exercise.

3. What risk factors place an adolescent at greater than average risk for developing iron deficiency anemia?

- Disadvantaged socioeconomic background
- Menorrhagia
- Pregnancy
- Family history of anemia or bleeding disorder
- Vegetarian or "fad" diets
- Intense lengthy physical training
- Malabsorption
- Chronic disease

4. How is iron deficiency anemia treated?

Treatment consists of oral iron supplementation with 5–6 mg of elemental iron per kg of body weight per day for at least 3 months. Low-dose oral iron supplementation may be needed throughout adolescence and even into adulthood, depending on individual risk factors.

COAGULATION DISORDERS

5. What is the most common inherited bleeding disorder?

Von Willebrand's disease is the most common inherited bleeding disorder, affecting at least 1% of the population. More than 20 subtypes of von Willebrand's disease have been identified, but the vast majority of patients have type I, which is characterized by a mild-to-moderate deficiency of plasma von Willebrand factor.

6. What are the most common clinical manifestations of von Willebrand's disease?

The most common clinical manifestations of von Willebrand's disease are epistaxis, ecchymoses, petechiae, menorrhagia, and postoperative bleeding. Symptoms of von Willebrand's disease may not become evident until adolescence. Recurrent epistaxis may be perceived as normal in a young child, whereas in adolescents it may lead to a more detailed diagnostic evaluation. Adolescents are more likely to undergo dental extractions than young children, and excessive postsurgical bleeding may develop for the first time. Menorrhagia is seen most commonly during adolescence.

7. How often is an inherited coagulation disorder responsible for menorrhagia in female adolescents?

Based on studies by Claessens and Cowell, about 20% of female adolescents with severe menorrhagia have some type of inherited coagulation disorder. Von Willebrand's disease was the most common inherited coagulopathy associated with menorrhagia in their study.

8. Discuss treatment options for an adolescent with von Willebrand's disease and bleeding.

1. **DDAVP** (1-deamino-8-D-arginine vasopressin). Intravenous or intranasal DDAVP is standard treatment for excessive bleeding in an adolescent with type I von Willebrand's disease. DDAVP stimulates the release of stores of von Willebrand's factor into the circulation. Because all patients do not respond to DDAVP, it is common practice to assess response to DDAVP before using it for the control of bleeding or for preoperative prophylaxis (DDAVP challenge).

2. **A factor concentrate containing von Willebrand's factor**. If a patient does not respond adequately to DDAVP or bleeding continues despite DDAVP, a factor concentrate containing von Willebrand factor should be infused intravenously.

3. When the site of bleeding or surgery is within the oropharynx, an antifibrinolytic known as **aminocaproic acid** (Amicar) can be administered orally.

4. **Estrogen supplements** or combination oral contraceptive pills (OCPs) are often prescribed to control excessive menstrual bleeding. Continuous OCPs may be used to decrease the frequency of menses.

5. In certain rare subtypes of von Willebrand's disease, **platelet transfusions** in addition to standard treatment may be helpful. This approach is used primarily in the treatment of rare patients with a deficiency of intraplatelet von Willebrand factor.

9. Are children older than 10 years who present with immune thrombocytopenic purpura (ITP) at increased risk for chronic ITP?

Yes. Other factors predisposing children to the chronic form of ITP include female gender, a longer than two-week history of purpura before diagnosis, no history of preceding viral illness, and a family history of autoimmune disorders. ITP may be an early manifestation of systemic lupus erythematosus.

10. What are treatment options for an adolescent with chronic ITP?

The most common forms of treatment include splenectomy, which has a 65–75% response rate, and pulse doses of corticosteroids, which have a 50% response rate. In patients who fail to respond to these interventions, intravenous gammaglobulin, danazol, or other immunosuppresive agents may be beneficial.

11. What types of liver disease occur in adolescent males with hemophilia?

Hepatitis C is the major cause of liver disease in the hemophilia population. Liver disease may first become evident in an adolescent male with hemophilia after he receives blood products throughout childhood.

12. What is the most common cause of thrombocytosis during childhood?

Infection is the most common cause of thrombocytosis and accounts for at least 25% of elevated platelet counts measured in children. Other causes of thrombocytosis include chronic inflammation, asplenia, iron deficiency, myeloproliferative disorders, tissue injury, hemolytic anemia, and malignancy.

13. What are some reasons for the increased incidence of thromboembolic problems during adolescence?

Thromboembolic problems are extremely rare in childhood, but when they occur, they occur most often in adolescents. The increasing frequency of thrombotic episodes with increasing age may be related to factors such as oral contraceptive use, cigarette smoking, and a concomitant rise in the incidence of autoimmune disorders. As many as two-thirds of children with systemic lupus erythematosus develop antiphospholipid antibodies, and about one-third of these experience thromboembolic complications.

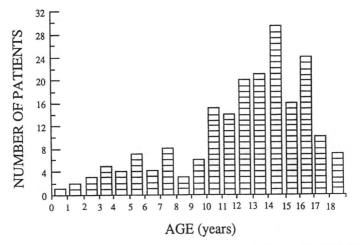

AGE (years)

Age distribution of deep vein thrombosis (DVT) and pulmonary embolism in 199 of 214 children. The sex distribution was equal. However, age dependency was demonstrated, with more adolescents than younger children being affected. The decline in later adolescent years reflects the referral of patients to adult clinics. (Adapted from David M, Andrew M: Venous thromboembolic complications in children. J Pediatr 123:339, 1993 with permission.)

14. Describe the clinical features of deep vein thrombosis (DVT).

Clinical features of DVT in a lower extremity include pain and swelling in the affected extremity, occasional fever, and, less frequently, abdominal or inguinal pain. Patients may have dyspnea and tachypnea if the DVT leads to a pulmonary embolus (PE), but PE is less common in adolescents than adults.

15. When an adolescent experiences a thrombotic problem, it is extremely important to evaluate the patient for inherited prothrombotic disorders (thrombophilia). List inherited disorders associated with an increased risk of clot formation.

An evaluation for inherited hypercoagulable disorders would include testing for the following:
- Factor V Leiden mutation
- Prothrombin gene variant (2210AG polymorphism)
- Methylenetetrahydrofolate reductase variant (C677T)
- Protein C deficiency
- Protein S deficiency
- Antithrombin-III deficiency
- Hyperhomocysteinemia

SICKLE CELL DISEASE

16. Are adolescents with sickle cell disease more likely to experience vasoocclusive painful crises than younger children?

Yes. During adolescence the frequency and severity of generalized vasoocclusive painful crises begin to increase. Both the intensity and length of each episode increase. About

20–25% of high-risk patients with sickle cell anemia develop recurrent severe painful episodes.

17. What is the most common cause of significant morbidity and mortality among adolescents with sickle cell disease?

Throughout adolescence pulmonary complications such as acute chest syndrome contribute most commonly to morbidity and mortality. Sickle cell lung disease occurs in all of the common sickle hemoglobinopathies, including hemoglobin SS disease, hemoglobin SC disease, and hemoglobin S–beta thalassemia. Acute pulmonary complications most often seen during adolescence include acute chest syndrome, pulmonary edema, and bone marrow/fat embolism. Of the acute pulmonary complications of sickle cell disease, the acute chest syndrome is the most common, occurring in 15–43% of all patients with sickle cell disease. Acute chest syndrome consists of a new pulmonary infiltrate on radiograph and may be accompanied by cough, dyspnea, chest pain, fever, and/or hypoxia. Among those who develop acute chest syndrome, there is a high rate of recurrence.

18. List indications for chronic red blood cell transfusion therapy in a patient with sickle cell disease.

Chronic transfusion therapy causes a 90% reduction in recurrence of thrombotic strokes. Neurovascular complications such as stroke occur in 10–20% of patients with sickle cell disease before the age of 20. Without intervention nearly two-thirds of these patients will have recurrent stroke within 3 years. The goal of chronic transfusion therapy is long-term maintenance of hemoglobin S below 30% while avoiding the hyperviscosity of overtransfusion. The optimal length of transfusion therapy for patients with neurologic complications is unknown. Similarly, patients with elevated velocities of cerebral blood flow, as measured by transcranial Doppler ultrasound, may experience a reduction in risk of stroke by receiving red blood cell transfusions on a chronic basis. Other indications for chronic transfusions are recurrent acute chest syndrome with chronic lung disease and chronic unremitting painful crises. Iron overload is a serious complication of chronic transfusion therapy.

19. When should hydroxyurea therapy be considered in an adolescent with sickle cell disease?

The indications for administration of hydroxyurea in a compliant patient with sickle cell disease are frequent painful crises requiring medical attention, recurrent acute chest syndrome, and recurrent episodes of priapism. When hydroxyurea is given on a daily basis to patients with clinically severe homozygous SS disease, approximately 80% experience clinical improvement. Careful monitoring of blood counts, liver function, and renal function is required. Because of potential teratogenic effects of hydroxyurea on the unborn fetus, hydroxyurea should not be administered to pregnant women. Patients receiving the medication should remain abstinent or use an effective method of birth control. The mechanisms through which hydroxyurea reduces clinical disease severity are not entirely clear but probably include an increase in fetal hemoglobin, reduction in white blood cell count, and, in some cases, reduction in platelet count.

20. How does sickle cell disease affect sexual maturation?

In girls with sickle cell disease, both the onset of menarche and progression through the Tanner stages of development are delayed. The mean age of menarche is 15–16 years with a delay of 2–3 years compared with unaffected girls. Male patients also have pubertal delays. They reach the various stages of sexual maturation approximately 2 years later than age-matched controls.

21. What is the best hormonal contraceptive for adolescents with sickle cell disease?

Depot medroxyprogesterone acetate (Depo Provera) is a good choice for many young women with sickle cell disease. It has been shown to decrease the incidence of painful crises in affected patients and may improve anemia by inducing amenorrhea. Many providers are uncomfortable prescribing combination oral contraceptive pills to sickle cell patients, because estrogen is known to increase the risk of thrombosis. Although no evidence indicates that the use of a low-dose oral contraceptive has any deleterious effects on young women with sickle cell disease, Depo Provera provides an estrogen-free alternative.

MALIGNANCIES

22. List the most common malignant tumors among adolescents.
According to the National Cancer Institute's Surveillance, Epidemiology and End Results (SEER) data from 1986 to 1995, the most common tumors among adolescents are Hodgkin's disease (16.1%), germ cell tumors (15.2%), central nervous system (CNS) tumors (10.0%), non-Hodgkin's lymphoma (7.6%), thyroid cancer (7.2%), malignant melanoma (7.0%), and acute lymphoblastic leukemia (6.4%).

23. What is the overall survival rate for adolescents with cancer?
The overall 5-year survival rate for adolescents with cancer from 1985 to 1994 was 77%. For some types of cancer (Hodgkin's disease, germ cell tumors, thyroid cancer, and melanoma), 5-year survival rates were 90% or higher.

24. Describe the typical presenting signs and symptoms of Hodgkin's lymphoma in an adolescent.
Eighty percent of patients with Hodgkin's lymphoma present with adenopathy on one or both sides of the neck—more commonly the lower rather than the upper portion of the neck. The involved lymph nodes are typically painless, firm, and nonmobile. About two-thirds of patients have some mediastinal adenopathy. Patients also may have fever, night sweats, and/or weight loss. Splenomegaly may be noted in a small group of patients with disseminated disease.

25. What is the survival rate for adolescents with Hodgkin's disease?
Patients with localized disease have a greater than 90% survival rate when treated with reduced radiation and limited chemotherapy. Children with advanced stage Hodgkin's disease have a 5-year disease-free survival rate of 70–90% after treatment with high-dose multiagent chemotherapy, often combined with low-dose radiotherapy.

26. What is the major late complication seen in female adolescents treated for Hodgkin's disease with radiation therapy to the chest?
The incidence of breast cancer is markedly increased.

27. Name the two most common types of bone tumors seen in adolescents.
Osteosarcoma and Ewing's sarcoma account for the vast majority of bone tumors in adolescents. The peak incidence for both tumors is in the second decade of life. The peak occurrence of osteosarcoma during the adolescent growth spurt suggests a relationship between rapid bone growth and the development of malignancy. Supporting evidence includes the finding that patients with osteosarcoma are taller than their peers; the disease appears earlier in girls, corresponding to an earlier onset of accelerated growth; and the disease occurs most often at the metaphyseal ends of the most rapidly growing bones. Sixty-four percent of all Ewing's sarcomas occur during the second decade of life. The disease occurs with a slightly greater frequently in males and is rare among African-Americans.

28. What are the clinical features of an adolescent with T-cell acute lymphocytic leukemia?
Patients with T-cell lineage acute leukemia are often older children and adolescents. They generally have high white blood cell counts at diagnosis and may have lymphomatous features

with mediastinal masses, hepatosplenomegaly, and bulky lymphadenopathy. There is also a higher incidence of CNS involvement.

29. Which congenital disorders predispose a child to the development of myelodysplasia during the first two decades of life?
In children and adolescents, nearly 40% of the cases of myelodysplasia are associated with constitutional chromosomal disorders (Down syndrome), gene deletion (neurofibromatosis type 1), congenital neutropenic disorders (Kostmann and Shwachman syndromes), and DNA repair defects (Fanconi anemia).

30. List three late complications of systemic corticosteroids as used in many chemotherapy regimens.
Three late complications of systemic corticosteroids include avascular necrosis of bone (especially of the femoral head), osteoporosis, and cataract formation.

31. List therapies applied to the treatment of cancer that may lead to infertility.
1. Radiation therapy is directly toxic to germ cells and Leydig cells in men. As a result, boys treated prepubertally with radiation for testicular leukemia/lymphoma are at extremely high risk for infertility and delayed sexual maturation associated with decreased testosterone levels. It is well-documented that radiation to the ovaries may lead to irreversible ovarian failure.
2. Alkylating agents such as cyclophosphamide and the nitroureas can decrease spermatogenesis in cancer survivors. Ovarian failure also has been associated with alkylating agents. Although such toxicity is dose- and age-dependent, morbidity is usually less in females than in males.

32. What two interventions can be employed in an attempt to preserve fertility in an adolescent with cancer who is about to start treatment with chemotherapy and/or radiotherapy?
Sperm banking is one attempt to preserve fertility in an adolescent male who is about to undergo chemotherapy. This should be done before the administration of any chemotherapy. Oophoropexy or surgical relocation of the ovaries can be used in adolescent females to preserve fertility when the ovaries would otherwise be in the field of radiation.

33. Is the outcome different for teenagers treated at a pediatric oncology center compared with adolescents treated at an adult oncology facility?
Based on research performed by Rauck and colleagues, adolescents between the ages of 15 and 19 years treated at pediatric oncology cooperative group institutions held a survival advantage when the diagnosis was acute lymphoblastic leukemia, acute myelogenous leukemia, osteosarcoma, or Ewing's sarcoma. In addition, most pediatric oncology centers have specialists from a variety of disciplines that are focused on the adolescent. Such specialists may include adolescent medicine physicians, pain management specialists, psychologists, child life specialists, reproductive medicine specialists, social workers, and pediatric surgeons.

34. What is the greatest cause of death beyond 5 years from diagnosis in long-term survivors of childhood cancer?
Recurrent tumor.

BIBLIOGRAPHY

1. Claessens EA, Cowell CA: Acute adolescent menorrhagia. Am J Obstet Gynecol 139:277–280, 1981.
2. Dunsmore KP: Acute lymphocytic leukemia in the adolescent: Diagnosis, treatment, and outcomes. Adolesc Med 10:407, 1999.
3. Embury SH, Hebbel RP, Mohandas N, Steinberg MH (eds): Sickle Cell Disease: Basic Principles and Clinical Practice. New York, Raven Press, 1994.

4. Hilgartner MW, Pochedly C (eds): Hemophilia in the Child and Adult, 3rd ed. New York, Raven Press, 1989.
5. Hord JD: Anemia and coagulation disorders in adolescents. Adolesc Med 10:359–367, 1999.
6. Rauck A, Fremgen AM, Hutchison CL, et al: Adolescent cancers in the United States: A National Cancer Data Base (NCDB) report [abstract]. J Pediatr Hematol Oncol 21, 310, 1999.
7. Ries LAG, Smith MA, Gurney JG, et al (eds): Cancer Incidence and Survival among Children and Adolescents: United States SEER Program 1975–1995. Bethesda, MD, National Cancer Institute, SEER Program. NIH Pub. No. 99-4649, 1999.
8. Russell EC, Dunn NL, Massey GV: Lymphomas and bone tumors: Clinical presentation, management, and potential late effects of current treatment strategies. Adolesc Med 10:419–435, 1999.
9. Winter SS, Mathew P, Vaughan RL, Foucar K: Myelodysplastic syndromes in the adolescent. Adolesc Med 10:401, 1999.

17. INFECTIOUS DISEASES

Katalin I. Koranyi, M.D.

IMMUNIZATIONS

1. What are the differences between protein conjugate and polysaccharide vaccines?

Conjugate vaccines are coupled with a carrier protein. They elicit immune response in young children under 2 years of age; decrease nasopharyngeal carriage of the organism, providing some protection for unimmunized people; and are T-cell dependent. When exposed to an antigen, they elicit an amnestic response with antibody production.

2. What are the current recommendations for reimmunizations with the 23-valent pneumococcal polysaccharide vaccine in adolescents?

The 23-valent polysaccharide pneumococcal vaccine does not induce immunologic memory, and serotype-specific antibody declines with time. Therefore, for patients over 10 years of age, the vaccine should be repeated every 5 years if splenic dysfunction or immunocompromise is present.

3. Is the meningococcal vaccine recommended routinely?

No. The currently licensed polysaccharide tetravalent meningococcal vaccine for serotypes A, C, Y, and W-135 is poorly antigenic in children under 2 years of age. Immunization is recommended for older children and adolescents in high-risk groups, including those with functional or anatomic asplenia or complement deficiencies. Because of the small but highly publicized outbreaks of meningococcal disease on college campuses, the American College Health Association recommends immunization of college students. The American Academy of Pediatrics recommends that college students and parents should be informed about the risks of disease and that the meningococcal vaccine should be readily available if requested. Research is under way for meningococcal conjugate vaccines, which would be effective in young children and provide long-lasting protection. Immunity with the available polysaccharide vaccine lasts for 5 years in vaccinated adults.

4. What agents are recommended for chemoprophylaxis in people exposed to a patient with invasive meningococcal disease?

The antimicrobials recommended by the Red Book 2000 include:

1. Rifampin, 600 mg orally every 12 hours for 2 days, *or*
2. Ceftriaxone, 250 mg intramuscularly as a single dose for persons over 12 years of age, *or*
3. Ciprofloxacin, 500 mg orally as a single dose

Rifampin is not recommended in pregnant women. Ciprofloxacin is not recommended for persons less than 18 years of age.

5. What are the current recommendations for hepatitis A vaccine?

The hepatitis A vaccine is recommended under the following circumstances:

1. Foreign travel by susceptible persons working in countries with intermediate or high rates of hepatitis A infection. For people 2 years of age and older, vaccine is preferable but immunoglobulin is an acceptable alternative.

2. For persons living in communities with consistently elevated hepatitis A rates, including Arizona, Alaska, Oregon, New Mexico, Utah, Washington, Oklahoma, South Dakota, Idaho, Nevada, and California.

3. Persons with chronic liver disease.

4. Homosexual and bisexual men.
5. Users of injection and noninjection illegal drugs.
6. Patients with clotting-factor disorders.
7. Persons at risk of occupational exposure, such as handlers of nonhuman primates.

6. What are the current recommendations for postexposure prophylaxis for hepatitis A?

After exposure to hepatitis A virus, immunoglobulin is recommended in the following circumstances:

1. For household and sexual contacts.
2. For newborn infants born to hepatitis A virus–infected mothers.
3. Child care staff, children, and household contacts.
4. Schoolroom exposure generally is not an indication when a single case occurs. However, immunoglobulin may be used if transmission within the school setting is documented.
5. In institutions and hospitals routine administration of immunoglobulin to hospital personnel caring for patients with hepatitis A is not indicated, unless an outbreak is documented.

7. What immunizations are recommended for adolescents over 11 years of age?

1. Hepatitis A vaccine is indicated for adolescents at increased risks of hepatitis A infection or its complications. Two doses are administered at 0 and 6–12 months.
2. Hepatitis B vaccine is recommended for adolescents not previously vaccinated. Three doses are given: at 0, 1–2, and 4–6 months. In September of 1999, the Food and Drug Administration (FDA) approved Recombivax HB for an alternate 2-dose schedule for children 11–15 years of age . The two doses of the 10-mg/ml adult formulation are given 4–6 months apart.
3. Influenza vaccine is recommended for adolescents who are at increased risk for complications caused by influenza or who have contact with persons at increased risk. The influenza vaccine is recommended annually from September to December.
4. A single dose of measles, mumps, and rubella vaccine (MMR) is indicated for adolescents who have not previously received two doses of vaccine.
5. Pneumococcal polysaccharide vaccine is indicated for adolescents at increased risk for pneumococcal disease or its complications.
6. Tetanus and diphtheria toxoids (Td) are recommended for adolescents not vaccinated within the previous 5 years. The vaccination needs to be repeated every 10 years.
7. Varicella virus vaccine is recommended for adolescents who have not been vaccinated previously and who have no reliable history of chickenpox. For adolescents over 13 years of age, two doses of the vaccine are given 4–8 weeks apart.

HUMAN IMMUNODEFICIENCY VIRUS (HIV) INFECTION

8. What is the role of the physician in educating adolescents about prevention of HIV infection?

Physicians should counsel adolescents about behaviors that place them at risk. Although abstinence from sexual intercourse and oral sex is the safest method of avoiding sexual exposure to HIV, it is impossible to predict which adolescents will remain abstinent. Education about safer sex should include the use of latex condoms and other barrier methods. Alternatives to sexual intercourse, such as masturbation and petting, should also be discussed with the adolescent. When an adolescent is diagnosed with a sexually transmitted infection (STI) such as herpes simplex or syphilis, information about the association between these infections and transmission of HIV infections should be given. An STI should serve as a marker for unprotected sexual intercourse. Discussions between the physician and adolescent should include dangers of sharing needles for injection of drugs or body piercing. Physicians should include HIV infection on the lists of risks associated with the use of alcohol, marijuana, cocaine, and other noninjection drugs, which impair judgment and increase the likelihood of unsafe sexual practices. Physicians need to inform adolescents that one-half of all new HIV infections in the United States occur in people between the ages of 13 and 24 years. Heterosexual transmission of HIV infection, particularly among female adolescents, is on the rise.

9. What is the role of the physician in testing of adolescents for HIV infection?
More than one-half of all HIV-infected adolescents are unaware of their HIV status and have not been tested. Therefore, the physician must discuss testing for HIV and refer the HIV-infected adolescent to appropriate medical care. Methods for the prevention of HIV transmission from the infected adolescent to others should also be addressed. A negative HIV test result provides an opportunity to counsel the adolescent in ways to prevent future high-risk behaviors. Retesting after 6 months is advisable in the context of recent high-risk behavior because HIV antibody may not appear for several months after infection. Recent advances in the treatment of HIV infection with combination drugs can relieve HIV-related symptoms and prolong survival. An HIV-positive female adolescent who becomes pregnant can reduce the risk of mother-to-child HIV transmission by taking antiretroviral therapy, including zidovudine (AZT). AZT can reduce the risk of transmission to the infant from 28% to 7%. Combination regimens of antiretroviral drugs have reduced the risks of HIV vertical transmission even further. Physicians should offer support and assistance to the adolescent in partner notification and help the adolescent to make disclosure of his or her HIV status.

10. Is the adolescent's consent to perform HIV testing sufficient?
Parental involvement in adolescent health care is desirable, but consent of the adolescent alone is sufficient for testing and treatment of suspected or confirmed HIV infection.

11. What is the physician's role in disclosing the HIV status of an adolescent?
1. The physician who intends to disclose information about the HIV status to sexual partners should inform the adolescent before testing.
2. Anonymous partner notification is available through the local health departments. Maintaining confidentiality is important.
3. HIV infection status should not be disclosed to school authorities without consent from the adolescent. After obtaining the adolescent's consent, the physician can play an important role in disclosure and education of school authorities and schoolmates. The physician should advocate for the special needs of adolescents for information, access to testing and counseling, and treatment of HIV infection.

12. What are the currently recommended indications for the initiation of antiretroviral drug therapy in the chronically HIV-infected adolescent or adult?
Therapy is indicated for patients who have low CD4 count (below 500/ml) or high viral load (HIV RNA over 20,000 copies/ml) and symptomatic patients with thrush, unexplained fever, or an AIDS-defining condition. Most experts observe an asymptomatic patient with a CD4 count of 350–500/ml. Asymptomatic patients with a CD4 count above 500/ml and HIV RNA (viral load) below 20,000 copies/ml are observed and followed by most experts; some physicians, however, initiate treatment.

13. What are the goals of HIV therapy?
1. Maximal and durable suppression of viral load
2. Restoration and preservation of immunologic function
3. Reduction of HIV-related morbidity and mortality

14. How do the physician and adolescent decide when to initiate treatment for HIV infection?
Decisions about initiation of HIV treatment should be made only after lengthy education and discussion with the adolescent about the risks and benefits of treatment. Factors that must

be considered include the willingness of the adolescent to make a lifetime commitment and the likelihood of adherence to the prescribed treatment regimen. Close follow-up and support should take place to assess adherence and response to therapy.

15. What toxicities may be associated with the treatment of HIV infection?

Potent combination antiretroviral therapy has resulted in marked decline in mortality due to HIV. Unfortunately, this decline comes at a significant cost because of HIV drug-related toxicities. HIV lipodystrophy syndrome includes peripheral wasting, central adiposity (increased abdominal girth and buffalo hump), insulin resistance and development of diabetes, and hyperlipidemia. The use of nucleoside reverse transcriptase inhibitors (NRTIs) has been associated with mitochondrial toxicities. The symptoms are similar to those of genetically based mitochondrial diseases and include neuropathy, myopathy, steatosis, lactic acidosis, and bone marrow suppression. The incidence of asymptomatic lactic acidemia in NRTI-treated patients is between 8% and 21%. Symptomatic lactic acidosis occurs at a considerably lower rate but carries significant morbidity and mortality. Fatal liver failure with lactic acidosis has been reported in three pregnant women treated with NRTIs (d4T and ddI-containing regimens). A study from France showed that 0.7% of children exposed to NRTIs before birth had confirmed or suspected mitochondrial toxicities. In the United States, a large-scale review of infants exposed to NRTIs in utero found no evidence of deaths due to mitochondrial toxicity.

16. Describe the management of lactic acidosis in HIV-infected patients.

1. Consider other possible causes of an elevated anion-gap, such as diabetic ketoacidosis, sepsis, or uremia.

2. For severally ill patients, bicarbonate and hydration should be administered intravenously.

3. Order serial measurements of serum lactate.

4. Withdraw offending agent(s) (NRTIs) immediately.

5. The benefit of vitamin supplementation (e.g., vitamins C, E, and K3; coenzyme Q; riboflavin), which has been used in a small number of patients, remains unclear.

INFECTIOUS MONONUCLEOSIS

17. What clinical syndromes are associated with Epstein-Barr virus (EBV) infections?

The most common syndromes associated with EBV infections include the following:

1. Infectious mononucleosis.
2. Chronic active EBV infection.
3. Cancers associated with EBV:
   • Nasopharyngeal carcinoma
   • Burkitt's lymphoma
   • Hodgkin's disease
   • Lymphoproliferative disorders, including X-linked lymphoproliferative disease
   • EBV and HIV have been associated with oral hairy leukoplakia, lymphoid interstitial pneumonitis (LIP), and non-Hodgkin lymphoma.

18. What are the common clinical manifestations of EBV mononucleosis?

The classic triad of fever, lymphadenopathy, and pharyngitis is present in over 50% of patients. Less often splenomegaly, palatal petechiae and hepatomegaly are present. If amoxicillin is given for the treatment of sore throat, a morbilliform rash develops in most patients.

19. What are the most common complications of EBV mononucleosis?

   • Hematologic complications, such as hemolytic anemia, thrombocytopenia, and aplastic anemia
   • Myocarditis
   • Hepatitis

- Genital ulcers
- Splenic rupture
- Rash
- Neurologic complications such as Guillain-Barré syndrome, encephalitis, and meningitis
- Upper airway obstruction

20. Describe the treatment of EBV mononucleosis.

Infectious mononucleosis is a self-limited disease; therefore, treatment is supportive. Saline gargles and analgesics are indicated for throat discomfort. In more severe cases, codeine or meperidine may be required. Short-courses of corticosteroids may be beneficial in severe cases of infectious mononucleosis with impending upper airway obstruction. Corticosteroid therapy may also be indicated in cases of thrombocytopenic purpura. Long-term effects of corticosteroids on the normal immune response to EBV are unknown. Contact sports should be avoided until the patient is fully recovered and the spleen is no longer palpable. Splenic rupture has been reported in 5 of 8,000 cases of infectious mononucleosis. Although acyclovir and ganciclovir inhibit EBV replication in vitro, they have little effect on the clinical course. Antiviral therapy is not recommended for acute infectious mononucleosis.

21. How is EBV mononucleosis diagnosed in the laboratory?

The diagnosis often can be made on the basis of clinical findings of fever, sore throat, and lymphadenopathy in the presence of lymphocytosis and atypical lymphocytes and a positive heterophil agglutination antibody test (monospot). Because younger children often have low heterophil antibody response, the monospot test may be negative. In this situation, the diagnosis is confirmed by the presence of antibodies to specific EBV antigens. Antibodies produced during primary EBV infections are directed against the viral capsid antigen (VCA). Both IgM and IgG antibodies are produced; IgM antibodies are transient, whereas IgG antibodies persist for life. Later in the disease antibodies against the early antigens (EAs) appear and gradually disappear after 6 months. Low levels of antibodies to the R component of the EA can be detected for years. During the convalescent phase antibodies against the nuclear antigen (EBNA) appear, taking 1–6 months to become detectable. Antibodies against EBNA remain present for life.

Serologic Findings in EBV Mononucleosis

Primary infection	VCA IgM: present
	VCA IgG: present
	Early antigen: present
	EBNA: absent
Convalescent or past infection	VCA IgG: present
	Early antigen: present (low) or absent
	EBNA: present
Reactivation	VCA IgG: present
	Early antigen: present
	EBNA: present

22. What is the period of communicability of infectious mononucleosis?

The period of communicability of infectious mononucleosis is unknown. The intermittent excretion of EBV in the saliva is lifelong. Close personal contact is required for transmission; hence, mononucleosis is sometimes known as the "kissing disease." Occasionally transmission of EBV by blood transfusion has been documented. Although the virus can survive for several hours outside the body, the role of fomites in transmission is not known. In lower social economic groups, infection occurs frequently at a young age, whereas in affluent social groups infection usually is delayed until adolescence or adulthood. Asymptomatic infection is the rule, particularly in the younger age groups. The incubation period of infectious mononucleosis is about 30–50 days.

23. Give your diagnosis for the following scenarios:
  (a) If EBV antibody testing shows the presence of anti-VCA IgG and anti-EBNA.
  The diagnosis is past infection. The presence of IgG antibody against VCA denotes acute, recent, or past infection. Antibody against the early antigen (EA) also is present during acute and recent infection. The detection of antibody against EBNA helps differentiate acute from past infection. In acute infection EBNA is absent, and in the case of recent infection antibody against EBNA may be present at a low level.
  (b) If the testing shows high VCA IgM and IgG and absent anti-EBNA.
  The diagnosis is primary acute EBV infection. IgM VCA antibody is present only during the acute stage of EBV infection, whereas antibody against EBNA appears during the convalescent stage and remains for life.

24. What is the differential diagnosis of infectious mononucleosis?
  EBV is the cause of heterophil-positive infectious mononucleosis and also of most cases of heterophil-negative infectious mononucleosis. Heterophil antibody is mainly IgM and appears during the first or second week of the illness. Typically it is absent in the serum of young children. Heterophil antibody with infectious mononucleosis causes agglutination of sheep red blood cells after absorption with guinea pig kidney antigens, but no agglutination is seen after absorption with beef red blood cells. In addition to EBV mononucleosis, other causes of heterophil-negative infectious mononucleosis include cytomegalovirus (CMV), rubella, adenovirus, human herpes virus-6, HIV, hepatitis A, and toxoplasmosis. Symptoms with these viruses are usually less severe than with EBV-induced mononucleosis.

PNEUMONIA

25. What agents commonly cause acute pneumonia?
  Not much information is available about the agents that cause community-acquired pneumonia because cultures obtained from the upper respiratory tract and sputum are insensitive. Although a positive blood culture usually confirms etiology, bacteremia is present in only about 10–20% of all cases of pneumonia. Collection of sputum is seldom successful in children.
  In children over 5 years of age, the common agents causing acute pneumonia are respiratory viruses, *Mycoplasma pneumoniae*, *Chlamydia pneumoniae*, and *Streptococcus pneumoniae*. Beyond the neonatal period respiratory viruses are the most frequent cause of pneumonia, including respiratory syncytial virus (RSV), influenza viruses, and parainfluenza viruses. RSV and influenza viruses are more common during the winter months, whereas parainfluenza viruses are more often seen during the autumn and spring.
  The atypical bacteria *M. pneumoniae* and *C. pneumoniae* are the most frequent causes of pneumonia requiring hospitalization in school-aged children. The transmission of *M. pneumoniae* among family members is slow, usually taking 3 weeks. It has been estimated that 6–19% of community-acquired pneumonia among adults and older children is due to *C. pneumoniae*. Beyond the neonatal period, the most common bacterial agent causing pneumonia in all age groups is *S. pneumoniae*. Pneumonia caused by *Haemophilus influenzae* is rare in countries where vaccination is routine. Occasionally, *Staphylococcus aureus* and *Streptococcus pyogenes* cause severe and prolonged pneumonia. Polymicrobial infection due to organisms from the mouth flora should raise the concern of aspiration. Tuberculosis should always be considered in the differential diagnosis of pneumonia in children and adults.

SINUSITIS

26. Describe the clinical manifestations of acute sinusitis.
  Sinusitis is a common complication of an upper respiratory tract infection, estimated to occur in approximately 5–10% of upper respiratory infections. The clinical manifestations are

varied, and the diagnosis is suggested by a constellation of symptoms. Persistent nasal discharge, cough, or both for over 10 days without signs of improvement points to the diagnosis of acute sinusitis. Severe symptoms, such as high fever and purulent nasal discharge for more than 3 days, also suggest acute sinusitis. Cough (which may be present in the daytime), halitosis, facial pain, and periorbital swelling on awakening may be present.

Subacute or chronic sinusitis is suspected when respiratory symptoms last more than 1 month. Because of mouth breathing, sore throat, especially in the morning, is a common complaint. Fever, nasal discharge, and headache are less common.

The physical examination of the patient with sinusitis is variable. Postnasal drainage may be seen. The nasal discharge is often purulent but also may be clear. There may be tenderness on palpation over the paranasal sinuses.

27. What organisms cause sinusitis?

The bacteriology of acute sinusitis (10–29 days) includes *S. pneumoniae, H. influenzae,* and *Moraxella catarrhalis.* Similar microbiology is seen in patients with subacute (30–120 days) and chronic (over 120 days) sinusitis. In addition to these three organisms, *S. aureus* and anaerobic bacteria from the oral flora may be cultured from sinus aspiration.

28. How do you treat sinusitis?

If symptoms are indicative of acute sinusitis, antimicrobial agents are the mainstays of management. For most cases of uncomplicated sinusitis, amoxicillin is the drug of choice. Because of the high frequency of penicillin-resistant *S. pneumoniae,* a high dose of amoxicillin (875 mg 2 times/day) is recommended for 10–14 days. In patients who fail amoxicillin therapy and those with chronic sinusitis, amoxicillin-potassium clavulanate or a second-generation cephalosporin is recommended. For patients hospitalized because of severity of symptoms, intravenous cefuroxime or ampicillin-sulbactam is recommended. Patients with recurrent or chronic sinusitis may need further evaluation, including consultation with an allergist, a sweat test for cystic fibrosis, quantitative immunoglobulins, and, in rare cases, mucosal biopsy to detect ciliary dyskinesia. Surgical intervention is rarely necessary, but in the presence of orbital or central nervous system complications (e.g., periorbital cellulitis, epidural or subdural empyema) sinus surgery should be performed.

ACUTE BRONCHITIS

29. Describe the clinical manifestations of acute bronchitis.

The prodromal phase lasts 1–2 days and is manifested by fever and upper respiratory symptoms, followed by tracheobronchial symptoms, which usually last 4–6 days and include fever, discomfort, and cough. During the recovery stage, which may last 1–2 weeks, cough and expectoration of phlegm are the likely symptoms.

30. What organisms cause acute bronchitis?

Viruses including respiratory syncytial virus (RSV), parainfluenza viruses, and influenza virus. *M. pneumoniae, C. pneumoniae,* and occasionally *Bordetella pertussis* can also cause bronchitis.

31. Describe the management of acute bronchitis.

Influenza vaccine given every fall may prevent bronchitis caused by influenza A or B viruses. Antiviral agents such as amantadine, rimantadine, ostelmavir, or zanamivir have been shown to reduce the severity and shorten the duration of influenza. Bronchitis due to *M. pneumoniae* or *C. pneumoniae* can be treated with a macrolide or doxycycline for patients 9 years of age or older. Inhaled bronchodilators have been shown to improve symptoms when there is a significant component of reactive airway disease.

PARVOVIRUS B19 INFECTIONS

32. What is the mode of transmission of parvovirus B19?

The most frequent mode of transmission is contact with respiratory secretion, but the virus can also be transmitted by percutaneous exposure to blood or blood products and by vertical transmission between mother and fetus. Most cases of parvovirus B19 infection are asymptomatic. By 15 years of age, approximately 50% of adolescents are seropositive, and more than 90% of elderly persons have measurable antibody against parvovirus B19.

33. Describe the clinical manifestations of parvovirus B19 infection.

Several syndromes have been recognized. Erythema infectiosum or fifth disease has been recognized for the longest time. Erythema infectiosum is characterized by the appearance of "slapped cheeks," followed by a lacy rash that may itch. Systemic symptoms are infrequent, but adults, particularly women, may have arthralgia or frank arthritis. The rash of erythema infectiosum may wax and wane for several days to weeks. Transient aplastic crisis with profound anemia and reticulocytopenia lasting 7–10 days occurs in patients with hemolytic anemia such as sickle cell disease. Chronic parvovirus B19 infection with persistent anemia lasting for several months to years occurs in immunocompromised patients. Parvovirus B19 infection during pregnancy can cause fetal hydrops and death. The risk of fetal death is between 2% and 6%.

34. What should you recommend to a pregnant adolescent who has been in contact with a child diagnosed with erythema infectiosum?

The physician should explain that about 50% of adolescents are already seropositive for parvovirus B19. In the event of seroconversion during pregnancy, the risks of fetal complications are relatively low. Fetal ultrasonography may be offered. A congenital syndrome has not been described with intrauterine parvovirus B19 infection.

LYME DISEASE

35. Identify the agent and mode of transmission of Lyme disease.

Lyme disease is caused by the spirochete *Borrelia burgdorferi*, which is transmitted by infected tick vectors.The occurrence of cases correlates geographically with the distribution of these vectors. *Ixodes scapularis* is found in the Eastern and Mid-Western United States, and *Ixodes pacificus* is found in the West. In the United States Lyme disease occurs in three distinct geographic regions: in the Northeast from Massachusetts to Maryland; in the upper Midwest, especially Wisconsin and Minnesota; and on the West Coast in northern California.

36. Describe the common clinical manifestations of Lyme disease.

Manifestations can be divided into three stages: early localized, early disseminated, and late disease. **Early localized disease** presents with the rash of erythema migrans at the site of the tick bite. It begins as a red macule or papule and expands over several days to a larger lesion with partial central clearing. Other manifestations such as fever, headache, myalgia, arthralgia, and neck stiffness may be present. If untreated, these symptoms may be intermittent for several weeks.

The second stage, **early disseminated disease**, is characterized by multiple lesions of erythema migrans. This rash usually begins 3–5 weeks after the tick bite and is similar to the primary lesion but smaller. The rash reflects the presence of spirochetes in the blood. Cranial nerve palsies, meningitis, arthralgia, myalgia, fatigue, and headache are common. The most common manifestations during the third stage, **late disease**, is recurrent pauciarticular arthritis affecting the large joints. Encephalopathy and polyradiculoneuropathy also occur during late disease. If Lyme disease is treated during the early stages, late manifestations are uncommon.

37. How is Lyme disease treated?
1. **Early localized disease**. The treatment of choice for adolescents is doxycycline, 100 mg 2 times/day for 14–21 days.
2. **Early disseminated and late disease**. For multiple erythema migrans the treatment is the same as for early disease, but the duration of treatment is extended to 21 days. For isolated facial palsy the same regimen is given for 21–28 days. For persistent or recurrent arthritis, carditis, meningitis, or encephalitis, the treatment is parenteral ceftriaxone or intravenous penicillin for 14–21 days.

TOXIC SHOCK SYNDROME

38. What causes toxic shock syndrome (TSS)?
TSS is caused by *S. aureus* or *Streptococcus pyogenes* (group A streptococci). In the case of *S. aureus*–mediated TSS, the strains usually produce toxic shock syndrome toxin-1 (TSST-1). When *S. pyogenes* causes TSS, at least one of five superantigen exotoxins (A, B, C, or others) has been implicated. These toxins act as superantigens that stimulate lymphocytes and endothelial cells to produce inflammatory mediators such as tumor necrosis factor and interleukin-1. Capillary inflammation and leakage lead to loss of intravascular volume and hypotension. The multiorgan system dysfunction is related to the degree of hypotension. Staphylococcal TSS is more likely to occur in younger people who do not have neutralizing antibody. Young women with vaginal colonization with toxin-producing *S. aureus* are at a higher risk of developing TSS, especially with tampon use. Invasive infections, such as pneumonia, osteomyelitis, or surgical wound infection, can be the source of the toxin-producing *S. aureus*. The recent increase of severe invasive disease due to *S. pyogenes* associated with strains of M types 1 or 3 that produce pyrogenic exotoxins has caused severe scarlet fever, necrotizing fasciitis, and TSS.

39. What are the criteria for diagnosing staphylococcal toxic shock syndrome?
1. **Major criteria** include fever of 102°F or higher, hypotension, and a rash of erythroderma with late desquamation. All three major criteria are required for the diagnosis of staphylococcal TSS.
2. Three of the following **minor criteria** are required for the diagnosis of staphylococcal toxic shock syndrome:
   • Evidence of inflammation, such as conjunctivitis or pharyngitis
   • Gastrointestinal tract manifestationsm such as vomiting or diarrhea
   • Muscle involvement manifested as myalgia or elevated creatine kinase level
   • Central nervous system abnormalities, such as disorientation or altered level of consciousness
   • Liver abnormalities with elevated bilirubin or transaminases
   • Renal abnormalities, such as elevated blood urea nitrogen
   • Decreased platelet count.
3. **Serologic tests** for Rocky Mountain spotted fever, leptospirosis, or measles, if obtained, must be negative. Blood, throat, and cerebrospinal fluid cultures must be negative except for a positive blood culture for *S. aureus*.

40. What are the risk factors for staphylococcal TSS?
For women risk factors include the use of tampons with menstruation, other vaginal foreign body, barrier contraception, or postpartum state. For both women and men risk factors include surgical wound infection and focal or systemic *S. aureus* infection.

41. What are the diagnostic criteria for streptococcal toxic shock syndrome?
1. Isolation of *S. pyogenes* from a normally sterile site, such as blood, cerebrospinal fluid, or tissue biopsy. The organism also may be isolated from a nonsterile site, such as throat, sputum or vagina.

2. Clinical signs of hypotension and two or more of the following signs: renal impairment, thrombocytopenia or disseminated intravascular coagulation, hepatic involvement, adult respiratory distress syndrome, generalized erythroderma that may desquamate, or soft tissue necrosis (including necrotizing fasciitis, myositis, or gangrene).

42. Describe therapy for staphylococcal or streptococcal TSS.

Treatment should be aggressive and must be initiated as soon as possible. Fluid management with vigorous expansion of the intravascular volume is paramount to prevent end-organ damage. Because of extensive capillary leak, edema is expected and is not caused by overhydration. Anticipatory management of multisystem organ failure, including the renal, respiratory, and cardiovascular systems, is equally important. Because it may be impossible to differentiate staphylococcal and streptococcal TSS, parenteral antimicrobial therapy at maximal doses directed against both organisms should be started immediately. Empiric antimicrobial therapy should include a beta lactamase-resistant antistaphylococcal antibiotic and a protein synthesis-inhibiting antibiotic, such as clindamycin. Clindamycin should not be used alone because 1–2% of *S. pyogenes* strains are resistant. In parts of the country where methicillin-resistant *S. aureus* is somewhat frequent, vancomycin is used for the initial empirical therapy. Length of therapy is generally 10–14 days.

TUBERCULOSIS

43. What is the difference between tuberculosis infection and disease?

Tuberculosis infection is defined as infection in a person who has a positive tuberculin skin test, no symptoms or physical findings, and normal chest radiograph. **Tuberculosis disease** is defined as disease in an infected person with symptoms, signs, or radiographic findings consistent with *Mycobacterium tuberculosis*. The clinical manifestations of tuberculosis may be pulmonary, extrapulmonary, or both. Clinical manifestations occur 1–6 months after infection and may include fever, cough, weight loss, and night sweats. The radiographic findings of the lungs can include lymphadenopathy, segmental or lobar pneumonia, pleural effusion, or miliary disease. Meningitis also can occur, especially in young children. Late manifestations occur 12 months or more after the initial infection and include diseases of the bones, joints, and skin. Reactivation of pulmonary tuberculosis can occur in adolescents.

44. How do you make the diagnosis of tuberculosis infection in asymptomatic people?

Tuberculin testing is the only practical tool for diagnosing tuberculosis infection in asymptomatic people. The Mantoux test contains 5 tuberculin units of purified protein derivative (PPD). Other strengths of Mantoux skin test should not be used. Multiple puncture or "tine" tests are no longer recommended. The indications for tuberculin skin testing for infants, children, and adolescents have changed in recent years. Routine skin test administration for populations at low risk is no longer recommended. The tuberculin skin test can be given during the same visits as immunizations, including live-virus vaccines. Previous immunization with bacille Calmette-Guérin (BCG) is not a contraindication to skin testing. The tuberculin skin test should be read 48–72 hours after placement.

45. What are the indications for tuberculin skin testing (PPD)?

1. Children for whom *immediate* tuberculin skin testing is indicated include contacts of persons with confirmed or suspected infectious tuberculosis, children with clinical or radiographic findings suggestive of tuberculosis disease, children immigrating from endemic countries, and children with travel history to endemic countries or close contact with persons from such countries.

2. Children who should have *annual* tuberculin skin testing are those infected with HIV, those living in households with HIV-infected persons, and incarcerated adolescents.

3. Tuberculin skin testing is indicated every *2–3 years* for children who are exposed to HIV-infected people, homeless people, residents of nursing homes, institutionalized or incarcerated adolescents or adults, users of illicit drugs, or migrant farm workers.

4. Children who should be considered for tuberculin skin testing at *4–6* and *11–16 years of age* are those whose parents immigrated from countries with high prevalence of tuberculosis or who have continued potential exposure by travel to endemic areas, and children and adolescents who have household contact with persons from endemic areas with unknown tuberculin status. Children without specific risk factors who reside in high-prevalence areas should also be tested. The physician should be aware of the rates of tuberculosis disease in specific areas of the city, because they may vary from one neighborhood to the next.

46. What is the definition of positive tuberculin skin test?

The tuberculin skin test should be read at 48–72 hours after placement by a physician or a specially trained person. The area of induration is carefully measured and recorded:

1. **Induration ≥ 5 mm** is considered positive in the following people:
   - Those in close contact with known or suspected contagious cases of tuberculosis disease
   - Those suspected of having tuberculosis disease, either by radiographic or clinical evidence
   - Those receiving immunosuppressive therapy or with immunosuppressive conditions, such as HIV infection
2. **Induration ≥ 10 mm** is considered positive in the following people:
   - Those at increased risk of disseminated disease, such as children younger than 4 years of age and children with medical conditions, including diabetes, chronic renal failure, or malnutrition
   - Those with increased exposure to tuberculosis disease, such as children born in or whose parents were born in areas in the world endemic for tuberculosis and children exposed to adults who are HIV-infected, incarcerated, or homeless
3. **Induration ≥ 15 mm** is considered positive in people 4 years of age or older with no risk factors.

47. When does tuberculin reactivity appear after infection with *M. tuberculosis*?

Positive tuberculin skin test appears 2–12 weeks after the initial infection. The median interval is 3–4 weeks.

48. What are the adverse effects of isoniazid (INH)?

Hepatotoxic effects from INH therapy are rare in adolescents. Peripheral neuritis or seizures caused by inhibition of pyridoxine metabolism are rare. Pyridoxine is recommended for adolescents on meat-deficient diets or malnourished adolescents, pregnant adolescents and women, and breast-feeding infants and their mothers. Routine determination of liver function tests in otherwise healthy adolescents is not recommended. However, in adolescents with severe tuberculosis, such as disseminated disease; adolescents with recent or concurrent liver disease; patients taking a high daily dose of INH; pregnant or postpartum girls; or adolescents with concurrent use of other hepatotoxic drugs, aminotransferase concentrations should be determined monthly during the first several months of treatment.

HEPATITIS B

49. What are the modes of transmission of hepatitis B virus?

- Transfusion of blood or blood products (now rare in the United States because of screening of blood donors and viral inactivation of certain blood products)
- Sharing of needles or syringes
- Mucous membrane or percutaneous exposure to blood or body fluids

- Sexual transmission (homosexual and heterosexual)
- Nonsexual transmission (Person-to-person spread may occur when a chronically infected person resides in a household. Transmission may result from contact of nonintact skin or mucous membranes with blood-containing secretions or saliva. Inanimate objects can also transmit the hepatitis B virus.)
- Vertical transmission from mother to infant during the perinatal period can occur and unfortunately results in chronic infection up to 90% of the infants if the mother is positive for hepatitis B surface antigen (HBsAg).

50. Who should receive hepatitis B immunization?
- All infants
- Adolescents who were not immunized during childhood
- Injection drug users
- Sexually active heterosexual men and women with more than one sex partner during the previous 6 months
- Men who have sex with men
- Contacts and sexual partners of HBsAg-positive people
- Health care personnel
- Residents and staff of institutions for developmentally disabled persons
- Patients on hemodialysis
- Patients who receive clotting factor concentrate
- International travelers to areas in which hepatitis B virus infection is endemic
- Inmates of correctional facilities

HEPATITIS C

51. Describe the clinical manifestations of hepatitis C virus infection.
Hepatitis C virus infection is clinically indistinguishable from hepatitis A or B infections. Acute infection may be asymptomatic, particularly in children. Overall the clinical manifestations tend to be mild, but persistent hepatitis C infection occurs in up to 85% of cases. Of these cases, chronic hepatitis develops in 60–70%; 10% develop cirrhosis. In the United States hepatitis C virus infection is the leading reason for liver transplantation. Some patients also develop primary hepatocellular carcinoma.

52. How is hepatitis C transmitted?
Hepatitis C generally is transmitted via contaminated blood products. Illicit intravenous drug use is a strong risk factor. Tattooing is also associated with increased risk of hepatitis C infection, and body-piercing with a shared or unclean needle also poses a theoretical risk. Although cases of sexually transmitted hepatitis C infection have been suspected, sexual activity is not a major means of transmission.

53. How is hepatitis C virus infection diagnosed?
The diagnosis is made by serologic assays. The first test was an enzyme-linked immunoassay (ELISA), but because of poor sensitivity and specificity (50% false-positive rate) it has been replaced by a second-generation ELISA that detects antibodies to both nucleocapsid and nonstructural proteins. Seroconversion occurs within approximately 4–6 weeks of onset of hepatitis. To confirm a positive ELISA, the recombinant immunoblot assay (RIBA) was developed. Polymerase chain reaction (PCR) assay for detection of the hepatitis C virus RNA is also available. This test detects the virus weeks before onset of liver enzyme abnormalities.

54. What treatment is available for hepatitis C virus infection?
A combination of interferon-alpha with ribavirin is approved for treatment of chronic hepatitis C virus infection in people over 18 years of age. This combination therapy results in

sustained response in about 40% of patients. Adverse reactions with interferon include fever, headache, and muscle aches. People infected with hepatitis C virus should be immunized against hepatitis A and B viruses.

BIBLIOGRAPHY

1. Cherry JD: Parvovirus infections in children and adults. Adv Pediatr 46:245–269, 1999.
2. Dabis F, Leroy V: Preventing mother-to-child transmission of HIV: Practical strategies for developing countries. AIDS Read 10:241–244, 2000.
3. Fauci AS, Bartlett JG, Goosby ER, et al: Guidelines for the use of antiretroviral agents in HIV-infected adults and adolescents. Available at www.hivatis.org (living document updated April 2001).
4. Georges P, Gardner P (ed): Standards for immunization practice for vaccines in children and adults. Infect Dis Clin North 15:9–19, 2001.
5. Katz BZ: Epstein-Barr virus (mononucleosis and lymphoproliferative disorders). In Long SS, Pickering LK, Prober CG (eds): Principles and Practice of Pediatric Infectious Diseases. Philadelphia, Churchill Livingstone, 1997, pp 1165–1176.
6. Landovitz RJ, Sax PE: NRTI-associated mitochondal toxicity. Aids Clin Care 13:43–45, 48, 2001.
7. McCracken GM: Diagnosis and management of pneumonia in children. Pediatr Infect Dis J 19:924–928, 2000.
8. Moellering RC, Mayer KM (eds): Antiretroviral therapy in the year 2000. Infect Dis Clin North Am 14:827–849, 2000.
9. Pickering LK, Georges P, Baker CJ, et al (eds): Meningococcal infections. In 2000 Red Book: Report of the Committee on Infectious Diseases, 25th ed. Elk Grove Village, IL, American Academy of Pediatrics, 2000, pp 396–401.
10. Pickering LK, Georges P, Baker CJ, et al (eds): Hepatitis B, hepatitis C. In 2000 Red Book: Report of the Committee on Infectious Diseases, 25th ed. Elk Grove Village, IL, American Academy of Pediatrics, 2000, pp 289–306.
11. Schambelan M: Metabolic and morphologic complications of HIV. Top HIV Med 8:4–8, 2000.

18. NEUROLOGY

Juliann M. Paolicchi, M.A., M.D., Ann Pakalnis, M.D.,
and S. Anne Joseph, M.D.

EPILEPSY IN ADOLESCENTS

1. What tests are indicated if seizures are suspected in an adolescent?

If the patient is evaluated in the outpatient setting for the possibility of a seizure disorder, a careful history should be followed by an electroencephalogram (EEG) and magnetic resonance imaging (MRI) of the head. The history is important, because a normal routine EEG can be found in 50% of people with epilepsy. Head MRI is the optimal test for detecting subtle brain anomalies that may be responsible for epilepsy, such as mesial temporal sclerosis (MTS), slow-growing neoplasms, and cortical dysplasia (a heterogeneous collection of neurons). The history also should include a frank discussion of alcohol and drug use. Further testing may be indicated by the history.

If the patient presents to the emergency department with a seizure, a careful history is important to determine the seizure type and possible cause. Laboratory studies should include serum electrolytes, glucose, and serum and urine toxicology screen. A head CT is indicated to rule out acute hemorrhage or stroke. A lumbar puncture should be performed if the patient is febrile, had a prolonged seizure or postictal state, or has a history of recent infection treated with oral antibiotics. If the patient returns to baseline, referral should be made for subsequent EEG and MRI. If not, admission to the hospital for observation and presumptive treatment with intravenous antibiotics and acyclovir for meningitis and herpetic meningoencephalitis, respectively, is warranted.

2. What specific factors contribute to seizure control in adolescents?

1. **Changes in body weight**. The pubertal growth spurt results in rapid changes in body weight that can lower the effective serum concentration of antiepileptic drugs (AEDs). More frequent monitoring of plasma levels and dose adjustments may be indicated to maintain adequate dosing.

2. **Patient compliance**. As adolescents become increasingly independent of parents, compliance may suffer. Adolescents may not take medication to avoid being "different" from peers. At the onset of adolescence, the patient must be counseled about the importance of taking medications regularly and must be given the responsibility of doing so in later adolescence. The threat of losing driving privileges becomes a strong incentive for drug compliance in older teens.

3. **Seizure-provoking behavior**. With increased independence comes an increase in sleep deprivation, stress, and alcohol and drug abuse. All of the above can lower the seizure threshold and result in poor seizure control.

4. **Natural history of patient's epilepsy type**. Some syndromes, such as benign rolandic epilepsy and typical absence epilepsy, remit in mid-adolescence. Other syndromes, such as juvenile myoclonic epilepsy and symptomatic focal epilepsies, may begin. Seizures in patients with more severe forms of epilepsy, such as temporal lobe epilepsy and Lennox-Gastaut syndrome, may become more intractable to medications at this time.

3. What are the restrictions on driving a car for an adolescent with epilepsy?

The conditions for obtaining a driver's license vary widely from state to state. The physician's role in this determination also varies. Check with the Department of Motor Vehicles (DMV) or the Epilepsy Foundation in the state where you practice to learn local requirements.

In general, the presence of epilepsy requires applicants for a driver's license to submit medical information about their condition and updates on their condition either annually or at the discretion of the DMV. The physician's role is often to verify such data. As of 2001, the states requiring physicians to report the names of people whom they treat for epilepsy include California, Delaware, New Jersey, Nevada, Oregon, and Pennsylvania. Most states require patients to be seizure-free for at least 1 year, but exceptions may be applicable if the seizures are nocturnal, involve a prolonged aura, or have occurred secondary to a physician-directed change or withdrawal of antiepileptic drugs (AEDs). Although the primary responsibility for reporting in most states lies with the patient, the physician may voluntarily contact the DMV with information about patients who in their opinion pose a threat to themselves and others by driving. It is recommended that the physician also inform the patient of his or her intention to do so.

On a practical point, if withdrawal of medications is considered, an optimal time to do so is before the adolescent begins driving. There is less risk if breakthrough seizures occur without AEDs, and the need for long-term treatment can be established the adolescent applies for a license.

4. What reproductive health concerns affect female adolescents with epilepsy?

Adolescent women with epilepsy must be counseled about the effects of their disease and medications on reproduction:
- Infertility is nearly 40% more common in women with epilepsy than in the general population.
- The risk of major birth defects in infants born to women with epilepsy is 4–8% compared with 2–4% in the general population.
- The failure rate of oral contraceptives may exceed 6% per year for women taking certain AEDs.
- The risk of polycystic ovary syndrome is increased in women with epilepsy; it is further increased in women taking valproic acid.
- Sexual dysfunction in women with epilepsy ranges from 14–50%, with deficits in libido and arousal reported.

5. What are the treatment recommendations for female adolescents with epilepsy who are of reproductive age?

- Contraceptive counseling. Prescribe an oral contraceptive pill containing 50 μg of estrogen for women taking carbamazepine, oxcarbamazepine, phenobarbital, phenytoin, and topiramate, all of which increase the metabolism of estrogen. Advise a barrier method if breakthrough bleeding occurs, indicating inadequate ovarian suppression. Alternatively, consider using a progestin-only contraceptive in such patients.
- Refer for gynecologic evaluation for sexual dysfunction, weight increase, excessive acne, hirsutism, or abnormal menstrual cycle lengths.
- Prescribe prophylactic folic acid: a minimum of 0.4 mg/day for women of child-bearing age and 4–5 mg/day for women at increased risk of neural tube defects.
- Recommend adequate daily intake of calcium and vitamin D.
- Refer to neurologist for close monitoring if the patient is pregnant or planning a pregnancy.

MIGRAINE AND OTHER HEADACHES

6. How are migraine headaches classified and diagnosed?

Migraine headaches affect up to 10% of children and adolescents, with a slightly increased prevalence in boys; in contrast, migraines affect about 20% of adults in the United States and are three times more common in women. In about 25% of women, migraines first appear at menarche. The International Headache Society has defined criteria for diagnosis of migraine in the pediatric population. Migraine tends to have a strong genetic predisposition; about 75% of patients have a positive family history. Inheritance appears to be polygenic, but recently a rare type of familial hemiplegic migraine was linked to chromosome 19.

7. What are the acute treatment options for migraine?

The over-the-counter analgesics acetaminophen and ibuprofen provide the mainstay of acute analgesic intervention for migraine. Recent studies suggest that both ibuprofen (10 mg/kg) and acetaminophen (15 mg/kg) are safe and effective compared with placebo; ibuprofen produces the best overall pain relief. For more severe pain symptoms, the triptan medications have been used in the pediatric population. These serotonin agonists display proven efficacy in adults; sumatriptan is generally the reference standard. The triptans have been shown to be safe in migraine with and without aura but are contraindicated in complicated migraine syndromes (see table).

Comparative Overview of the Triptans*

	SUMATRIPTAN (IMITREX)	RIZATRIPTAN (MAXALT)	NARATRIPTAN (AMERGE)	ZOLMITRIPTAN (ZOMIG)
Company	Glaxo Wellcome	Merck	Glaxo Wellcome	Zeneca
Formulations	Injection, nasal spray, tablet	Tablet, orally disintegrating tablet (MLT)	Tablet	Tablet
Usual adult dose	50 mg tablet 20 mg nasal spray 6 mg sub-cutaneously	10 mg	2.5 mg	2.5 mg
Onset: pain relief at 30 minutes	10–12% tablet 27% nasal spray 63% subcutaneously	20%	8–10%	15–18%
Efficacy: pain relief at 2 hours	50–61% tablet 55–64% nasal spray 81–82% subcutaneously	67–77%	48%	62–65%

* Source of information: medication package inserts.

8. When should prophylactic treatment be considered?

In general, if migraine headaches are severe and associated with disability, such as frequent school absences, prophylactic medication should be considered—usually in patients with at least 3–4 headaches per month. Medications with some benefit include the tricyclic antidepressants and the beta-blockers such as propranolol. Recent studies suggest that some AEDs, such as divalproex sodium, topiramate, and gabapentin, may be helpful in migraine prophylaxis.

Nonpharmacologic therapies, such as biofeedback and relaxation therapy, have proven efficacy. Preliminary studies of dietary additions, such as riboflavin and feverfew, suggest few side effects and questionable benefit. Stress and fatigue are major exacerbating factors in pediatric migraine. Diet, poor sleep hygiene, and chronic mild dehydration are also contributing factors.

9. How are tension-type headaches diagnosed?

Tension headaches have nonmigrainous features, usually with bilateral pain that is constant; initially, however, they may be episodic and related to stress. The International Headache Society criteria for diagnosis of tension headache are as follows:
- Pressing or tight quality
- Mild intensity, which inhibits but does not prevent daily activities
- Bilateral distribution
- Not aggravated by routine physician activity

Episodic tension headaches occur less than 15 days/month, whereas chronic tension-type headaches occur more than 15 days/month. About 10–15% of children suffer from recurrent tension-type headaches.

10. What are the treatment options for tension-type headaches?

Anxiety and stress can be major contributors, and referral for counseling can be helpful. Nonpharmacologic therapies, such as biofeedback and relaxation therapy, are beneficial. A thorough eye exam excludes visual problems, such as new-onset myopia. Episodic headaches respond well to ibuprofen or acetaminophen; however, when taken frequently, these drugs may lead to rebound headaches or induce chronic daily headaches.

For chronic headaches, low-dose amitriptyline is effective and well-tolerated. It may need to be continued for up to 6 months, then slowly tapered. Sedation, dry mouth, and weight gain can be bothersome side effects. Divalproex sodium (10–30 mg/kg/day) also may be effective in treating chronic headaches. Weight gain and alopecia are reported side effects. Hepatic abnormalities are rare at such low doses.

TOURETTE SYNDROME AND TIC DISORDERS

11. What are tics? How are they classified?

Tics are involuntary, sudden, stereotyped, repetitive, purposeless movements or vocalizations that wax and wane. They can increase with anxiety, stress, excitement and fatigue and usually disappear with sleep. Although involuntary, they are briefly suppressible, which can lead to an overwhelming inner tension or a build-up of anxiety. Tic disorders are classified based on the type of tics and how long they wax and wane from the time of onset. **Transient tic disorder of childhood** is the mildest and most common tic disorder, affecting up to 5% of school children. It is characterized by a waxing and waning pattern of either motor or vocal tics or a combination of both for less than 1 year. **Chronic motor tic disorder** consists of motor tics that have had a waxing and waning pattern of more than a year. **Chronic vocal tic disorder** consists of repetitive vocal tics that have had a waxing and waning course for more than 1 year. A waxing and waning pattern of both motor and vocal tics for more than 1 year constitutes **Gilles de la Tourette syndrome**. It is now believed that the tic disorders are a spectrum of a single condition, with transient tic disorder at one end and Tourette syndrome at the other.

12. What associated conditions can be seen in patients with a tic disorder?
• Attention deficit disorder
• Learning disability
• Obsessive-compulsive disorder
• Behavior and mood disorders
• Speech and language problems
• Sleep disorders
• Disturbed auditory discrimination
• Impaired visual-perceptual performance
• Impaired visual-motor skills

13. How is Tourette syndrome diagnosed and managed?

No blood tests, scans, or ancillary tests can confirm Tourette syndrome. The diagnosis is purely clinical. Once tics have been documented, the first step is to classify the tic disorder. The next step is to delineate comorbid problems. The impact of the tics and comorbid problems on daily function is then determined. The common long-term goal is to enable the patient to succeed in life. Each patient is unique, and not everyone requires treatment. Therefore, it is important to determine which symptom, if any, disrupts daily social and academic activities. General management is then tailored to target those symptoms.

14. Can any medications cure tics?

No. Pharmacologic treatment for tics is purely symptomatic and not curative. Medications that can suppress tics include neuroleptics, clonidine, anticonvulsants, and antidepressants.

Neuroleptics used in the treatment of tics include haloperidol, pimozide, fluphenazine, and risperidone. Haloperidol reduces tics in 70% of treated patients, but over 50 % of patients receiving it complain of side effects. Only 25% of patients report significant improvement without side effects. Haloperidol therapy is usually begun with 0.25 mg at night for the first week and increased as needed by 0.25 mg per day on a weekly basis. Total daily doses of 1.5–2.5 mg/day are usually therapeutic. Pimozide treatment usually is begun with 1 mg given daily at bedtime. On a weekly basis, the dosage is increased by 1 mg until symptom relief is obtained or intolerable side effects occur (maximal daily dose = 10 mg). The Food and Drug Administration continues to caution against the use of pimozide in children below the age of 12 years.

15. Are stimulant medications, such as methylphenidate, contraindicated in the treatment of attentional difficulties in patients with Tourette syndrome?
Stimulants are not absolutely contraindicated in the management of attention-deficit disorder in persons with Tourette syndrome. On occasion, however, they can exacerbate tics. If other medications, such as clonidine or antidepressants, are ineffective in improving attention or cause intolerable side effects, a cautious trial of stimulants may be considered.

ADOLESCENT SLEEP DISORDERS

16. Why is sleep important?
The physiologic role of sleep is yet unknown. However, there is a clear biologic need for both rapid-eye-movement (REM) and non-REM sleep. If a person is selectively deprived of REM sleep by systematic awakenings, a rebound of REM sleep occurs to levels higher than normal when undisturbed sleep is once again permitted. Selective deprivation of non-REM sleep produces the opposite rebound phenomenon during the recovery period. If subjects are deprived of all sleep, the first recovery night is marked by excessive non-REM sleep, and rebound REM is delayed until the second or third recovery night. A primary function of non-REM sleep may be to facilitate conservation of metabolic energy and thermal regulation. However, there is little agreement about the role of REM sleep. In clinical practice, a wide range of behavioral, psychiatric, and medical disorders can disturb sleep. In turn, sleep disturbances can influence many behavioral and physiologic systems and worsen already existing behavior and mood problems.

17. How much sleep does an adolescent require?
The total sleep requirement varies among adolescents; some require more sleep than others. The quality of sleep has a more significant impact than duration. The average person needs a period of sleep with at least 5–7 uninterrupted cycles. Each cycle consists of a progression from stage 1 to stage 5 sleep and takes approximately 90 minutes. In general, sleep requirements tend to decrease gradually from the neonatal period to adulthood. However, as teenagers move from early to late adolescence, they actually require more rather than less sleep. Unfortunately, social norms that require teenagers to stay up later at night to complete school work and to get up early to get to school put the average adolescent at risk for inadequate sleep.

18. What are the most common sleep-related symptoms in adolescents?
Inability to awaken on time in the morning, daytime sleepiness, and insomnia are some of the presenting symptoms of sleep disorders in adolescents.

19. What are the causes of daytime sleepiness in an adolescent?
Excessive daytime sleepiness may arise from inadequate amounts of nocturnal sleep, disturbed nocturnal sleep, increased sleep requirements despite adequate nocturnal sleep, or circadian disorders. Inadequate amounts of nocturnal sleep usually are seen in adolescents when

the combination of social schedules or school work and extracurricular activities leads to late nights and early mornings that significantly diminish the number of hours of sleep. The catch-up sleep of naps and late awakenings on weekends and holidays can worsen the situation by leading to erratic schedules and even later nights. Disturbed nocturnal sleep can arise from obstructive sleep apnea syndrome, chronic medical problems that disrupt sleep directly or secondarily from drugs used in treatment, use of drugs or alcohol, or withdrawal from drugs or alcohol. Two conditions that may be seen in adolescents with pathologic daytime sleepiness include narcolepsy and a poorly understood condition called Kleine-Levin syndrome. Circadian rhythm sleep disorders result from a defect in the patient's indigenous circadian clock (e.g., with blindness or hypothalamic dysfunction) or from the limited capacity of the intrinsic clock to adjust to scheduling demands of social and work schedules or during travel (jet lag). In mood and anxiety disorders, insomnia and/or disturbed sleep may be prominent symptoms.

20. Describe narcolepsy and cataplexy.

Narcolepsy-cataplexy is a sleep disorder characterized by an abnormally short latency from sleep onset to REM sleep. REM sleep is attained in less than 20 minutes rather than the usual 90 minutes. In narcolepsy-cataplexy, irresistible sleep attacks occur during the day. Normal REM is characterized by vivid dreams and decreased muscle tone. In narcolepsy these two phenomena may occur during the day. The classic combination of narcolepsy-cataplexy consists of daytime sleep attacks, cataplexy (sudden loss of muscle tone), sleep paralysis, and dream imagery when falling asleep or awakening (hypnagogic and hypnopompic hallucinations). The classic combination may not be present in all cases. Particularly in teenagers, sudden sleep attacks during the day may be the only symptom. Cataplexy is typically provoked by laughter, anger, or sudden emotional change. If a cataplectic attack lasts long enough, full sleep can follow. The diagnosis of narcolepsy requires evaluation in the sleep laboratory. Treatment focuses on education, counseling, and adherence to a regular schedule to obtain optimal sleep (often including scheduled daytime naps), use of short-acting stimulants for treatment of daytime sleepiness, and use of REM suppressant medications, such as protriptyline, when cataplexy is a major problem.

21. Describe Kleine-Levin syndrome.

Kleine-Levin syndrome consists of excessive somnolence, hypersexuality, and compulsive overeating in adolescent boys. Symptoms usually are episodic, with cycles lasting from 1 to 30 days. The onset may follow a flu-like illness or injury with loss of consciousness. The symptoms usually disappear spontaneously in late adolescence or early adulthood. The diagnosis is made on clinical grounds after organic causes, such as hypothalamic tumors, central nervous system infections, and strokes, have been ruled out. Treatment consists of supportive care and reassurance. In selected cases of severely affected patients, trials of stimulant medications, lithium carbonate, phenytoin, valproic acid, and carbamazepine with antidepressants have been effective.

22. What is delayed sleep phase syndrome?

Delayed sleep phase syndrome (DSPS) is extreme difficulty in initiating sleep at a conventional hour of the night. Once the person is asleep, however, the sleep pattern and requirement are normal and not disrupted. Thus, patients have great difficulty in awakening on time in the morning. Daytime sleepiness, especially before midday, may be the main complaint. A survey of adolescents suggested a prevalence greater than 7%. Despite as much sleep deprivation as peers and attempts to change and maintain sleep patterns consistent with scheduling demands, patients with DSPS experience severe and persistent difficulty with sleep onset. There are no rapid methods to treat this condition. Chromotherapy sometimes is used in combination with hypnotics. Chromotherapy consists of daily three-hour delays of bedtime and arising until the patient's sleep schedule is realigned with the desired social schedule. Once this goal has been accomplished, the schedule has to be strictly followed seven days a week, or relapse is likely.

23. How are the parasomnias classified?

Parasomnias are a group of undesirable nonepileptic events that appear during sleep or are exacerbated by sleep. They usually consist of behavioral or autonomic activity. The International Classification of Sleep Disorders groups parasomnias under the categories of arousal disorders, sleep-wake transition disorders, parasomnias usually associated with REM sleep, and other parasomnias (see table).

Parasomnias

AROUSAL DISORDERS	SLEEP–WAKE TRANSITION DISORDERS	PARASOMNIAS USUALLY ASSOCIATED WITH REM SLEEP	OTHER PARASOMNIAS	
Sleepwalking (somnam-bulism)	Rhythmic move-ment disorder*	Nightmares*	Sleep bruxism	Primary snoring*
Sleep terrors (pavor noc-turnus, incubus)	Sleep starts	Sleep paralysis*	Sleep enuresis	Infant sleep apnea
Confusional arousals*	Sleep talking*	Impaired sleep-related penile erections*	Sleep-related abnormal swalling syndrome	Congenital central hypoventilations syndrome
	Nocturnal leg cramps*	Sleep-related painful erections*	Nocturnal par-oxysmal dys-tonia	Sudden infant death syndrome
			Sudden unex-plained noc-turnal death	Benign neonatal sleep myoclonus

* Parasomnias seen in adolescents.

BIBLIOGRAPHY

1. American Sleep Disorder Association: The International Classification of Sleep Disorders: Diagnostic and Coding Manual. Rochester, MN, American Sleep Disorders Association, 1990.
2. Dahl RE: The development of disorders of sleep. Adv Pediatr 45:73, 1988.
3. Erenberg G: Pharmacologic therapy of tics in childhood. Pediatr Ann 17:395, 1988.
4. Hamalianen M, Hoppu K, Valkeila E, Santavuori P: Ibuprofen or acetaminophen for the acute treatment of migraine in children: A double-blind, randomized, placebo-controlled, crossover study. Neurology 48:103, 1997.
5. Hershey AD, Powers SW, Bentti AL, de Grauw T: Effectiveness of amitryptilene in the prophylactic management of child headaches. Headache 40:539, 2000.
6. Lance JW, Goadsby P (eds): Mechanism and Management of Headache, 6th ed. Boston, Butterworth-Heinemann, 1998.
7. Maytol J, Young M, Shechter A, et al: Pediatric migraine and the International Headache Society (IHS) criteria. Neurology 50:1729, 1988.
8. Pakalnis A: New avenues in treatment of pediatric migraine: A review of the literature. Fam Pract 18:101, 2001.
9. Singer HS: Tic disorders. Pediatr Ann 22:22–29, 1993.
10. Thorpy M J, Glovinsky PB: Parasomnias. Psychiatr Clin North Am 10:623, 1987.
11. Wyllie E (ed): The Treatment of Epilepsy: Principles and Practices. Philadelphia, Lea & Febiger, 1993.

19. RENAL SYSTEM

Martin A. Turman, M.D., Ph.D., and John D. Mahan, M.D.

PROTEINURIA AND HEMATURIA

1. What in a urinalysis can indicate an underlying renal condition?

The presence of hematuria, proteinuria, glucose, nitrites, or leukocyte esterase can suggest a renal or urinary tract problem.

Hematuria is proved by demonstration of red blood cells (RBCs) on microscopic examination of the urine when the dipstick is positive for "blood." Free hemoglobin, myoglobin, and red pigments (porphyria, beets, blackberries, vegetable dyes, and phenolphthalein) can cause a urine dipstick to turn positive for blood in the absence of true hematuria. Hematuria may arise from inflammatory, structural, or traumatic renal conditions.

Proteinuria on the dipstick actually means increased levels of urinary albumin. Other tests for urine protein (e.g., Comassie blue) can be done in the laboratory to detect all urine proteins. Proteinuria may indicate glomerular or tubular disease or may be a variant of normal (e.g., orthostatic proteinuria).

Glucose may appear in the urine as a result of diabetes mellitus or renal tubular dysfunction.

Nitrites appear when certain bacteria (most gram-negative but few gram-positive bacteria) are able to convert nitrates in the urine to nitrites over time. Not all bacteria can make this conversion, but when positive, the test is highly specific for the presence of large numbers of bacteria in the urine (or consumption of nitrite-laced hot dogs or contaminated well water).

Leukocyte esterase detects esterases released from white blood cells (WBCs) in the urine. This test can be positive in the presence of urinary tract infection but is not highly specific because it also can be positive with inflammatory renal conditions such as nephritis or vaginal WBCs washed into the urine.

Clinitest positivity is often confusing to the clinician and generally indicates presence of glucose, fructose, galactose, pentose, lactose, penicillins, cephalosporins, or ascorbic acid in the urine.

2. What is the most common cause of proteinuria in adolescents?

Orthostatic proteinuria. In this benign disorder, an abnormally high amount of protein is excreted while the patient is upright and active, but excretion returns to normal when the patient is supine. The patient can have 4+ protein on a urine dipstick with orthostatic proteinuria, but if a full 24-hour urine is collected, the total protein excretion is always < 1.5 gm/day. It is most common in tall, thin adolescents and is present in as many as 5% of healthy adolescents.

When proteinuria is detected, a careful history and exam should be obtained. If the patient does not have signs or symptoms of a more worrisome causes of proteinuria (e.g., hypertension, hematuria, edema) and the review of systems is negative for signs of a systemic illness, the patient may have orthostatic proteinuria. If the patient has proteinuria *and* hematuria or hypertension, a form of glomerulonephritis is most likely and a more thorough evaluation is required.

3. How can orthostatic proteinuria be diagnosed?

1. The simplest method is to obtain a spot urine protein/creatinine on a first morning void. The adolescent should empty the bladder completely before going to bed and then, in the morning before other activities, provide a urine sample. The urine protein/creatinine should be < 0.2.

2. The family can be given urine dipsticks and a urine chart; they can then record the results from several first morning and afternoon urine samples. The morning samples should be negative or indicate trace protein, whereas the afternoon samples are more positive.

3. Collect a split 24-hour urine, in which two urine collections are obtained—one from urine produced while the patient is upright and one when the patient is supine. The supine urine should have < 40 mg/M^2/hr of protein. This test is difficult for an adolescent to do accurately.

If the tests confirm that the patient has orthostatic rather than persistent proteinuria, no further work-up is needed. However, it may be prudent to check a first morning urine at the patient's annual exam to be sure that persistent proteinuria or concomitant hematuria has not developed.

4. Can an adolescent have minimal-change nephrotic syndrome?

Nephrotic syndrome is defined as the presence of high grade (nephrotic range) proteinuria, hypoalbuminemia, hyperlipidemia, and edema. If an otherwise healthy adolescent presents with the acute onset of nephrotic syndrome, he or she has about a 25% chance of having minimal-change nephrotic syndrome rather than one of the forms of nephrotic syndrome with a poorer prognosis (e.g., focal segmental glomerulosclerosis, membranoproliferative glomerulonephritis, or membranous glomerulopathy). Proteinuria is considered in the nephrotic range if the spot urine protein/creatinine is > 2.0.

5. What can cause non–nephrotic-range proteinuria in an adolescent other than orthostatic proteinuria?

Once orthostatic proteinuria has been excluded, transient proteinuria should be ruled out. Fever, strenuous exercise, dehydration, and exposure to cold induce transient low-grade (1+ to 2+) proteinuria. If the patient has proteinuria over several weeks, the proteinuria is termed persistent. A thorough evaluation is warranted, including measurement of serum creatinine, albumin, and complement studies (C3 and C4) and a renal ultrasound. A renal biopsy may be needed. This evaluation probably will reveal one of the following disorders:

- Anatomic abnormalities (e.g., dysplasia, renal scars from reflux nephropathy or pyelonephritis)
- Focal segmental glomerulosclerosis, membranoproliferative glomerulonephritis, or membranous glomerulopathy
- Chronic glomerulonephritis (e.g., IgA nephropathy, Alport syndrome, lupus nephritis)
- Tubular disorders (e.g., from exposure to nephrotoxic drugs, such as aminoglycosides or heroin)
- Severe hypertension
- Long-standing diabetes mellitus

6. How do you know whether the adolescent obtained an accurate and complete 24-hour urine collection?

Measure the creatinine index, i.e., the amount of creatinine excreted in a 24-hour period per kilogram of body weight. The normal range is 18–24 mg/kg/day for older adolescents and adults, depending on muscle mass. Females have lower creatinine excretion than males, and obese patients have less excretion per kg. For younger children the expected creatinine excretion can be estimated from the formula: $15 + (0.5 \times age)$ [yr] ± 3 mg/kg/day. A lower-than-expected value implies that some urine was missed (a common problem for adolescents thinking about things other than collecting urine). A higher-than-expected value suggests that either the patient is very muscular or accidentally collected more than 24 hours of urine.

7. How common is asymptomatic hematuria in adolescents?

No good studies define the incidence and prevalence of hematuria specifically in adolescents. However, it is probably as frequent in adolescents as in school-aged children: 0.17–0.4% incidence for new onset per year and 0.5–2.0% prevalence for the total age group.

In the asymptomatic child it is important to determine that hematuria is persistent (over the span of weeks to months) before engaging in a detailed investigation. The American Academy of Pediatrics (AAP) recommends one screening urinalysis in adolescence, although the benefit of this approach is not certain.

8. What causes persistent isolated microscopic hematuria in adolescents?

Persistent hematuria means that the presence of hematuria has been documented over several weeks. **Isolated** hematuria means hematuria without proteinuria, hypertension, or signs of a systemic illness. Be sure that the urine samples were not collected within 4 or 5 days of a female patient's menstrual period. Causes include the following:

- Urinary tract infection
- Hypercalciuria: detected by determining a spot urine calcium/creatinine ratio (normal = < 0.2). Patients with hypercalciuria often have a family history of kidney stones.
- Benign hematuria: also frequently familial; therefore both parents' urine should be checked for hematuria.
- IgA nephropathy: may include episodes of gross hematuria with upper respiratory tract infections.
- Anatomic abnormalities of the kidneys (e.g., polycystic kidney disease, hydronephrosis).
- Sickle cell trait or disease
- Coagulopathy: especially with bleeding from minor trauma or a family history of coagulopathy.

The most common cause of hematuria in adolescent girls is urinary tract infection, although this is usually accompanied by dysuria, frequency or urgency. Hypercalciuria is the most common cause in boys.

9. Describe an appropriate work-up for persistent microscopic hematuria in an adolescent.

The initial laboratory evaluation for persistent microscopic hematuria should include a urine culture, urine calcium/creatinine, renal ultrasound, and, when indicated, coagulation studies and hemoglobin electrophoresis.

10. What tests should be obtained to evaluate an adolescent with a kidney stone?

Laboratory tests

- A 24-hour urine for calcium, oxalate, citrate, uric acid, and creatinine and a urine screening test for homocysteine to rule out cystinuria. An even more thorough evaluation can be obtained by sending the urine to a laboratory that specializes in performing "stone-risk profile," in which the laboratory measures supersaturation of constituents such as calcium oxalate and uric acid. One such laboratory is Litholink (1-800-338-4333).
- Serum calcium to test for hypercalcemia, creatinine to rule out renal insufficiency, electrolytes to exclude renal tubular acidosis, alkaline phosphatase to evaluate bone resorption, and N-parathyroid hormone to exclude hyperparathyroidism.

Imaging studies

- To evaluate for presence of a stone, the most sensitive method is a spiral computed tomography (CT), in which 0.5-cm cuts through the kidney are obtained in less than 5 minutes and no IV contrast is needed. Spiral CT is most sensitive for detecting small stones and also nicely demonstrates anatomic abnormalities. Other causes of pain, such as appendicitis, may be detected incidentally.
- A renal ultrasound also can be obtained, but it is not as sensitive as spiral CT for the detection of small stones. It also requires skilled operators who may not be as readily available after hours.

Intravenous pyelography (IVP) is the classic study for kidney stones but requires an IV infusion. In addition, some stones are not radiopaque, and sometimes the contrast obscures the stone, making it difficult to visualize. IVP also involves intravenous contrast that can cause an allergic reaction or contrast nephropathy (if the patient has antecedent renal disease or is dehydrated).

GLOMERULONEPHRITIS

11. What clinical features suggest the possibility of acute glomerulonephritis (GN) in an adolescent?

Hematuria (particularly with RBC casts or dysmorphic RBCs), proteinuria, edema, oliguria, hypertension, and renal insufficiency are classic features of GN. The more features that are present, the more likely that GN is the cause.

12. If a patient presents with acute glomerulonephritis, how do you determine whether it is poststreptococcal acute glomerulonephritis (PSAGN)?

The most common cause of acute onset of tea-colored urine, hematuria, and proteinuria is PSAGN. PSAGN has the best long-term prognosis of all causes of acute GN. There are three criteria for making the diagnosis:

1. A group A beta-hemolytic streptococcal infection must be documented by culture (either skin or throat infection) or serology. The most common serologic test is the antistreptolysin (ASO) titer. However, this test is not highly sensitive for detecting previous skin infections. The anti-DNAse B assay is better for this purpose.

2. The serum complement C3 must be decreased. The test must be given when the patient is first seen because serum C3 stays low for only a short time.

3. The C3 must normalize after 4–8 weeks. If the C3 does not become normal within 8 weeks, the diagnosis is most likely *not* PSAGN and is more likely to be lupus nephritis, membranoproliferative glomerulonephritis, or a form of parainfectious GN, such as the GN associated with chronic hepatitis.

Although adolescents with PSAGN should continue to improve over time and have a great prognosis, they can have significant morbidity during the acute phase. Thus, they must be closely monitored for hypertension and fluid retention. Hypertension can cause seizures, strokes, or other complications. Patients with PSAGN also can develop significant, albeit usually transient, renal failure with electrolyte abnormalities; this problem should be tested at presentation.

13. What are the risks to an adolescent who takes nonsteroidal anti-inflammatory drugs (NSAIDs)?

Gastritis is the most common risk of frequent NSAID use. Rarely, nephritis can develop and be associated with acute hypertension and renal failure. Surprisingly, the urine analysis is often benign or shows only a few red blood cells or white blood cells despite significantly elevated creatinine and severe hypertension. Therefore, it is important to ask about NSAID use in an ill adolescent with evidence of renal disease. Excessive NSAID use may be seen in adolescents involved in sport activities.

URINARY TRACT INFECTION

14. When should renal imaging studies be obtained for an adolescent with a urinary tract infection (UTI)?

Male adolescents rarely have urinary tract infections unless they have an anatomic lesion. Thus, any male with a documented UTI needs imaging studies (renal ultrasound and voiding cystourethrogram [VCUG]) to rule out posterior urethral valves, bladder abnormalities, or obstruction.

Female adolescents who develop mild urinary tract infection or cystitis do not need imaging studies initially. If the girl has an episode of pyelonephritis (flank pain and fever) or multiple episodes of cystitis, a more thorough evaluation with imaging studies may be warranted.

15. What are the risk factors for recurrent episodes of cystitis in adolescent girls?

1. Family history of recurrent UTI (in more than one family member) associated with increased adherence of specific gram-negative bacteria to bladder epithelial cell glycoproteins.

2. Anatomic abnormality, such as ureteropelvic obstruction or ureterocele, that prevents normal bladder emptying.

3. Constipation. Impacted stool can interfere with normal bladder emptying. Studies in patients with normal renal anatomy, recurrent cystitis, and constipation demonstrate that if the constipation is treated, the UTI frequency is greatly diminished.

4. Sexual activity. Antibiotic prophylaxis given nightly or before sexual intercourse may prevent recurrent infections. Urinating immediately after sexual intercourse also can prevent this type of cystitis.

5. Bladder dysfunction
- Irritable bladder syndrome. If a girl has small volumes of accidental urine leakage during the day, frequently does not sense the need to void, and then suddenly has a strong sense of urgency, irritable bladder syndrome or dyssynergia may be present and may respond to bladder retraining (voiding on schedule every 3–4 hours) or anticholinergic medication.
- Lazy bladder syndrome. If a girl has developed the habit of holding urine to the point that the bladder is overdistended and has lost its normal ability to contract, the bladder may empty by overflow incontinence. On VCUG the bladder is found to be large and smooth-walled.
- Neurogenic bladder. The patient may have a tethered cord or other neurologic abnormality that leads to inadequate innervation of the bladder. On VCUG the bladder usually appears contracted and trabeculated.

16. What are possible causes of pyuria in a teenager?

The most likely cause of pyuria is a urinary tract infection. However, if the urine culture is negative, several other explanations are possible:
- The patient may have received antibiotics that masked UTI.
- The patient may have urethritis rather than cystitis. A history of sexual activity and evaluation for sexually transmitted infections is warranted if a urine culture is negative.
- The patient may have cystitis caused by a fastidious organism, such as *Ureaplasma* sp. or a virus, that does not grow well under normal culture conditions. The microbiology laboratory can culture the urine on several different media to help rule out this possibility. Another fastidious organism that can cause pyuria is tuberculosis (TB). Therefore, a TB skin test should be placed in patients who have other risk factors for TB.
- Interstitial nephritis, either idiopathic, allergic, or in association with a glomerulonephritis, such as lupus nephritis, can cause pyuria as well as white blood cell casts.
- The white blood cells may come from inflammation adjacent to the bladder, as with appendicitis.

HYPERTENSION

17. How is hypertension defined in an adolescent?

The National High Blood Pressure Education Program Working Group on Hypertension Control in Children and Adolescents recently published an update of the 1987 Task Force Report on High Blood Pressure Control in Children and Adolescents. They clarified the definition and evaluation of pediatric hypertension, shifted the focus from secondary to primary hypertension, and underscored the relationship of childhood hypertension and high normal blood pressure values to adult hypertension. The new normal curves relate blood pressure to age *and* height and are the gold standard for determining the significance of measurements in adolescents. This report is also a treasure trove of important information about blood pressure measurement and etiologies in children.

18. How do you determine if a teenager really has hypertension?

First, be sure that the correct-size cuff is used. Many large adolescents need a large adult cuff or even a thigh cuff to fit properly on their arms. The inflatable bag of the cuff should be 20% wider than the diameter of the limb and at least two-thirds the length of that segment of the extremity. A cuff that is too small gives falsely elevated blood pressure values. Secondly, determine whether the patient has "white coat" hypertension, i.e., the hypertension is due to anxiety from being at the doctor's office. This problem can be assessed by multiple measurements at home with a cuff that has been tested for accuracy in the office. Many insurance companies now pay for a home blood pressure cuff to help with such an assessment. If the home cuff cannot be obtained, the school nurse or local fire station can obtain blood pressures measurements. If none of the above resources can be arranged, a 24-hour ambulatory monitor can be prescribed. If 20% or more of the home systolic or diastolic measurements are greater than the 95th percentile for the patient's height and age, and the mean blood pressure readings are > 95th percentile of mean blood pressure for age, hypertension is diagnosed.

Blood Pressure Levels for the 90th and 95th Percentiles of Blood Pressure for Boys Aged 10–17 Years by Percentile of Height

AGE (YR)	BLOOD PRESSURE PERCENTILE*	SYSTOLIC BLOOD PRESSURE BY PERCENTILE OF HEIGHT (mmHg)[†]							DIASTOLIC BLOOD PRESSURE BY PERCENTILE OF HEIGHT (mmHg)[†]						
		5%	10%	25%	50%	75%	90%	95%	5%	10%	25%	50%	75%	90%	95%
10	90th	110	112	113	115	117	118	119	73	74	74	75	76	77	78
	95th	114	115	117	119	121	122	123	77	78	79	80	80	81	82
11	90th	112	113	115	117	119	120	121	74	74	75	76	77	78	78
	95th	116	117	119	121	123	124	125	78	79	79	80	81	82	83
12	90th	115	116	117	119	121	123	123	75	75	76	77	78	78	79
	95th	119	120	121	123	125	126	127	79	79	80	81	82	83	83
13	90th	117	118	120	122	124	125	126	75	76	76	77	78	79	80
	95th	121	122	124	126	128	129	130	79	80	81	82	83	83	84
14	90th	120	121	123	125	126	128	128	76	76	77	78	79	80	80
	95th	124	125	127	128	130	132	132	80	81	81	82	83	84	85
15	90th	123	124	125	127	129	131	131	77	77	78	79	80	81	81
	95th	127	128	129	131	133	134	135	81	82	83	83	84	85	86
16	90th	125	126	128	130	132	133	134	79	79	80	81	82	82	83
	95th	129	130	132	134	136	137	138	83	83	84	85	86	87	87
17	90th	128	129	131	133	134	136	136	81	81	82	83	84	85	85
	95th	132	133	135	136	138	140	140	85	85	86	87	88	89	89

* Blood pressure percentile was determined by a single measurement.
[†] Height percentile was determined by standard growth curves.

Blood Pressure Levels for the 90th and 95th Percentiles of Blood Pressure for Girls Aged 10–17 Years by Percentile of Height

AGE (YR)	BLOOD PRESSURE PERCENTILE*	SYSTOLIC BLOOD PRESSURE BY PERCENTILE OF HEIGHT (mmHg)[†]							DIASTOLIC BLOOD PRESSURE BY PERCENTILE OF HEIGHT (mmHg)[†]						
		5%	10%	25%	50%	75%	90%	95%	5%	10%	25%	50%	75%	90%	95%
10	90th	112	112	114	115	116	117	118	73	73	73	74	75	76	76
	95th	116	116	117	119	120	121	122	77	77	77	78	79	80	80

(*Table continued on next page.*)

Blood Pressure Levels for the 90th and 95th Percentiles of Blood Pressure for Girls Aged 10–17 Years by Percentile of Height (cont.)

AGE (YR)	BLOOD PRESSURE PERCENTILE*	SYSTOLIC BLOOD PRESSURE BY PERCENTILE OF HEIGHT (mmHg)[†]							DIASTOLIC BLOOD PRESSURE BY PERCENTILE OF HEIGHT (mmHg)[†]						
		5%	10%	25%	50%	75%	90%	95%	5%	10%	25%	50%	75%	90%	95%
11	90th	114	114	116	117	118	119	120	74	74	75	75	76	77	77
	95th	118	118	119	121	122	123	124	78	78	79	79	80	81	81
12	90th	116	116	118	119	120	121	122	75	75	76	76	77	78	78
	95th	120	120	121	123	124	125	126	79	79	80	80	81	82	82
13	90th	118	118	119	121	122	123	124	76	76	77	78	78	79	80
	95th	121	122	123	125	126	127	128	80	80	81	82	82	83	84
14	90th	119	120	121	122	124	125	126	77	77	78	79	79	80	81
	95th	123	124	125	126	128	129	130	81	81	82	83	83	84	85
15	90th	121	121	122	124	125	126	127	78	78	79	79	80	81	82
	95th	124	125	126	128	129	130	131	82	82	83	83	84	85	86
16	90th	122	122	123	125	126	127	128	79	79	79	80	81	82	82
	95th	125	126	127	128	130	131	132	83	83	83	84	85	86	86
17	90th	122	123	124	125	126	128	128	79	79	79	80	81	82	82
	95th	136	126	127	129	130	131	132	83	83	83	84	85	86	86

* Blood pressure percentile was determined by a single measurement.
[†] Height percentile was determined by standard growth curves.
Adapted from National High Blood Pressure Education Program Working Group on Hypertension Control in Children and Adolescents. Update on the 1987 Task Force report on high blood pressure in children and adolescents: A working group report from the National High Blood Pressure Education Program. Pediatrics 98:649, 1996.

19. What evaluation is indicated for an adolescent with persistent hypertension?

After a thorough history and physical examination, with particular emphasis on family history and lifestyle risk factors (see question 20), all adolescents with hypertension should have a urinalysis and assessment of serum creatinine, electrolytes and calcium. A renal ultrasound to exclude structural renal disorders also should be obtained. Additional studies should be based on the history and physical examination.

20. Describe the appropriate treatment for mild asymptomatic hypertension in an adolescent.

Certain lifestyle risk factors sometimes can be modified to correct mild hypertension in the adolescent. Examples include obesity, sedentary lifestyle, high caffeine intake (especially colas and other sodas), use of over-the-counter decongestants, high salt intake, smoking, illicit drugs (e.g., amphetamines, cocaine), and stimulant weight-loss drugs. Prescribed drugs that also may contribute to hypertension include corticosteroids, birth control pills, stimulant drugs (e.g., methylphenidate), some antidepressants, and cyclosporine. If hypertension does not respond to attempts at lifestyle changes in a defined period of time, antihypertensive medications should be used.

21. Which medications are used most commonly to treat hypertension in adolescents?

As in adults, angiotensin convertase enzyme (ACE) inhibitors, such as enalapril and benazepril, and long-acting calcium channel blockers, such as amlodipine, are the usual choices. Diuretics are used if needed but often cause side effects (e.g., weakness, muscle cramps) that make their use in active adolescents less desirable.

22. To which renal diseases are African-American adolescents especially prone?

African Americans are more likely to have salt-sensitive hypertension, and their hypertension is often less responsive to ACE inhibitors and angiotensin II receptor inhibitors.

African Americans with persistent proteinuria have a high likelihood of having focal segmental glomerulosclerosis (FSGS). FSGS is more aggressive and more likely to lead to end-stage renal disease in African Americans than in whites. African Americans are less likely to have hypercalciuria or kidney stones than whites.

BIBLIOGRAPHY

1. Daniels SR: Consultation with the specialist: The diagnosis of hypertension in children: An update. Pediatr Rev 18:131–135, 1997.
2. Dodge WF, West EF, Smith EH, et al: Proteinuria and hematuria in schoolchildren: Epidemiology and natural history. J Pediatr 88:327–347, 1976.
3. Eddy AA, Schnapper HW: The nephrotic syndrome: From the simple to the complex. Semin Nephrol 18:304–316, 1998.
4. Fitzwater DS, Wyatt RJ: Hematuria. Pediatr Rev 15:102–109, 1994.
5. Johnson CE: New advances in childhood urinary tract infections. Pediatr Rev 20:335–342, 1999.
6. Kay JD, Sinaiko AR, Daniels SR: Pediatric hypertension. Am Heart J 142:422–432, 2001.
7. Loening-Baucke V: Urinary incontinence and urinary tract infection and their resolution with treatment of chronic constipation in childhood. Pediatrics 100:228–232, 1997.
8. Lohr JHA: Use of routine urinalysis in making a presumptive diagnosis of urinary tract infection in children. Pediatr Infect Dis J 10:646–650, 1991.
9. Mahan JD, Turman MA, Mentser MI: Evaluation of hematuria, proteinuria and hypertension in adolescents. Pediatr Clin North Am 44:1573–1589, 1997.
10. National High Blood Pressure Education Program Working Group on Hypertension Control in Children and Adolescents: Update on the 1987 Task Force Report on High Blood Pressure in Children and Adolescents: A Working Group Report from the National High Blood Pressure Education Program. Pediatrics 98:649–658, 1996.
11. Stapleton FB: Clinical approach to children with urolithiasis. Semin Nephrol 16:389–397, 1996.
12. Todd JK: Prevention of urinary tract infections in children. Report Pediatr Infect Dis 7:29–30, 1997.

20. RHEUMATOLOGY

Gloria C. Higgins, Ph.D., M.D.

PHYSICAL FINDINGS AND LABORATORY SCREENING

1. What signs and symptoms raise suspicion of a rheumatologic disorder?
Recurrent fever without a source
Arthritis
Purpuric rash
Chronic or recurrent rash on cheeks or other sun-exposed areas
Periungual inflammation
Rash on the eyelids, knuckles, knees, and elbows
Chronic dry mouth or dry eyes
Recurrent oral or nasal ulceration
Muscle weakness
Cold and poorly perfused extremities
Areas of thickened, "woody," or "hide-bound" skin

2. How is arthritis distinguished from arthralgia?
Arthritis must be distinguished from arthralgia (pain in the joint), which has a much broader differential diagnosis. Arthritis usually is associated with demonstrable swelling within the joint capsule due to effusion and/or synovial thickening. If joint swelling is not evident, patients with arthritis have warmth localized to the area of the joint or painful limitation of motion of the joint.

3. Name the four categories of diseases that should be considered in an adolescent with arthritis.
1. Infectious (e.g., septic arthritis, osteomyelitis, Lyme disease, parvovirus B19, postinfectious arthritis)
2. Orthopedic (e.g., trauma or mechanical derangements, including anterior knee pain syndromes)
3. Neoplastic (e.g., primary bone tumors, leukemia, lymphoma)
4. Rheumatologic (e.g., juvenile rheumatoid arthritis, lupus, dermatomyositis, other vasculitic syndromes)

4. What screening tests can aid in the diagnosis of a rheumatologic disorder?
Most patients with rheumatic disorders have laboratory abnormalities. For example, most patients with lupus have cytopenia on complete blood count or abnormal urinalysis in addition to a positive antinuclear antibody (ANA) test. Most patients with dermatomyositis have elevated creatine kinase or transaminases. Notable exceptions to this rule include juvenile rheumatoid arthritis, scleroderma, Raynaud's phenomenon, and Sjögren's syndrome. Patients with these disorders may have entirely normal screening labs, but they have typical histories and/or physical evidence of disease. Appropriate initial screening tests for rheumatologic disorders and their mimics are listed below. Of course, the lab evaluation should fit the presenting signs and symptoms.

Screening Lab Evaluation for Rheumatic Disorders

Complete blood count with differential and platelets
Erythrocyte sedimentation rate
C-reactive protein
Urinalysis
Aspartate aminotransferase, alanine aminotransferase, creatine kinase,
  blood urea nitrogen, creatinine
Throat culture, antistreptolysin O
Antinuclear antibody
Rheumatoid factor
X-ray of painful area
Chest x-ray

---

5. What infectious causes of acute arthritis should be especially considered in adolescents?

Monoarticular arthritis of acute onset should be considered septic arthritis until proved otherwise. Arthrocentesis for bacterial culture is indicated in such cases. *Staphylococcus aureus* is the most common bacterial pathogen causing septic arthritis in children. Arthritis due to sexually transmitted diseases becomes more prevalent after puberty.

In adolescence, the incidence of arthritis due to *Neisseria gonorrhoeae* is higher than that due to staphylococci. Gonococcal arthritis often begins as a migratory tenosynovitis that finally "settles" in one, or sometimes two, joints. Because of the difficulty in culturing the organism from joint fluid, all possible sites (genital tract, throat, rectum, and blood) should be cultured. Treatment with appropriate antibiotics leads to resolution of the arthritis.

Chlamydia trachomatis infection also should be considered in adolescents with arthritis alone or in association with eye pain or redness or rashes. Culture, antigen, or DNA tests of appropriate sites are indicated. Treatment of the underlying infection usually results in resolution of arthritis, although in some cases the arthritis can be chronic.

Parvovirus B-19 infection in adolescents and young adults can cause acute onset of polyarticular, symmetric arthritis that resembles polyarticular juvenile rheumatoid arthritis (JRA) or rheumatoid arthritis. The typical rash and "slapped-cheek" erythema of childhood fifth disease are usually absent. The arthritis may be either transient or chronic. Diagnosis is made by the presence of IgM antibodies against parvovirus B19 early in the disease.

ANTINUCLEAR ANTIBODIES AND RHEUMATOID FACTOR

6. When is it appropriate to check for antinuclear antibody (ANA)?

The ANA test helps to evaluate patients who are suspected, on the basis of history, physical exam, and initial lab testing, to have lupus, JRA, dermatomyositis, or another rheumatologic condition. A positive ANA also can be found in patients with autoimmune liver disease, viral infections, and neoplasia. However, in patients who have no objective abnormalities on physical exam and no abnormalities other than a low positive ANA on laboratory screening (see table in question 4), the likelihood of a rheumatologic disorder is low.

7. What does an ANA test measure?

The ANA test is a screening test that detects antibodies against a large number of different nuclear components (various proteins, nucleic acids, and protein-nucleic acid complexes). Antibodies against certain nuclear components are associated with certain rheumatologic disorders. However, the significance of most of the antibody specificities that can give a positive ANA test is unknown.

8. Can the ANA test be positive in healthy children and adolescents?

A low positive ANA test is not uncommon in healthy persons. Methods of doing the ANA test are not uniformly standardized. The frequency of positive ANA in healthy people depends on the age of the people tested, the method used to perform the test, and the lab where the test is conducted. As a rough estimation, about 10% of normal, healthy children have a positive ANA test, usually of low titer.

9. Who is most likely to have a positive ANA test of no clinical significance?

Antinuclear antibodies are found with greater frequency among healthy close relatives of patients with lupus and other rheumatologic diseases compared with the general population. Patients with a recent viral infection are also more likely to have a positive ANA.

10. How is the ANA test performed?

The most common method is the indirect immunofluorescent assay, using permeabilized cells (usually the HEp-2 cell line) as a substrate. The dilution of patient serum used for screening is usually 1:40. This dilution is chosen because of the high number of healthy people who have a positive ANA test at lower dilutions. If the test is positive at the screening dilution, the serum is further tested in a series of doubling dilutions (e.g., 1:80, 1:160, 1:320). The titer is reported as the highest dilution that gives a positive nuclear immunofluorescence. Other methods give ANA results as "units." Positive ANAs reported in "units" are more difficult to interpret, because their sensitivity and predictive value have not been as well studied in children.

11. Does the titer of ANA predict the presence of a rheumatologic disease?

Statistically, most people with a positive ANA of relatively low titer do not have a rheumatologic disorder. A low-titer ANA (1:40, 1:80) is found in healthy people more often than a high-titer ANA. Even high-titer ANAs can be caused by viral infections and certain medications and occasionally are found in normal individuals. Conversely, some patients with lupus or JRA may have low levels of antinuclear antibody.

12. What may cause a positive rheumatoid factor in adolescents?

Rheumatoid factor is an autoantibody against the Fc (constant region) of IgG. Rheumatoid factors may be of any immunoglobulin class, but IgM rheumatoid factor is routinely measured. Any condition associated with chronic antigen stimulation causing antibody production can give rise to anti-IgG antibody (rheumatoid factor). Examples include the following:
- Rheumatoid arthritis and seropositive polyarticular JRA
- Other rheumatologic disorders (including systemic lupus erythematosus, mixed connective tissue disease, scleroderma, and Sjögren's syndrome)
- Viral diseases (Epstein-Barr virus, cytomegalvirus, influenza, human immunodificiency virus, and viral hepatitis)
- Chronic bacterial or spirochetal infections (subacute bacterial endocarditis, tuberculosis, syphilis, Lyme disease)
- Chronic liver disease
- Chronic pulmonary disease
- Neoplasms
- Cryoglobulinemia
- Sarcoidosis

JUVENILE RHEUMATOID ARTHRITIS AND SPONDYLOARTHROPATHIES

13. Which types of JRA affect teenagers?

JRA is a family of inflammatory disorders that share chronic arthritis as a predominant feature. Any type of JRA can affect adolescents: polyarticular (5 or more joints), pauciarticular (4 or fewer joints), or systemic (systemic signs and symptoms with polyarticular arthritis, also called Still's disease). According to the American College of Rheumatology definition, onset of JRA is before age 16 years. By definition, patients with arthritis beginning at age 16 years or older have seropositive or seronegative rheumatoid arthritis, spondyloarthropathy, or adult-onset Still's disease. JRA is also known as juvenile idiopathic arthritis, a name that better characterizes this group of disorders as diverse and mostly different from the rheumatoid arthritis that occurs in adults.

14. Does the rheumatoid factor have to be positive in adolescents with JRA?

Certainly not. Among adults with rheumatoid arthritis, rheumatoid factor is positive in about 75%. In JRA, rheumatoid factor is positive in only 10% overall and is more often negative than positive even among children with polyarticular arthritis.

15. What lab abnormalities are common in adolescents with JRA?

Some patients with JRA have no lab abnormalities at all. However, anemia and elevated acute phase reactants (erythrocyte sedimentation rate, C-reactive protein) are frequently found. Positive rheumatoid factor defines a subgroup of patients with JRA (see question 14) who tend to have arthritis that is more severe and resistant to treatment. Positive antinuclear antibody may be found, but it is more common in younger patients with pauciarticular arthritis (type I pauciarticular JRA).

16. What is the role for HLA B-27 testing in the diagnosis of JRA?

HLA B-27 is a normal histocompatibility marker that is present in about 8% of the Caucasian population; it is less common in other racial groups. People with the B-27 allele statistically have a higher incidence of arthritis involving the spine and sacroiliac joints (spondyloarthropathy). However, HLA B-27 is not diagnostic for any kind of arthritis or rheumatologic condition and is not appropriate to use as a screening test.

17. What is the difference between JRA and spondyloarthropathy?

Type II pauciarticular JRA primarily involves the large joints of the lower extremities, usually in an asymmetric distribution. Inflammation at entheses, where tendons attach to bone (especially at the insertions of Achilles' tendons, patellar tendons, and plantar fascia), is common. Patients in this group are usually over age 9 years, and males are affected more frequently than females. Such patients also may fulfill criteria for seronegative enthesopathy and arthropathy (SEA) or spondyloarthropathy. Some develop ankylosing spondylitis and inflammation of the sacroiliac joints and of the ligamentous attachments of the spine.

18. Describe four kinds of inflammatory arthritis that can mimic JRA.

1. **Psoriatic arthritis**. The skin lesions of psoriasis are not necessarily severe in patients who develop arthritis. Nail-pitting can be a clue. Enthesopathy is common. Arthritis of the distal interphalangeal joints is more common in psoriatic arthritis than in JRA.

2. **Enteropathic arthritis**. Arthritis occurs in up to 20% of patients with inflammatory bowel disease and, especially in patients with Crohn's disease, may precede intestinal symptoms. Enthesopathy is common. Anemia and heme-positive stools can be clues.

3. **Post-infectious arthritis**. Most patients have a history of a recent streptococcal throat, upper respiratory infection, or acute enteritis. The arthritis usually resolves within 6 weeks. In patients with poststreptococcal arthritis, rheumatic fever should be carefully ruled out. Arthritis following enteric infection with *Salmonella enteritidis*, *Shigella flexneri*, *Yersinia enterocolitica*, or *Campylobacter* sp. is usually described by the term *reactive arthritis*.

4. **Lyme arthritis**. Arthritis in one or several joints may begin weeks to months after untreated *Borrelia burgdorferi* infection. The arthritis is usually pauciarticular and episodic, with each episode lasting for up to several weeks. In most cases it resolves completely after the infection is treated with appropriate antibiotics. The DNA of *B. burgdorferi* has been demonstrated in synovial fluid, but cultures are rarely positive, perhaps because of the fastidious nature of the organism. In the minority of patients who develop chronic arthritis despite antibiotic treatment, an autoimmune pathogenesis is plausible.

LUPUS

19. What are the two kinds of lupus?

Cutaneous lupus, which does not involve internal organs, and systemic lupus erythematosus (SLE). Cutaneous lupus may be of the discoid type, with round lesions that usually leave scars, or the subacute cutaneous type, in which the rash resembles that of SLE. Conversely, a discoid-type rash can be present in patients with SLE.

20. How is SLE diagnosed?

SLE is a syndrome of autoimmunity that is diagnosed by a collection of physical signs and abnormal laboratory test results. The American College of Rheumatology (ACR) criteria serve as a guide, because almost all patients with SLE have four or more criteria at some point during the disease. However, not all patients meet the criteria when they first present with symptoms. It is also important to remember that the ACR criteria do not describe all the common manifestations of lupus—only those that were found to be statistically the most specific and sensitive for disease.

21. How can one remember the ACR criteria for SLE?

A useful device is to "divide and conquer." The criteria can be divided into the following groups:

Four mucocutaneous manifestations
1. Malar rash
2. Photosensitive rash
3. Discoid rash
4. Oral or nasopharyngeal ulcers

Four systemic manifestations
1. Arthritis
2. Serositis (pleural or pericardial effusion)
3. Renal disorder (nephritis or nephrosis)
4. Neurologic disorder (seizures or psychosis)

Three lab abnormalities
1. Hematologic disorder (cytopenias)
2. Abnormal titers of ANA
3. Immunologic disorder (anti-DNA, anti-Smith, or antiphospholipid antibody)

22. Describe the typical presentation of SLE.

SLE manifests in many different ways; there is no typical presentation. Many common presenting signs and symptoms, occurring in various combinations, are represented in the ACR criteria above. In addition, lupus patients frequently have unexplained fevers, weight loss, severe fatigue, myalgia, arthralgia, lymphadenopathy, vasculitic rash particularly on the fingers, myositis, alopecia, and Raynaud's phenomenon. Internal organ involvement also frequently manifests as pulmonary parenchymal disease, cardiac valvular disease, and mild hepatitis. All these manifestations were not considered specific or sensitive enough for inclusion in the ACR criteria.

23. Is a positive ANA a prerequisite for the diagnosis of systemic lupus?

ANA-negative lupus is rare, accounting for approximately 2% of adult patients. A negative ANA raises greater concern for the presence of conditions that may mimic lupus and makes the diagnosis more problematic.

24. A 13-year-old girl has low-grade fevers, arthritis, and extreme fatigue. Screening laboratories reveal anemia, elevated erythrocyte sedimentation rate, and a positive ANA. What other lab tests are indicated to investigate the possibility of lupus?

- Anti–double-stranded (native) DNA
- Anti-Sm (anti-Smith; not to be confused with anti-SM, which stands for anti-smooth muscle)

- Anti-ribonucleoprotein (RNP)
- Anti-SSA and anti-SSB
- Direct Coombs' test
- Complements C3 and C4
- Rapid plasma reagin (RPR), prothrombin time, partial thromboplastin time, and anticardiolipin antibodies

25. What conditions may mimic SLE in teenagers?

Chronic infection (including hepatitis B and C), neoplasms, mixed connective tissue disease, and systemic vasculitides (including Wegener's granulomatosis, microscopic polyangiitis, and polyarteritis nodosa) may be confused with SLE in teenagers. Idiopathic autoimmune cytopenias and idiopathic nephritis or nephrotic syndrome may be difficult to distinguish from lupus, because they can be initial manifestations of SLE.

26. Does lupus occur in teenage males?

The reported female-to-male ratio in adults with systemic lupus is in the range of 8:1 to 10:1. In early childhood, the sex ratio is more nearly equal. With increasing age and onset of puberty, the female-to-male ratio increases to approach the adult ratio. About 15% of all cases of lupus have onset before adulthood.

27. How can the lupus anticoagulant cause a prolonged PTT, yet predispose to thrombosis?

Antiphospholipid antibodies (aPLA) are a heterogeneous family of autoantibodies that can be present in people with or without rheumatic disorders or symptoms of thrombosis. The lupus anticoagulant activity of certain antiphospholipid antibodies refers to their ability to prolong the PTT by binding to the phospholipid–prothrombin complex used in the test-tube reaction. False-positive serologic tests for syphilis (RPR or Venereal Disease Research Laboratory Test) result from the binding of aPLA to cardiolipin used as the test antigen. Most enzyme-linked immunosorbent assays for aPLA use a combination of cardiolipin and β_2-glycoprotein I as the antigen. The pathogenesis of arterial and venous thrombosis due to aPLA is not completely understood but is at least partly due to inhibition of the anticoagulant activity of β_2-glycoprotein I.

MYOSITIS

28. How does myositis present?

Postinfectious myositis usually presents as acute onset of severe leg pain. The patient usually has a history of a recent illness compatible with viral infection. The inflammatory myopathy of rheumatic diseases (including juvenile dermatomyositis, polymyositis, mixed connective tissue disease, and lupus) is usually of more insidious onset, and muscle weakness is almost always more prominent than pain. Actual weakness should be differentiated from generalized malaise and fatigue by manual muscle testing. Truncal and symmetric proximal extremity weakness typically occurs first; distal muscle weakness may appear later in the course of untreated or treatment-resistant disease.

29. Describe the typical rashes of juvenile dermatomyositis (JDMS).

The typical rashes of JDMS are heliotrope rash and Gottron's papules. The heliotrope rash is a purplish discoloration of the eyelids, often with capillary prominence and swelling. Gottron's papules are discrete pink papules on the knuckles, usually over the proximal interphalangeal and metacarpophalangeal joints. Often the skin around the papules is erythematous and scaly. Other areas that typically have a red, scaly rash are the cheeks and the extensor surfaces of the knees and elbows. Periungual swelling and erythema also are common in dermatomyositis. Generalized erythroderma is sometimes found.

30. What is the difference between dermatomyositis and polymyositis?

By definition, no rash is associated with polymyositis. Because idiopathic inflammatory polymyositis is much less common in children and adolescents than dermatomyositis, the appearance of muscle weakness without a typical JDMS rash necessitates careful evaluation for neurologic, infectious, and neoplastic causes. On the other hand, unlike dermatomyositis in adults, JDMS is almost never associated with neoplastic disease. Some difference in pathophysiology of the two conditions can be inferred by their different histologic characteristics. In dermatomyositis, small-vessel vasculitis is a prominent feature of involved muscle and other tissues, including the gastrointestinal tract, but in polymyositis the inflammation is more localized to muscle.

31. Explain elevated transaminases in patients with myositis.

When a muscle cell is damaged, its intracellular enzymes are released into the blood. These enzymes include creatine kinase (CK), aspartate transaminase (AST), alanine transaminase (ALT), aldolase, and lactate dehydrogenase (LDH). One or more of these enzymes is elevated in almost all patients with myositis. In muscle disease, AST is likely to be more abnormal than ALT. However, in any patient with elevated transaminases, both muscle and liver disease should be considered.

CHRONIC PAIN DISORDERS

32. Do children and adolescents have fibromyalgia?

Fibromyalgia is a noninflammatory disorder that is defined in adults by a combination of symptoms: chronic and widespread musculoskeletal pain, nonrestorative sleep, and fatigue. Symptoms of headaches and bowel irritability are common. The cause of the symptoms of fibromyalgia is not known. By definition, other causes of these symptoms, such as endocrine and autoimmune disorders, must be ruled out. There is considerable controversy over the diagnosis of fibromyalgia in children and adolescents. The terms *disproportional musculoskeletal pain disorder* or *pain amplification syndrome* may be preferable. Disproportional musculoskeletal pain disorder can occur with or without tender points in children and adolescents.

33. What do tender points have to do with fibromyalgia?

In adults with fibromyalgia, nine bilateral sites that are most consistently tender have been identified. A description of these sites may be found in many textbooks and articles. A positive exam consists of at least mild tenderness at 11 of the 18 sites palpated with a force of 4 kg. Operationally, this amount of force is just below that at which normal people experience tenderness. Experience is required to palpate with the proper amount of force.

34. What causes disproportional musculoskeletal pain syndrome?

Injury or viral infections, common in adolescents, may predate the onset of a chronic pain syndrome, but causality cannot be shown. In some studies of adults with fibromyalgia, mediators of pain were increased in the central nervous system. However, no consistent abnormalities in muscle or nerve physiology, muscle or tendon histology, or mediators of inflammation have been identified to explain this finding. The symptoms of widespread pain are believed to result from an interplay of physiologic and psychological factors, including disordered sensory processing (altered nociception) and response to stress, that results in a lowering of pain threshold.

35. Which adolescents are at highest risk for disproportional musculoskeletal pain?

This condition is most common in Caucasian females before adolescence or in early adolescence, with peak age onset around 12–13 years. Family history often reveals an adult role model for chronic musculoskeletal pain.

36. What is the treatment for disproportional musculoskeletal pain syndrome?

There are few studies of treatment for disproportionate pain syndromes in children and adolescents. The most commonly recommended treatment is similar to that used for adults with fibromyalgia: (1) education and enlistment of the patient to participate actively in treatment; (2) graduated aerobic exercise; (3) improvement of the quality of sleep, often using low-dose amitriptyline; and (4) stress management and/or counseling to identify and resolve emotional stressors.

37. Describe the syndrome of disproportional localized pain known as reflex sympathetic dystrophy (RSD) or reflex neurovascular dystrophy (RND).

Hyperalgesia, usually in a distal extremity, and allodynia (exquisite sensitivity to normally nonpainful stimuli) are characteristic of RSD. The pain is always in a nonanatomic distribution (not in the distribution of a nerve root or peripheral nerve). The patient often holds the affected extremity in an unusual position and is unable to use it because of pain. *Sympathetic* refers to localized dysautonomia, manifested by poor perfusion, coolness, and dusky or mottled skin with generalized puffiness. Occasionally, sweating is increased. *Dystrophy* describes the condition of the affected limb after prolonged disuse, whereupon thinning of the skin, increased hair growth, muscle atrophy, and sometimes osteopenia occur.

The *reflex* portion of the name describes the favored hypothesis for the pathophysiology of this disorder—establishment and perpetuation of an abnormal reflex arc between the affected extremity and spinal pain fibers. A previous injury serves as a precipitating event in some, but by no means all, cases. As in patients with widespread disproportional musculoskeletal pain syndrome, psychological stressors play an important role in many patients. Cases in which the symptoms recur during times of stress have been well described.

38. What conditions must be ruled out before a diagnosis of RSD can be entertained?

RSD can sometimes be confused with a localized allergic reaction (e.g., to an insect bite), venous thrombosis, or cellulitis. Osteomyelitis and arthritis usually can be be ruled out by lack of localization to a specific bone or joint. Leukemia with bone pain can occasionally mimic RSD but almost always shows abnormalities on plain x-ray or complete blood count. Nerve entrapment syndromes can be distinguished by their distribution. Painful peripheral neuropathy is rare and generally associated with other manifestations of rheumatic disease.

39. Describe the treatment for RSD.

A combined approach using education, desensitization therapy, local and systemic pain control, physical therapy, and psychotherapy is most effective. Hospitalization in a rehabilitation unit is required for severe cases. Sympathetic blockade is sometimes helpful. The longer the symptoms have persisted before institution of appropriate therapy, the less favorable the prognosis.

RAYNAUD'S PHENOMENON

40. An adolescent complains of episodes of coldness and color change in hands and/or feet. What conditions should be considered?

The patient may have Raynaud's phenomenon, which is due to reversible vasospasm of the peripheral blood vessels, usually in response to environmental stimuli. Other causes of these symptoms include sympathomimetic drugs; external pressure on the arterial supply, as in thoracic outlet syndrome; blood hyperviscosity syndromes; and excessive cooling of the skin due to hyperhidrosis. Raynaud's phenomenon can involve all or some digits of an affected extremity, and often the color of the affected digit is clearly demarcated during an attack.

41. What is the triphasic color change sequence of Raynaud's phenomenon?

1. White (pallor) due to hypoperfusion
2. Blue (cyanosis) due to hypoxemia
3. Red (hyperemia) due to reperfusion

Although not all patients with Raynaud's phenomenon exhibit all phases of the sequence, if pallor is absent the diagnosis is doubtful.

42. How does one determine whether Raynaud's phenomenon is primary or secondary to a rheumatologic condition?

Raynaud's phenomenon can exist as an isolated idiopathic condition (primary Raynaud's phenomenon), which infrequently leads to serious morbidity. Factors that increase the likelihood of the development of a rheumatic disorder in patients who initially present with Raynaud's phenomenon include nailfold capillary abnormalities and a positive antinuclear antibody test. The most commonly associated disorders include lupus, systemic sclerosis, mixed connective tissue disease, and dermatomyositis. Raynaud's phenomenon associated with a rheumatologic disorder tends to be more severe than primary Raynaud's phenomenon and is more likely to be associated with digital ulceration and infarction.

SCLERODERMA

43. Describe the types of scleroderma that can be found in adolescents.

Scleroderma in children and adolescents is most commonly of the localized type, which includes morphea (plaques) and linear scleroderma. Localized scleroderma usually involves only the skin and subcutaneous tissues, although underlying muscle and bone may be affected. In contrast, systemic sclerosis involves internal organs such as the lungs, kidneys, and gastrointestinal tract. The two types of systemic sclerosis are diffuse systemic sclerosis and limited systemic sclerosis or **CREST** syndrome (**c**alcinosis, **R**aynaud's phenomenon, **e**sophageal dysmotility, **s**clerodactyly, and **t**elangectasia).

44. How are autoantibodies used in the diagnosis of scleroderma?

Autoantibody testing is neither highly sensitive nor highly specific for scleroderma or its subsets. No autoantibody test is diagnostic. A positive ANA test is common in scleroderma. Antinuclear antibodies in a nucleolar pattern tend to be associated with localized scleroderma whereas in a centromeric distribution they tend to be associated with CREST syndrome. Anti-Scl 70 (antitopoisomerase 1) is associated with diffuse scleroderma.

45. Describe the natural history of localized scleroderma.

Localized scleroderma rarely involves internal organs or develops into a diffuse systemic sclerosis. Usually, the lesions begin as areas of induration in a linear or plaque-like distribution. Over time the skin acquires pigmentary changes and becomes hardened or tight. These changes may extend into the underlying subcutaneous tissues, with atrophy of fat and muscle. Scleroderma lesions crossing joint lines may result in fixed contractures, limitation of flexion, or both. Over the course of several years, the affected areas tend to soften but may never return to normal.

BIBLIOGRAPHY

1. Athreya BH (ed): Pediatric Rheumatology. Rheumatic Disease Clinics of North America, vol. 23, no. 3. Philadelphia, W.B. Saunders, 1997.
2. Cassidy JT, Petty RE: Textbook of Pediatric Rheumatology, 4th ed. Philadelphia, W.B. Saunders, 2001.
3. Greene WB (ed): Essentials of Musculoskeletal Care, 2nd ed. Rosemont, IL, American Academy of Orthopedic Surgeons, 2001.
4. Hochberg MC, for the Diagnostic and Therapeutic Criteria Committee of the American College of Rheumatology: Updating the American College of Rheumatology revised criteria for the classification of systemic lupus erythematosus. Arthritis Rheum 40:1725, 1997.

5. Isenberg DA, Miller JJ (eds): Adolescent Rheumatology. London, Martin Dunitz, 1999.
6. Koopman WJ (eds): Arthritis and Allied Conditions, 13th ed. Philadelphia, Lippincott Williams & Wilkins, 1997.
7. Roubey RA: Update on antiphospholipid antibodies. Curr Opin Rheumatol 12:374–378, 2000.
8. Simms RW: Fibromyalgia syndrome: Current concepts in pathophysiology, clinical features, and management. Arthritis Care Res 9:315–328, 1996.

21. SPORTS MEDICINE

Barbara J. Long, M.D., M.P.H., and Diane M. Straub, M.D., M.P.H.

SPORTS PARTICIPATION

1. What are the benefits of regular physical activity and sports participation for adolescents?

The many potential benefits of regular physical activity include improved cardiovascular health, improved muscle and bone strength, maintenance of appropriate weight and body composition, and improved psychological well-being. Specific psychological changes include improved self-confidence and reduction in symptoms related to stress, anxiety, and mild depression. Participation in organized sports also teaches the concepts of goal setting, teamwork, and self-discipline.

2. What risks are associated with participation in regular physical activity and sport?

Risks include musculoskeletal system injuries (e.g., fractures, ligamentous sprains, muscular strains, and overuse injuries) and specific medical problems (e.g., heat illness, exacerbation of respiratory or cardiovascular problems, and neurologic problems such as concussions). However, the risks of these adverse events can be greatly reduced by adhering to standard recommendations for sport-specific equipment, rules and safety regulations, appropriate levels of training and conditioning, supervision by knowledgeable adults, adequate preparticipation screening, and appropriate treatment and rehabilitation of injuries. The benefits of participating in regular physical activity far outweigh the potential risks. Even individuals with preexisting medical or musculoskeletal problems can participate in a wide range of activities modified to compensate for any limitations. In fact, in many instances participation in regular or modified physical activity can be an important complement to medical management of other medical or musculoskeletal conditions.

3. What are the key objectives of a preparticipation sports physical?

The American Academy of Pediatrics, the American Academy of Family Physicians, and several national sports medicine societies collaborated on a publication entitled *Preparticipation Physical Evaluation.* This is an excellent guide for providers who are involved in preparticipation physicals. In accordance with this monograph, the primary objectives of the preparticipation physical are to (1) detect conditions that may limit participation, (2) detect conditions that may predispose the individual to injury, and (3) comply with legal and insurance requirements. The preparticipation physical is also a valuable opportunity to assess general health and counsel the individual on other issues that often impact the morbidity and mortality of adolescents (e.g., substance use, violence, sexual activity, and motor vehicle and other accidents).

4. What is "sudden cardiac death," what are its causes in adolescent athletes, and what are the key components of screening?

Sudden cardiac death is a nontraumatic, nonviolent, unexpected event resulting from sudden cardiac arrest within 6 hours of a previously witnessed state of normal health. It occurs in approximately 1 in 200,000 high school athletes annually. Causes (in order of decreasing incidence) include hypertrophic cardiomyopathy, congenital coronary artery anomaly, myocarditis, right ventricular cardiomyopathy, idiopathic left ventricular (LV) cardiomyopathy, mitral valve prolapse, conduction system disease, aortic dissection, dilated cardiomyopathy, and coronary artery disease.

Because many of these etiologic causes do not have any clinical findings, taking a good history is particularly important to help identify those at risk. Historical clues include personal history of syncope, fatigue, dyspnea, chest pain, murmur, and high blood pressure. Significant family history includes cardiac death at age $\leq$ 50 years, cardiomyopathy, Marfan's syndrome, long QT syndrome, and other arrhythmias.

The cardiovascular exam should include brachial blood pressure in the sitting position, femoral arterial pulses, precordial auscultation in both the supine and standing positions (with specific attention to murmurs consistent with LV outflow obstruction), and noting any physical findings suggestive of Marfan's syndrome. Auscultation while the patient is performing a Valsalva maneuver increases LV outflow obstruction and, therefore, is a useful technique to enhance the detection of murmurs that require further evaluation. Echocardiogram and electrocardiogram (EKG) are not cost-effective screening tools in the absence of a concerning personal or family history.

5. Is weight training safe for adolescent athletes?

Weight training is a safe activity for all ages if the athlete has learned appropriate techniques under the supervision of a knowledgeable adult. In the prepubescent athlete, muscle bulk and hypertrophy is not an achievable goal due to the low levels of androgenic hormone (testosterone). Weight training will however promote neuromuscular training and some gains in muscular strength. In this age group the focus should be on developing proper technique, and the program should consist of low-weight, high-repetition exercises. Weight training during puberty and adolescence should continue to focus on proper technique and the development of a program that will promote muscle strength, endurance, and flexibility. Programs should focus on achieving balance between opposing muscle groups (e.g., hamstrings–quads) in order to enhance sport performance. Weight training should be differentiated from bodybuilding, in which the focus is on the development of increased muscle mass and definition and which may or may not lead to enhanced sport specific performance. Because bodybuilding requires the use of higher weights and lower repetitions, it is usually recommended only for the skeletally mature athlete.

6. Is weight training safe for female adolescents?

Females can benefit from weight training by gaining increased muscle strength and endurance. A weight-training program should focus on proper technique, achieving a balance between muscle groups, and maintaining flexibility. Females will not be able to achieve the same degree of muscle hypertrophy or bulk as their male counterparts because of their lower levels of testosterone. However, their improved muscle strength and endurance can enhance sport performance and potentially decrease the risk of injury. Improved muscle tone and definition also enhances the adolescent's body image and sense of well-being.

7. How can you counsel the athlete who wants to "bulk up" or gain weight for his or her sport?

"Bulking up" or gaining lean body mass is achieved through both proper nutrition and a resistance or weight-training program. The adolescent's body type and pubertal stage must be taken into consideration. The body type, or **somatotype** (ectomorph, mesomorph, or endomorph), provides a general guide to the athlete's genetic profile and is useful when establishing realistic goals regarding expected outcome or body composition. The stage of pubertal development is also important when counseling teens interested in bulking up. Young men experience a weight spurt just after the attainment of peak height velocity; young women's will occur approximately 6 months after their peak height velocity. Muscle bulk occurs around 3–6 months later, and muscle strength requires another 6 months. Additionally, young people are most susceptible to fractures and sprains during peak linear growth because of concurrent ligamentous laxity. Thus, advice should take into account physical development (pubertal stage) and emphasize safety, using low weights and frequent repetitions, during early to mid adolescence. Late adolescents may work safely on strength and bulk by using higher weights and performing fewer repetitions. In all athletes, proper nutrition is an important component to muscle building. In order to gain weight, 500–1000 additional calories above expenditure need to be consumed daily. These calories should include carbohydrate, fat, and protein sources. This can sometimes be difficult to accomplish especially in those athletes involved in endurance sports. Eating more times per day and adding high-density snacks between meals can be useful. Input from a nutritionist in designing a healthy plan can be extremely valuable.

8. How do I know if a prescription medication is okay for an athlete who is being drug tested for an athletic competition?

Substances banned for competition generally fall within the following categories: stimulants, anabolic agents, diuretics, street drugs, and peptide hormones and analogues. Additionally, there are sport-specific restrictions. The best way to determine if a medication is allowed is to *obtain the information directly from the governing organization for the sport.* For those sports governed by the U.S. Olympic Committee, a comprehensive guide, compiled from information from the International Olympic Committee Medical Commission and the U.S. Anti-Doping Agency, is available at www.usantidoping.org. A telephone hot line is also available at (800) 233-0393. For National Collegiate Athletic Association (NCAA) sports, a comprehensive list is provided on the following website: www.ncaa.org/sports_sciences/drugtesting/banned_list.html

NUTRITION AND SPORTS-RELATED ILLNESS

9. What are the differences among heat cramps, heat stress, heat exhaustion, and heatstroke?

These terms describe the continuum of problems associated with heat-related illness and exertional hyperthermia.

Heat cramps. Although commonly referred to as "heat cramps," muscle cramping can occur at any temperature and represents the exercising muscle's response to fatigue. It can also be precipitated by the depletion of total body sodium due to excessive sweating or to intake of excessive amounts of salt-free fluids during prolonged endurance activities. Symptoms include muscle cramps, fatigue, tachycardia, and weakness.

Heat stress. This term indicates a mild elevation of body temperature associated with tachycardia, elevated blood pressure, and symptoms associated with fatigue and mild dehydration.

Heat exhaustion. The key features here are hypovolemia and a body temperature between 100.4° and 104°F ($< 40°C$). Symptoms include orthostasis, profuse sweating, clammy skin, dizziness, syncope, headache, nausea, and lack of coordination.

Heatstroke. This is a medical emergency; features include body temperature $> 104°F$, hypovolemia, hypotension, loss of coordination and inability to walk, loss of consciousness, and finally shock with multisystem involvement.

10. How does dehydration affect sports performance?

Insufficient hydration at baseline and the development of dehydration during physical activity cause significant declines in performance. Changes in performance level can begin at as little as 2% dehydration, which is below the level at which individuals perceive thirst. Thus, the athlete needs to begin participation in a well-hydrated state and to continuously and systematically consume fluids during participation instead of waiting until he or she is thirsty.

11. What are the recommendations for fluid intake associated with physical activity and sport?

The amount of fluid required during participation depends on many factors such as intensity of sport, duration of participation, level of conditioning, and ambient or environmental conditions. The goal is to match fluid intake with the amount of fluid lost due to sweating. To ensure appropriate hydration, it is important that athletes maintain good nutrition and hydration in the 24 hours prior to participation. In addition, recommendations include prehydration, or fluid intake prior to participation, which ensures a well-hydrated status at baseline. Several hours before the activity, the athlete should drink 400–600 ml (13–20 oz) of water or sports drink. This amount of time will allow any excess fluid to be removed by the kidneys as urine prior to participation. The athlete should then drink 6–12 oz of fluid approximately 10–20 minutes prior to activity and every 15–20 minutes during activity. Body weight before and after activity also can be used to gauge hydration status; after exercise at least 20 oz of fluid should be consumed for every pound of weight lost during physical activity.

12. What is the best sports drink to use?

For most activities lasting less than 60 minutes, cold water is adequate. However, for activities lasting longer than 1 hour, a sport drink containing glucose (carbohydrate source) and salt is indicated. The optimal amount of carbohydrate and salt content varies based on individual differences, the intensity and duration of activities, and the environmental conditions. The American College of Sports Medicine recommends 4–8% carbohydrates (4–8 gm per 100 ml) and 0.5–0.7 gm of sodium per liter, which can be found in a variety of commercial sports drinks. Because these drinks are often more palatable to adolescents than plain water, they are frequently used to improve overall consumption of fluids. Additionally, the use of drinks with appropriate levels of glucose and salt helps avoid gastrointestinal (GI) upset and diarrhea, which is not acceptable to the adolescent athlete or, for that matter, any age athlete.

13. How can I counsel my patients regarding the use of dietary supplements?

Athletes of all ages look for any and all ways to improve their performance. Health care providers need to be familiar with commonly available supplements, their advertised benefits, and their potential risks. Scare tactics and blanket condemnation of all supplements tend not to work with adolescents and can adversely affect the athlete's perception of the physician's credibility. Counseling should focus on whether the athlete is maximizing all aspects of his or her current training program including appropriate nutrition, proper hydration, and appropriate sport-specific training and conditioning. Athletes need to "buy into" the value of maximizing these core areas of their training program before they buy into the variety of supplements available.

14. Do anabolic steroids work? What are the side effects?

Although anabolic steroids have been shown to increase muscle mass and strength, they are also associated with a long list of potential reversible and irreversible side effects including:
- Premature closure of growth plates (irreversible)
- Acne
- Testicular atrophy
- Clitoromegaly, hirsutism, and voice deepening in females (irreversible)
- Psychological changes, alterations in mood
- Hepatocellular disease
- Hepatocellular cancer
- Abnormal lipid problems
- Hypertension
- Gynecomastia (males)
- Alopecia

15. What is exercise-induced bronchospasm (EIB)?

Also known as exercise-induced asthma, EIB is an exacerbation of airway reactivity with exercise seen in many adolescent asthmatics. Possible mechanisms include heat loss or water loss from the airway and airway rewarming. Diagnosis is made by history and exam. A typical pattern is a 5–10-minute period of normal bronchodilation that occurs at the start of activity, followed by a progressive bronchoconstriction peaking at 10 minutes after cessation of the activity, with spontaneous remission in 30–60 minutes. There also may be late phase bronchoconstriction 4–12 hours after exercise. Treatment includes control of baseline asthma, adequate warm-up, avoiding dry cold air (using masks and scarves if necessary), and the use of a short-acting beta agonist 20 minutes prior to exercise. Other treatment options include the use of mast cell stabilizers (cromolyn sodium), longer acting beta agonists (salmeterol), and leukotriene-receptor antagonists (montelukast).

16. What sports are best for my patients with asthma?

With proper management, most athletes with asthma can participate in any sport. The following sports, however, are considered less asthmagenic: tennis, gymnastics, wrestling, football, baseball, and martial arts (due to lower minute ventilation requirements) and swimming, water polo, and diving (due to a warmer, more humid exercise environment). Sports that pose higher risk (more asthmagenic) include long distance running, cycling, basketball, soccer, and rugby (high minute ventilation requirements) and ice hockey, ice skating, and cross-country skiing (colder, dryer climatic conditions).

17. What is the female athlete triad?

The female athlete triad recognizes the interrelationship among disordered eating, amenorrhea, and osteoporosis. Disordered eating is represented by a wide spectrum of behaviors including inadequate caloric intake (inadequate energy intake for expenditure); restrictive eating (e.g., "forbidden" foods, episodic fasting, and chronic voluntary starvation); bingeing and purging; use of diet pills, laxatives, diuretics, vomiting, and excessive exercise; and the *Diagnostic and Statistical Manual of Mental Disorders*, 4th edition (DSM-IV) diagnoses of anorexia nervosa and bulimia nervosa. Amenorrhea is defined as the absence of menarche by age 16 in the presence of secondary sexual characteristics or the absence of three or more consecutive cycles after menarche. The mechanism is thought to be hypothalamic in origin, which results in low estrogen levels and subsequent osteoporosis similar to postmenopausal women.

18. How does one screen for the female athlete triad in the clinical setting?

Screening for the triad can be done during the preparticipation physical examination by eliciting information regarding dietary practices, menstrual irregularities, and history of stress fractures and by noting vital signs (including body mass index) and physical stigmata of disordered eating (e.g., lanugo hair, parotid gland enlargement, tooth enamel changes). This diagnosis also should be considered when female athletes present for the clinical evaluation of stress fractures or menstrual irregularities. Families may bring their adolescents into the office because of concern regarding disordered eating patterns, weight change, decreased athletic performance, or symptoms of depression. Effective treatment should employ a multidisciplinary approach including a physician, a nutritionist, and a psychologist or psychiatrist. Given the powerful influence of the coach upon the adolescent athlete, he or she can be a valuable asset in the treatment plan and should be enlisted early on as part of the treatment team.

19. What sports are frequently associated with the development of eating disorders?

Sports in which appearance, size, and body shape are emphasized, such as gymnastics, ballet, diving, figure skating, and distance running, have been associated with a higher prevalence of disordered eating patterns and frank eating disorders. Athletes involved in sports that have weight classes or requirements, such as wrestling, martial arts, and crew, are also at risk.

INJURIES

20. What is meant by the Q angle?

The quadriceps (Q) angle describes the alignment of the quadriceps, patella, and tibial tuberosity. The angle is measured as the intersection of a line drawn from the anterior superior iliac crest to the patella and a line from the tibial tuberosity, which bisects the patella. Women have a wider pelvis and therefore have greater Q angles than men. Q angles in males are usually 8–10°, and in females it ranges from 12 to 15°. Excessive Q angles (> 20°) increase the lateral forces on the patella and may predispose the athlete to anterior knee pain, patellar subluxation, and overuse injuries of the lower extremity.

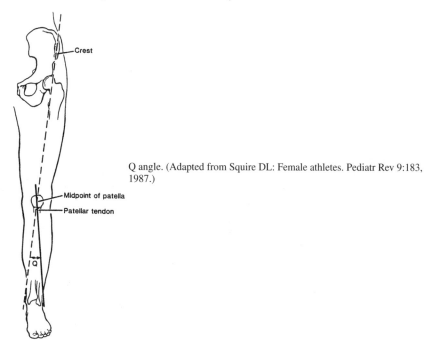

Q angle. (Adapted from Squire DL: Female athletes. Pediatr Rev 9:183, 1987.)

21. Are female athletes at greater risk for ligamentous injuries than male athletes?

Females have been experiencing an increased incidence of ligamentous injuries, especially anterior cruciate ligament (ACL) injuries of the knee, compared to males. This is an issue that has received a great deal of attention and study. Current thinking regarding possible etiologic factors for ACL injury in females includes (1) increased ligamentous laxity, (2) biomechanical factors such as increased pelvic width and resultant increased Q angle, (3) decreased quadriceps strength or quadriceps–hamstring strength imbalance, and (4) errors in technique.

22. What can be done to prevent ACL injuries?

ACL injuries frequently are noncontact, noncollision, hyperextension injuries. They often occur as part of a landing or deceleration or as part of a planting or cutting move. Keeping the knees bent on landing and using a gradual deceleration–acceleration move instead of a planting or cutting move can reduce the occurrence. Also, strength training of the quadriceps and hamstring muscles, focused on improving both strength and balance between the opposing muscle groups, is thought to decrease the risk of injury. Because fatigue is associated with a decrease in proper technique and muscular performance, general conditioning to improve endurance also may be helpful.

23. What are overuse injuries?

Activity and training place stress on the body across all systems. A positive training effect occurs when the body responds to an appropriate level of training or stress by adapting to a higher level of strength or increased performance capacity (e.g., improved aerobic and anaerobic conditioning, muscle strength or endurance, and increased bone density or strength). If, however, the stress or workload is greater than the body's ability to adapt by increased strength, then the system begins to fail and an overuse injury occurs. The involved body part begins to break down, leading to loss of strength, decreased performance, and pain. Often in response to pain, a change in technique occurs, which leads to further injury. This cycle of overload, pain, and injury leads to the development of an overuse injury. As opposed to acute injuries, or macro trauma (e.g., ACL rupture), overuse injuries result from repetitive micro-trauma to bone, ligaments, or musculotendinous junctions (e.g., stress fractures, tendinitis, tendinosis).

24. What are the risk factors for the development of overuse injuries?
Changes across several parameters are thought to set the stage for overuse syndromes. These can include changes in frequency, intensity, playing surface, footwear, technique, or the addition of another activity. Biomechanical malalignment or abnormalities may cause some individuals to be more susceptible to overuse injuries given similar stresses or changes in activity levels.

25. What is the approach to treatment of overuse injuries?
The first step in treatment is to correctly identify the site of injury (bone, ligament, or tendon) based on the history and clinical exam. A detailed history from the athlete determining the risk factors noted above and the location, quality, and timing of pain related to activity will guide your physical exam and in many instances suggest the appropriate diagnosis. The next step in treament is to alleviate the symptoms by eliminating the pain-producing activity and recommending active rest. **Active rest** involves limiting or reducing pain-producing activities and recommending other nonpainful activities that help maintain conditioning. The use of local icing and nonsteroidal anti-inflammatory drugs (NSAIDs) also can be an important part of the treatment plan. The definitive treatment takes the form of a rehabilitation program that corrects any muscle weakness, muscle imbalance, and inflexibility. Evaluation and correction of any technique or training errors are also needed to avoid recurrence of the overuse syndrome.

26. What are the common causes of chronic anterior knee pain in adolescent athletes?

Activity Related	Nonactivity Related
Patellofemoral syndrome	Juvenile rheumatoid arthritis
Osgood-Schlatter syndrome	Reactive arthritis
Patellar tendinitis	Neoplasm
Quadriceps tendinitis	
Osteochrondritis dissecans	
Pes anserine bursitis	

27. What is patellofemoral syndrome (PFS)?
There are many different causes of anterior knee pain and various systems of classification. PFS is anterior knee pain related to increased or excessive load on the patellofemoral joint. This increased load can be related to malalignment, weakness, or imbalances or inflexibilty of the dynamic joint stabilizers (muscles) or the static joint stabilizers (ligaments). The end result is that the patella tracks abnormally, causing chronic inflammation and pain. PFS frequently presents as an overuse injury following an increase or change in activity. It also can occur following acute trauma to the patella. Symptoms of PFS include diffuse anterior knee pain aggravated by activity, climbing or descending stairs, and prolonged sitting ("theater sign").

28. How is patellofemoral syndrome treated?
Treatment is similar to other overuse syndromes. Pain control is the first step. Pain-producing activity should be decreased or eliminated. Icing and NSAIDs can be helpful. More definitive treatment is directed at correcting the abnormal tracking and excessive load on the

patellofemoral joint. Strenghtening of the vastus medialis obliquus (VMO) portion of the quadriceps can improve patellar tracking. Strengthening and stretching both the quadriceps and hamstrings is a key part of the rehabilitation. As with all overuse injuries, changes in training intensity, frequency, type, and technique are important. Running shoes should be evaluated for degree of wear and biomechanical fit. If available, a physical therapist or athletic trainer can be invaluable. PFS that fails to respond to conservative care should be evaluated further by an orthopedist.

29. Does stretching decrease the risk of musculoskeletal injury?

The benefits of regular stretching include increased flexibility, maintenance of flexibility, and improved biomechanical functioning, with subsequent enhancement of athletic performance. Although all of these benefits have traditionally been thought to lead to a decrease in injuries, the research in this area remains unclear. The optimal timing of stretching related to exercise also has been a point of controversy. Vigorous stretching right before exercise may not be of particular benefit because of the potential for muscle fatigue or strain. Current recommendations for the preactivity regimen focuses on the warm-up period, which should consist of 10–15 minutes of low-intensity activities (walking, jogging, calisthenics) done to the point of starting to sweat. Following the activity or athletic event, stretching can be incorporated as part of the cool-down period. Stretching 2–3 times a week *is* an important component of any training or fitness program. It can be done either as part of the cool-down period after exercise or at other times unrelated to exercise. For adolescents, stretching while talking on the phone or watching TV can be a convenient way to incorporate it into their routines.

30. What is the most common sports-related acute musculoskeletal injury?

Ankle sprains.

31. What is the most common mechanism of ligamentous damage to the ankle?

The most common mechanism of injury is inversion of the ankle joint, which damages the lateral ligaments (anterior talofibular, calcaneofibular, and posterior talofibular ligament).

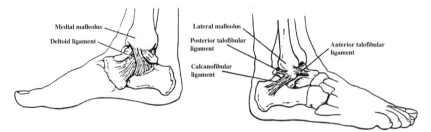

Ankle ligaments. (Adapted from Harvey J: Ankle injuries in children and adolescents. Pediatr Rev 2:217, 1981.)

32. How are ankle sprains graded?

The grading of ankle sprains is helpful only to assist in describing the degree of injury and estimating prognosis and length of rehabilitation. Ankle sprains are commonly graded as mild, moderate, or severe or grade I, II, III, or IV.

Grade I sprain: Stretching with perhaps partial tearing of the anterior talofibular ligament. There is minimal pain, tenderness, or swelling and no instability.

Grade II sprain: A complete disruption of the anterior talofibular ligament. There is increased pain, swelling, ecchymosis, decreased range of motion, and subjective and objective instability (objective instability can be assessed by the anterior drawer test and talar tilt test). The calcaneofibular ligament can be partially disrupted in a grade II sprain.

Grade III sprain: Damage to all three ligaments (anterior talofibular, calcaneofibular, and posterior talofibular) with significant pain, loss of range of motion, and instability.

Grade IV sprain: Associated with an eversion or external rotation mechanism of injury, with or without dorsiflexion. Superficial and deep portions of the deltoid ligament (medial ankle), anterior and posterior talofibular ligaments, and interosseous ligaments can be involved.

Orthopedic referral should be considered for grades III and IV sprains.

33. What are the Ottawa ankle rules and how are they used?

The Ottawa ankle rules were created to assist physicians in determining the need for x-rays when evaluating patients with ankle sprains. Ankle x-rays are recommended when there is pain in the malleolar region and

1. Bony tenderness at the posterior edge or tip of the lateral malleolus *or*
2. Bony tenderness at the posterior edge or tip of the medial malleolus *or*
3. The inability to bear weight (for a minimum of four steps) immediately after the injury and in the emergency department

These rules are useful for identifying patients who have significant fractures (bone fragment > 3 mm). Injuries of the growth plate can occur in younger adolescents, but, because of the presence of bony tenderness, these injuries meet the criteria for radiography.

34. What is the initial treatment for a sprained ankle?

As in most activity-related injuries, the mainstay of treatment is the RICE method: rest, ice, compression, and elevation. The most important step to speed recovery is to compress the ankle as soon as possible after the injury to minimize swelling. A horseshoe-shaped felt pad or a rolled athletic sock can be used around the malleolus to provide appropriate compression over the injured ligament(s). Icing for 20 minutes at a time should be encouraged as often as possible during the initial postinjury period to assist in minimizing edema and pain. Range-of-motion exercises (within a pain-free range) should be started as soon as possible, usually after the first 24–36 hours. Crutches should be used until the patient is able to bear weight.

35. How soon can the adolescent athlete return to participation after a sprained ankle? What are the key elements of an ankle rehabilitation program?

There are four phases of rehabilitation. The length of time spent in each phase is related to the severity of injury, the promptness and appropriateness of initial treatment, compliance with the treatment program, and motivation of the athlete. Overall rehab time can range from 2 weeks to 2–3 months.

- **Phase 1: Stabilization (or prevention) of edema**. Includes focal compression, icing, elevation, and limited range-of-motion exercises. This phase is usually the first 2–3 days following the sprain.
- **Phase 2: Range of motion exercises**. This phase should focus on regaining full pain-free range of motion of the ankle joint. The patient should limit these exercises to the pain-free range. Drawing the alphabet with the injuried foot, using the big toe as a pointer, is an easy way to instruct the patient and provides the full range of movement of the ankle joint. Straight-ahead activities such as walking and stationary cycling can be started during this phase.
- **Phase 3: Strengthening**. Begin with isometric contractions and advance to resistance training. Straight-ahead activities should be continued, and light jogging can be added as tolerated. The use of an Aircast, elastic ankle support, or lace-up brace during activity is useful to provide additional support while the supporting joint stabilizers (ligaments and muscles) are undergoing healing and strengthening.
- **Phase 4: Balance retraining (proprioception retraining)**. This phase is extremely important, yet is frequently overlooked by the athlete. Loss of appropriate proprioception can lead to reinjury. Balance training can include activities such as standing on one foot, toe raises, running figure eights, or working directly with an athletic trainer or physical therapist.

36. How can I help the adolescent with "weak ankles" who has recurrent ankle sprains?
Many recurrent ankle sprains occur when sprains have been incompletely rehabilitated. It is important to focus on strengthening the supporting muscles and regaining balance. If available, an athletic trainer or physical therapist can be extremely helpful in instructing the athlete and monitoring the rehabilitation program. The athlete who fails conservative treatment with aggressive rehabilitation should be referred to an orthopedist.

37. What is "little league elbow"?
This term refers to a constellation of injuries produced by excessive medial tension or lateral compression (valgus) forces characteristic of throwing athletes. Other susceptible athletes include golfers, gymnasts, tennis players, wrestlers, weight lifters, and even violinists. The most common of these syndromes consists of medial elbow and volar forearm pain related to the use of the wrist flexor and pronator teres muscles. This is commonly called medial (humeral) epicondylitis (although it may be more properly referred to as flexor/pronator tendinitis). The most common mechanism of injury is repetitive valgus stress at the elbow. Medial tension tends to cause extra-articular injuries including flexor-pronator strain or tendinitis, ulnar collateral ligament sprain, ulnar traction spurring, or ulnar neuritis. Lateral compression overload typically results in intra-articular injuries such as capitellar osteochondrosis, radial head deformity, loose body formation, and degenerative joint disease.

38. What are the symptoms of flexor-pronator tendinitis and how is it diagnosed?
The hallmark symptom is medial elbow pain related to use of the wrist flexor and pronator teres muscles. In the case of neuritis, radiation of pain to the ulnar forearm and hand and paresthesias of the fourth and fifth digits may be present. Stiffness after activity and limitation of motion are common. Hallmark signs include point tenderness over or just distal to the medial humeral epicondyle (the bony attachment of the flexor carpi and pronator teres tendons) and pain with resisted wrist flexion or forearm pronation. The most sensitive and specific sign of ulnar nerve sensory dysfunction is impaired two-point discrimination over the palmar surfaces of the small finger and ulnar half of the ring finger. In lateral compression syndromes, there is typically lateral joint line tenderness and lateral elbow pain when valgus stress is applied during flexion and extension of the elbow. Clinical diagnosis is sufficient to make the diagnosis of flexor-pronator tendinitis in a skeletally mature athlete; otherwise, radiographs are indicated. Cortical thickening, hypertrophy of the medial epicondyle, and alteration of the trabecular pattern reflect physiologic adaptation to repetitive valgus stress and must be differentiated from pathologic processes.

39. How is flexor-pronator tendinitis treated?
Initial treatment is symptomatic and anti-inflammatory. Relative rest (with sling, if necessary), ice, and NSAIDs are the mainstays of therapy. Oral corticosteroid medication may be indicated if neuritis is present. Rehabilitation includes limited-arc, fast-contraction, light-resistance wrist flexion exercises with a Theraband. Subsequently the athlete advances to heavy-resistance wrist flexion and forearm pronation exercises. Correction of faulty technique and gradual resumption of activity complete the rehabilitation.

40. What is Osgood-Schlatter syndrome?
Osgood-Schlatter syndrome is a form of patellar tendinitis or apophysitis occurring at the insertion of the patellar tendon on the tibial tuberosity in the skeletally immature athlete. This is more appropriately considered an overuse syndrome than a disease. It usually presents gradually after a change in activity or athletic environment (e.g., running or jumping on hard surfaces). It is more common in boys and often presents during or shortly after a growth spurt. The main symptom is pain localized to the tibial tuberosity that is exacerbated by running, jumping, and squatting. In addition to localized tenderness, the exam often reveals localized swelling accompanied by warmth, erythema, and sometimes limited knee flexion. Radiographs may reveal

fragmentation of the bony attachment of the tendon and bone formation within the patellar tendon.

41. How is Osgood-Schlatter syndrome treated?

Initial treatment is relative rest (discontinuation of the pain-producing activities), ice, anti-inflammatory medications, and quadriceps isometric exercises. Subsequent therapy should focus on restoration of normal quadriceps strength, endurance, and flexibility with gradual return to activities. The use of an Osgood-Schlatter pad, a device that pads the tibial tuberosity in a horseshoe distribution, thus protecting it from direct pressure, is helpful and effective. Referral is necessary only when conservative treatment fails.

42. What is "jumper's knee"?

Jumper's knee is the common name given to patellar tendinitis. This overuse injury is common in athletes who are involved in sports with a lot of jumping and sudden acceleration and deceleration, such as basketball, volleyball, and sprinting. The mechanism involves excessive overload placed on the extensor mechanism consisting of the quadriceps muscle, quadriceps tendon, and patellar tendon. Pain is localized to a portion of patellar tendon at the inferior pole of the patella, the body of the tendon, or the insertion of the tendon on the tibial tuberosity. Acute treatment follows the general approach to an overuse injury: relative rest with avoidance of pain-producing activity, icing, and a short course of anti-inflammatory medication. Definitive treatment and rehabilitation focus on a stretching and strengthening program for both the quadriceps and hamstring muscles.

43. What are the components of the rotator cuff and what is the individual function of each?

The rotator cuff is composed of four muscles easily remembered by the mnemonic SITS: supraspinatus, infraspinatus, teres minor, and subscapularis. The supraspinatus is responsible for the first 30° of abduction of the shoulder; the infraspinatus and the teres minor externally rotate and the subscapularis internally rotates the shoulder.

44. What is the shoulder impingement syndrome?

The shoulder impingement syndrome probably accounts for most cases of chronic shoulder pain in athletes and represents varying degrees of injury and subsequent inflammation, atrophy, and insufficiency of the rotator cuff and related structures. The mechanism of injury is forced or repetitive muscle action leading to subsequent tendinitis. Activity-related pain also can represent impingement of inflamed tendons and bursae between the humeral head and coracoacromial arch, usually secondary to insufficiency of the stabilizing muscles of the shoulder, which allows displacement of the humeral head when the arm is moved. The hallmark symptom is deep, aching shoulder pain generally referred to the lateral area of the arm. The usual presentation is of gradual onset of pain initially postexercise, followed by progressive pain with activity, and finally resulting in constant, aching pain present even at night and exacerbated by routine activities of daily living. Physical exam will reveal point tenderness over involved structures, pain with specific muscle testing, subacromial tenderness, and a positive impingement sign (grimacing or pain with passive horizontal flexion and internal rotation of the involved shoulder—with the elbow "up" and in front of the patient). Signs of glenohumeral instability also may be present, including limitation of motion, abnormal patterns of glenohumeral or scapulothoracic motion, pain and crepitus with motion, and muscular atrophy and weakness or frank instability. Imaging is indicated with a positive impingement sign to evaluate for degenerative or acute changes in the glenohumeral joint.

45. What is the treatment and rehabilitation for shoulder impingement syndrome?

Initial treatment is routine RICE therapy, emphasizing relative rest (with a sling if there is pain with activities of daily living); useful adjuncts may include electrogalvanic stimulation and ultrasound. Definitive treatment is usually appropriate rehabilitation. Presence and direction of glenohumeral instability will determine initial rehab. With anterior instability, the emphasis is on the adductors and internal rotators, and with posterior instability, the external rotators and posterior deltoid are emphasized. After these muscles are fully restored (full strength and no pain, apprehension, or instability with shoulder motion), complete shoulder rehabilitation commences. Sport-specific functional drills are appropriate only when full and pain-free shoulder motion is achieved. As with all overuse syndromes, training errors should be addressed. Referral is indicated if disabling pain, apprehension, or frank instability persists despite complete rehabilitation and appropriate activity modification.

46. How does one approach a patient who has had his or her "bell rung" during sport?

The Centers for Disease Control and Prevention (CDC) estimates an incidence of approximately 300,000 sports-related concussions annually. **Concussion** is defined as a traumatically induced alteration in mental status, with or without loss of consciousness. The sports medicine community has not achieved consensus on classification and treatment. The following are the currently recognized grading systems: American Academy of Neurology, Cantu, Colorado, Virginia Neurological Institute, and Torg. Perhaps the simplest are the Colorado guidelines:

- **Grade 1**: Confusion (having their "bell rung") without post-traumatic amnesia or loss of consciousness
- **Grade 2**: Confusion with amnesia, but no loss of consciousness
- **Grade 3**: Loss of consciousness

47. What is second impact syndrome and why is it important?

Following head trauma, there is a period of time during which there is loss of autoregulation of the cerebral fluid. If the athlete suffers a second impact during this time, even with minimal trauma, massive cerebral edema can result. This is the reason for the development of return-to-play guidelines. These guidelines are based on the severity of the initial head trauma and provide guidelines for how long an athlete needs to be asymptomatic before being allowed to return to play.

48. What are the Colorado guidelines for evaluation, treatment, and return to play after experiencing a head injury?

Remove the athlete from the contest and examine him or her immediately. The term *symptomatic* refers to headache, dizziness, impaired orientation, impaired concentration, or memory dysfunction and includes evaluation at rest and with provocative testing.

- **Grade 1**: May return to play after 20 minutes of observation if asymptomatic. If symptomatic after the injury, the athlete can return when asymptomatic for 1 week. If it is the second concussion, the athlete can return in 2 weeks if asymptomatic for 1 week.
- **Grade 2**: Thorough neurologic evaluation with frequent re-examination over the subsequent 24 hours by direct medical observation or explicit written instructions given to the family to detect any evolving intracranial pathology. May not resume play until asymptomatic for 1 week. If symptomatic after the injury, consider hospital admission. If not admitted, a computed tomography (CT) scan is required if still symptomatic 1 week postinjury. For a second concussion, no play until a minimum of 1 month postinjury and 1 week without symptoms.
- **Grade 3**: Transport from the field by ambulance to the nearest hospital with cervical spine immobilization, if indicated. A thorough neurologic evaluation should be performed on an emergent basis; imaging should be considered. Admission is strongly recommended and is required for any signs of pathology. Neurologic status should be followed until symptoms resolve. Imaging is recommended if symptoms worsen or persist longer than 1 week. May return to play after 1 month only if asymptomatic at rest and with exertion for 2 weeks. If this is a second episode or if there are any imaging

abnormalities or intracranial pathology, the athlete is out for the season and should be strongly advised to consider noncontact sports.

If this is the third concussion, the athlete is out for the season; with three grade 3 concussions, strongly advise a noncontact sport.

49. What is a "burner" or "stinger"?

Stingers or burners are common terms for brachial plexus injuries. They occur most commonly in football but can occur in any setting in which the neck is laterally hyperextended. In fact, it has been reported that up to 50% of football players sustain such an injury during their playing careers. Most injuries are thought to be neurapraxias, or temporary disruption of nerve function with full recovery minutes afterward. However, symptoms may persist, indicating some degree of axonal degeneration. Mechanism of injury is stretching of the brachial plexus by forcible depression of the ipsilateral shoulder, usually with lateral flexion of the neck to the contralateral side, as can occur during blocking or tackling. Symptoms include severe, burning, unilateral pain associated with paresthesias and weakness. The pain usually starts at the shoulder and radiates to the hand; the intense pain usually abates within seconds. Numbness, tingling, and weakness generally last several minutes.

50. How should burners or stingers be evaluated and treated?

Evaluation should *always* include consideration of spinal cord injury; red flags include bilateral involvement, loss or alteration of consciousness, and neck pain. Guidelines for return to play include no pain and full range of motion of the neck, no neurologic abnormalities (including deep tendon reflexes, strength, and sensory exam), a negative Spurling test (while the patient extends head and flexes laterally, the examiner applies gentle pressure on the forehead), and no associated injuries. Persistent weakness of the deltoid, supraspinatus, infraspinatus, and biceps muscles are consistent with a more severe injury. Recurrent or unresolving burners require further investigation (to rule out cervical stenosis or other abnormality), and, again, the presence of bilateral symptoms *always* necessitates evaluation. Radiographs, electromyographic examination, referral, and physical therapy may be indicated. Prevention includes the following protective equipment for football: neck roll, lifter, and cowboy collar.

51. What are spondylolysis and spondylolisthesis?

Spondylolysis is a radiographically demonstrable defect in the pars interarticularis of the vertebral arch, due either to stress fracture or to developmental defect. *Spondylolisthesis* is the anterior displacement of one vertebral body on another as a result of spondylolysis or abnormal elongation of the pars interarticularis. Either condition may or may not be symptomatic. Injury is thought to be due to repetitive extension loading of the lumbar spine, as occurs frequently in dancing, football (especially linemen), gymnastics, and weight training. The main symptom is low-back pain exacerbated or induced by activity, characteristically with hyperextension of the lumbar spine. It is usually unilateral and well localized. On physical exam, the pain is reproduced with one-leg-standing lumbar extension on the leg ipsilateral to the fracture. Hyperlordosis, hamstring tightness, and, in severe cases, sciatica are often seen with spondylolisthesis. Radiographic examination reveals the "Scottie dog sign," in which the dog's ear, snout, and foreleg represent, respectively, the superior articular facet, lateral process, and inferior articular facet; spondylolysis is represented by the presence of a radiolucent "collar." Bone scan may be helpful in the setting of a normal radiograph to determine acuity of the fracture.

52. How are spondylolysis and spondylolisthesis treated, and when should they be referred to an orthopedic surgeon?

The mainstay of treatment is strict avoidance of pain-producing activity. Adjuncts include abdominal strengthening and hamstring stretching. Sports participation is permitted if the patient is symptom free and vertebral displacement is less than 25% of the width of the vertebral body. Referral is indicated if symptoms do not respond to conservative treatment or if vertebral displacement is greater than 25%. Any skeletally immature athlete with spondylolysis is at risk for spondylolisthesis and should be followed radiographically until growth is complete; youth between the ages of 9 and 14 years and girls are at greatest risk.

BIBLIOGRAPHY

1. American College of Sports Medicine Position Stand: Exercise and fluid replacement. Med Sci Sports Exerc 29:i–vii, 1996.
2. Anderson SJ, Sullivan JA (eds): Care of the Young Athlete. Rosemont, IL, American Academy of Orthopaedic Surgeons and American Academy of Pediatrics, 2000.
3. Casa DJ, Armstrong LE, Hillman SK, et al: National Athletic Trainers' Association position statement: Fluid replacement for athletes. J Athletic Training 35:212–224, 2000.
4. Garrick JG, Web DR: Sports Injuries: Diagnosis and Management, 2nd ed. Philadelphia, W.B. Saunders, 1999.
5. Harries M, Williams C, Stanish W, Micheli L (eds): Oxford Textbook of Sports Medicine, 2nd ed. New York, Oxford University Press, 1998.
6. Otis C, et al: ACSM position stand on the female athlete triad. Med Sci Sports Exer 29:i–ix, 1997.
7. Plint AC, Bulloch B, Osmond MH, et al: Validation of the Ottawa ankle rules in children with ankle injuries. Acad Emerg Med 6:1005–1009, 1999.
8. Sallis RE, Massimino (eds): ACSM's Essentials of Sports Medicine. St. Louis, Mosby, 1996.

III. Reproductive Health

22. BREAST HEALTH AND DISORDERS IN ADOLESCENT FEMALES

Patricia S. Simmons, M.D.

1. What is important to know about adolescents' breasts?

The answer is: the "other stuff." Good people with good intentions have introduced screening for breast cancer into the adolescent population. In addition to examining adolescents for breast masses, many doctors, nurses, advocacy groups, and schools encourage and teach teenagers to do breast self-examinations (BSEs). In many locations it has become a standard of care. The problem lies in applying an early detection tool developed for adults, who are at significant risk for breast carcinoma, to a population that is not. Although breast carcinoma can occur in the young, it is exceedingly rare. There are 15 case reports in the child and adolescent literature, but the risk is less than one per million population.

However, those who care for adolescent girls are likely to encounter other breast problems and should know how to recognize them and how to help their patients. The more common problems include breast discharges, abnormal appearances, injury, and masses.

2. In an adolescent girl, what is a breast mass most likely to be?

The most common masses in the adolescent female breast are fibrocystic changes, which are diagnosed clinically, and fibroadenomas, which are diagnosed surgically. A breast abscess may present as a mass, but it is usually distinguishable clinically by the presence of symptoms and signs characteristic of infection, including erythema, tenderness, and warmth over the mass itself. Simple cysts, lymph nodes, hematomas, hemangiomas, and fat necrosis may present as a mass in the breast. Less common tumors include papillomatosis, papillomas, and cystosarcoma phyllodes.

3. What is cystosarcoma phyllodes?

This uncommon tumor may occur during adolescence and mimic a fibroadenoma. It may enlarge, suggesting giant fibroadenoma or malignancy. Although the histopathology is usually benign, some of these tumors become malignant. Therefore, they should be completely excised, and patients should be followed for recurrence and malignancy for many years.

4. How common is breast cancer in adolescents?

The likelihood that a mass in an adolescent breast is cancer is extremely low. Because many breast masses resolve spontaneously, only a fraction of patients undergo surgery; in such patients, malignancy accounts for 0–5% of masses. Only 0.2% of breast cancers in women present before age 20 years. In a population-based study, the incidence of breast cancer under age 18 years was found to be zero per million.

5. Are the presentation and prognosis of breast cancer similar in adolescents and adults?

No. Breast cancer in female adolescents is more likely to be a malignancy other than adenocarcinoma (the most common breast cancer in adults). Rhabdomyosarcoma, lymphoma, neuroblastoma, and leukemia have been reported. There are case reports of breast adenocarcinoma presenting in childhood and adolescence, but their natural history may be different from that experienced by adults. Breast adenocarcinoma in children and adolescents is so rare that optimal management and natural history are not established.

6. When an adolescent presents with a breast mass, how should she be evaluated?
Begin with a thorough history, which should include symptoms of infection, trauma, and risk factors for malignancy as well as duration (if the patient has been aware of the mass) and presence of constitutional symptoms. In addition to blunt trauma, the patient should be asked about piercing and areolar hair plucking, which can lead to hematoma or mastitis. Risk factors for malignancy during adolescence include presence of constitutional symptoms not attributable to mastitis, prior malignancy, chest wall radiation, and genetic predisposition. Although a breast mass in an otherwise healthy adolescent is unlikely to be malignant, even in the face of a family history of breast cancer, the history helps to address the patient's and family's anxiety and to explain her risk appropriately.

7. What are the key elements of the physical examination?
The physical examination should seek findings suggestive of malignancy (lymphadenopathy, hepatosplenomegaly) and focus on the characteristics of the mass. Fibrocystic changes may present as single or multiple cystic or rope-like, freely moveable structures that are mildly or non-tender. They may occur anywhere in the breast, and, though usually bilateral, may present in only one breast. Fibroadenoma occurs most commonly in the upper outer quadrant. It is freely moveable, nontender, and not associated with overlying skin changes. Although usually singular, multiple fibroadenomas may present in one or both breasts. Infections (mastitis with or without abscess formation) have the expected characteristics of erythema, warmth, tenderness, and induration and may be associated with systemic symptoms and/or axillary lymphadenopathy.

8. How should an apparently benign mass be followed?
When a mass has the characteristics of a cyst, fibrocystic changes, or fibroadenoma, it is generally appropriate to re-examine the patient 1 or 2 months later through the course of a menstrual cycle. Simple cysts may resolve spontaneously or persist until drained. Masses secondary to fibrocystic changes may resolve or evolve into more fibrocystic findings. Fibroadenoma is likely to persist for only 1–2 months, but many resolve over the course of several months. A growing mass or a mass associated with other symptoms and findings requires further evaluation.

9. What type of imaging is best for evaluating a breast mass in adolescents?
Ultrasonography. Ultrasound images of cysts and fibroadenomas have well-recognized characteristics that are likely to lead to a definitive diagnosis. Ultrasound demonstrates a useful degree of specificity and sensitivity in identifying not only the clinically detected mass, but also additional masses, as in multiple fibroadenomas or fibrocystic mastopathy. Ultrasound is also useful in determining the presence of abscess in patients with mastitis who do not respond adequately to antibiotics.

Ultrasound-guided needle aspiration of cysts is effective and atraumatic, although some cysts recur. Masses with worrisome clinical or ultrasound characteristics can be diagnosed safely and accurately through ultrasound-guided core needle biopsy. For patients with known or suspected malignancy, ultrasound-guided core needle biopsy or open excisional biopsy may determine the diagnosis or recurrence of cancer. For such patients, additional imaging with computerized tomography (CT) or magnetic resonance imaging (MRI) is indicated.

10. What role does mammography play in screening or diagnosis during adolescence?
Not much, if any. Mammography is the standard screening modality for breast cancer in adults. Application of this tool to teenagers is not appropriate for a number of reasons. First,

breast adenocarcinoma is rare in adolescence. Second, the tissue characteristics of the adolescent breast render mammography less sensitive. The young breast is more dense with relatively less fat and more stroma than the older breast. Finally, the adolescent's breast may be too small to be positioned adequately in the imaging port. The current standard of practice is to initiate mammographic screening at 25 years of age for women at high risk for breast cancer.

Imaging modalities other than mammography are more sensitive and specific in diagnosing breast masses in adolescents. When imaging is needed to diagnose a breast mass, ultrasonography is preferred. In patients with known or malignant disease, CT or MRI is indicated.

11. What are the indications for surgery in the adolescent with a breast mass?
- Recurring cyst after needle aspiration
- Growing mass(es) that may disfigure the breast
- Known or suspected cystosarcoma phyllodes
- Suspected papilloma or papillomatosis
- Abscess

12. How should fibroadenoma be managed?
There is neither uniform agreement nor consistent practice in terms of whether fibroadenomas should be surgically removed. Many fibroadenomas spontaneously resolve or fail to progress. If they are not growing, do not distort the breast, and have no worrisome features, surgical excision is not necessary. If the diagnosis is in question, ultrasound-guided core needle biopsy is an alternative to excisional biopsy for some patients. Surgical excision is indicated when the fibroadenoma is large and/or growing because such tumors can lead to distortion of the breast and some progress to malignancy in later years. An adolescent whose self-image suffers because of readily palpable or visible masses may benefit from excision of large fibroadenomas.

Although patient or parental anxiety can be extreme and persuasive, care should be taken so that clinical insecurity does not lead to an uninformed decision about excision. Balanced judgment with a well-informed patient and family may not lead to an entirely consistent practice, but it is preferable to either "removing it because it's there" or "leaving it alone because it's benign" as the sole basis for the decision.

13. Other than evaluating or excising masses, what are the indications for breast surgery in adolescents?
Other conditions besides masses may necessitate surgery, including juvenile or virginal hypertrophy, gross asymmetry, amastia, or hypomastia. Gross asymmetry and even unilateral or bilateral amastia can be addressed in adolescence to create growth rather than waiting for full maturity. A recent article by Chadbourne et al. nicely addresses reductive mammoplasty for breast hypertrophy.

14. How do adolescents get mastitis?
Mastitis most commonly occurs in lactating women. Abrasions, hematomas, lacerations, piercing, and areolar hair plucking can lead to mastitis, sometimes with abscess formation. Like cellulitis elsewhere on the body, however, mastitis can occur as a result of trauma or even without known cause.

Usually the diagnosis of mastitis is obvious; it presents as a warm, tender, indurated area of the breast. Exudate associated with a break in the skin may be present. An abscess may be suspected if fluctuation is present or response to appropriate medical therapy is incomplete. Patients may have systemic symptoms of infection.

15. How is mastitis treated?
Removal of foreign bodies, cleansing of broken areas of skin, warm compresses, and systemic antibiotics with close follow-up are recommended. Skin flora (*Staphylococcus* and

Streptococcus species), especially in the presence of a foreign body or break in the skin, are likely pathogens. Gram-negative bacteria also may be responsible. Therefore, a broad-spectrum antibiotic such as amoxicillin-clavulanic acid is usually the first choice. An abscess is likely to require incision and drainage.

16. What causes breast discharge in adolescents?

Galactorrhea

• Lactation of pregnancy: during pregnancy, after delivery or abortion
• Not associated with pregnancy: primary hypothyroidism, idiopathic disorder, hyperprolactinemia/prolactinoma, nipple stimulation, drugs.

Non–lactose-containing discharge: benign duct secretion

Bloody discharge

• Benign, spontaneous
• Trauma
• Papillomatosis or papilloma

17. Describe the work-up for a nipple discharge.

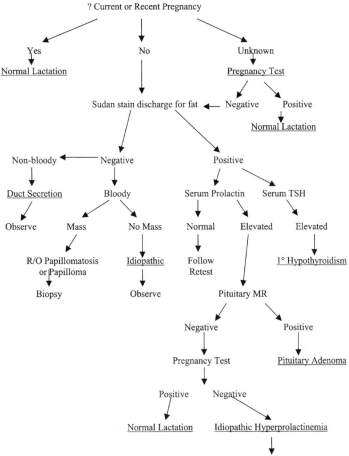

TSH = thyroid-stimulating hormone, MR = magnetic resonance imaging

Keep in mind also that medications, particularly certain psychotropics, can be associated with mild elevations in prolactin and therefore may cause galactorrhea.

18. Should adolescents be taught BSE?

Ideally, all medical practices, including anticipatory guidance, should be data-driven. No data determine the value of BSE in adolescents. Some argue that it is worth teaching BSE to adolescents to establish future behavior. However, compliance with BSEs is low among adolescents. Since time with adolescent patients is limited, caretakers should weigh the relative values of the areas on which to concentrate. Consider the patient's risk for a particular problem as well as the potential for a positive effect of anticipatory guidance.

Subgroups of adolescents, however, are at higher risk for breast cancer at a young age, including those with a history of malignancy or chest wall radiation and those with a genetic predisposition. Even in the absence of compelling data, most argue that any practice that may facilitate early detection of cancer is logical, including teaching BSE to higher-risk patients.

19. Should the breasts be examined as part of general or health maintenance adolescent visits?

Yes. The most important part of the exam is visual inspection for Tanner stage, asymmetry, anomaly, or skin, areolar, or nipple abnormalities. Asymptomatic galactorrhea is uncommon, but gentle pressure to elicit any discharge is simple to perform. Palpation for masses is reasonable. If BSE is to be taught, the healthy maintenance visit is an efficient and logical time to do so. More importantly, it is an opportune time to educate patients about breast health: why you are or are not going to teach BSE; sensitive approach to significant asymmetry or anomalies; and discussion of the risks of piercing and, in patients at risk, nipple trauma (e.g., cold exposure and friction for athletes).

20. Should teenagers be tested for the hereditary breast cancer gene (*BRCA1*)?

Maybe. Caregivers must ask several questions of themselves, their patient, and her family:
- Is this a research or clinical situation?
- Who wants to know? Why?
- Who should consent if the patient is a minor?
- Does the patient understand the implications of testing?
- How will the knowledge help her?
- Could this knowledge be harmful?
- If testing offers potential benefit, is this the right time for the patient?

Because the ethics of genetic testing of minors are evolving as clinical and research experience matures, an individualized approach is best to test and meet the interests of patients, their families, and medical science.

BIBLIOGRAPHY

1. Chadbourne EB, Zhang S, Gordon MJ, et al: Clinical outcomes in reduction mammaplasty: A systematic review and meta-analysis of published studies. Mayo Clin Proc 76:503–510, 2001.
2. Elger BS, Harding TW: Testing adolescents for a hereditary breast cancer gene (BRCA1). Arch Pediatr Adolesc Med 154:113–119, 2000.
3. Garcia CJ, Espinoza A, Dinamarca V, Navarro O, et al: Breast ultrasound in children and adolescents. Radiographics 20:1605–1612, 2000.
4. Neinstein LS, Atkinson J, Diament M: Prevalence and longitudinal study of breast masses in adolescents. J Adolesc Health 14:277–281, 1993.
5. Simmons PS: Diagnostic considerations in breast disorders of children and adolescents. Obstet Gynecol Clin North Am 19:91–102, 1992.
6. Simmons PS: Breast disorders in adolescent females. Curr Opin Obstet Gynecol 13:459–461, 2001.
7. Simmons PS, Wold LE: Surgically treated breast disease in adolescent females: A retrospective review of 185 cases. Adoles Pediatr Gynecol 2:95–98, 1989.

8. Simmons PS: Breast disorders in adolescents. In Sanfilippo J, Muram D (eds): Pediatric and Adolescent Gynecology, 2nd ed. Philadelphia, W.B. Saunders, 2001, pp 603–620.

9. Simmons PS, Melton J: Incidence of breast cancer in female children and adolescents. Presented at the World Congess of Pediatric and Adolescent Gynecology. Helsinki, June 2–3, 1998.

10. Templeman C, Hertweck SP: Breast disorders in the pediatric and adolescent patient. Obstet Gynecol Clin North Am 27:19–34, 2000.

11. Weinstein SP, Conant EF, Orel SG, et al: Spectrum of ultrasound findings in pediatric and adolescent patients with palpable breast masses. Radiographics 20:1613–1621, 2000.

23. GYNECOLOGY

Geri D. Hewitt, M.D.

HISTORY AND PHYSICAL EXAMINATION

1. How do you obtain a gynecologic history from a teenage girl?

A physician has to be patient with younger patients, not only because these girls may come to the visit with tremendous anxiety about what will happen there, but also because they typically come armed with their mothers. The dynamic between an adolescent, her parent(s), and the clinician can be a tricky one, and the expectations regarding the patient's care and confidentiality should be made clear to everyone from the onset. Adolescent women usually present with a specific gynecologic complaint allowing the clinician to focus the evaluation accordingly. Important aspects of the interview include the history of the present complaint, complete medical history, menstrual history, sexual and contraceptive history, and psychosocial history.

2. When taking the history, to whom should you talk—the mother or the patient?

Typically the patient is interviewed with the parent present. Questions should be directed to the patient, and the clinician should wait for the patient's response. The patient's parent may need to expand on certain responses or fill in details of the patient's history, but it should be clear that the patient is expected to answer questions about her concerns and her health, a task most girls can accomplish by the age of 14. All girls should be given an opportunity to speak to the clinician alone, in order to complete the sexual history as well to address any questions they may not want to ask in front of their parents. An explanation of patient confidentiality should be provided simultaneously to both patient and parent.

3. How do you prepare an adolescent for a gynecologic exam?

With great patience, a complete gynecologic examination can be performed successfully in adolescent women. The patient should be asked if she wants her parent or a chaperone present during the examination. If the examiner is male, a chaperone is mandatory. Helpful hints for the clinician include patience, numerous explanations, and interrupting the examination if the patient expresses pain. The examination should begin with height, weight, and vital signs. The patient should disrobe privately and put on a gown. A general examination should be performed before beginning the breast and pelvic exam. The breast examination should elicit any masses or abnormal nipple secretions and determine the Tanner stage. The breast exam is a tremendous opportunity to instruct the patient on self-examination of her breasts.

4. What are the steps of the pelvic examination?

The pelvic examination should begin with examination of the vulva and Tanner staging of the pubic hair. The clitoris and hymenal opening should be evaluated. Examination of the vagina and cervix is performed using either a Huffman adolescent or Peterson speculum. Any vaginal discharge present should be swabbed for wet mount microscopic evaluation. Rarely is it difficult to insert the speculum if the patient is either sexually active or practiced at using tampons and if she is relaxed during the examination. Lubricant should not be placed on the speculum if a cytologic smear is to be performed. All adolescents who are sexually active should have annual Papanicolaou (Pap) smears. If indicated, cervical DNA probes for sexually transmitted disease (STD) screening should be performed prior to obtaining the Pap smear. After the speculum examination is completed, attention is turned to the bimanual examination. One lubricated finger should be placed inside the vagina with the other hand placed on the abdomen to palpate both the uterus and adnexa. A rectal or rectovaginal examination, if indicated, completes the evaluation.

MENSTRUAL DISTURBANCES

5. What is a normal menstrual cycle pattern?
Regular, ovulatory menstrual cycles occur every 21–35 days (counted from the first day of the menses to the first day of the next menses), last 7 days or less, and result in a total blood loss less than 80 ml.

6. What percentage of menstrual cycles are anovulatory in the adolescent? When do clinicians need to intervene?
Patients often will not have normal menstrual cycles for the first couple of years after menarche because of the immaturity of the hypothalamic-pituitary-ovarian axis. Up to 82% of cycles the first year after menarche and 28% of cycles the fifth year after menarche are anovulatory. Most adolescents having irregular bleeding the first year or two after menarche do not require intervention. If the abnormal bleeding pattern persists longer than 4 years, diagnostic and therapeutic intervention is required.

7. What is oligomenorrhea? What are the most common causes of oligomenorrhea?
Oligomenorrhea is defined as irregular bleeding episodes occurring at intervals of greater than 42 days. The most frequent cause of oligomenorrhea is anovulation. If the oligomenorrhea is accompanied by acne or hirsutism, it may represent polycystic ovarian syndrome (PCOS), chronic anovulation accompanied by hyperandrogenism and insulin resistance. Other causes of oligomenorrhea include pregnancy and recurrent functional ovarian cysts.

8. What is the most common reason adolescents present with excessive vaginal bleeding?
Anovulation is the most common reason that adolescents present with heavy, irregular bleeding. This type of bleeding represents dysfunctional uterine bleeding (DUB, abnormal bleeding in the presence of a normal uterus).

9. How do you evaluate a patient with presumed dysfunctional uterine bleeding?
DUB is a diagnosis of exclusion, and patients who present with abnormal bleeding must be evaluated for other causes. The evaluation should be tailored to the age of the patient and whether or not she has ever been sexually active. Physical examination may include a speculum exam to evaluate the cervix and look for any signs of trauma or foreign objects, cervical cultures and a Pap smear to rule out cervicitis and cervical dysplasia, and a bimanual examination to evaluate for fibroids, adnexal masses, and pelvic inflammatory disease. Complete blood count (CBC) and coagulation studies are necessary to quantify the amount of bleeding and to rule out a coagulopathy. A pelvic ultrasound may be indicated for further evaluation of any suspected uterine or adnexal abnormalities.

10. How do you treat a patient with DUB?
The treatment of a patient with DUB varies depending on the clinical scenario. If the patient is asymptomatic with normal vital signs and a normal hemoglobin despite having irregular, heavy bleeding, she can be managed with either low-dose oral contraceptive pills or with cyclic medroxyprogesterone acetate (10 mg a day for 10–12 days each month). If the patient has asymptomatic anemia, she should be given oral ferrous sulfate to replace iron loss in addition to the medical management of her irregular bleeding.

11. What if a patient with DUB has very brisk vaginal bleeding and orthostatic hypotension?
This patient would require IV fluid hydration and rapid cessation of her vaginal bleeding. Anovulatory bleeding can be stopped quickly (usually in less than 24 hours) by a variety of

medical regimens including IV conjugated estrogens (25 mg IV every 6 hours), four low-dose oral contraceptive pills taken over 24 hours, and high doses of medroxyprogesterone acetate (up to 40 mg in 24 hours). The vast majority of patients can be managed medically without surgical intervention. If the patient continues to bleed despite aggressive medical intervention, dilation and curettage may be indicated. Patients with profound, symptomatic anemia may require blood transfusion. Clotting studies ideally should be obtained prior to blood transfusion or initiation of hormonal therapy. After the acute bleeding episode is under control, patients need to be maintained on a regimen to control abnormal bleeding that may occur as a result of withdrawal from the acute therapy (especially the IV estrogen). If they are not placed on a maintenance regimen, abnormal bleeding is likely to recur. Appropriate regimens include cyclic low-dose contraceptive pills and cyclic medroxyprogesterone acetate.

12. What concerns should a clinician have for a patient who presents with very heavy ovulatory cycles (menorrhagia)?

Patients who give a history of extremely heavy ovulatory cycles, particularly those requiring blood transfusion, should be evaluated for bleeding abnormalities. Up to 25% of adolescents with acute menorrhagia at menarche have a bleeding abnormality, von Willebrand's disease (VWD) and thrombocytopenia being the most common. A personal or family history of bleeding problems raises further concern for an inherited coagulopathy.

13. What are some of the blood dyscrasias that may present with menorrhagia?

Menorrhagia may be the presenting symptom for a wide range of bleeding abnormalities including idiopathic thrombocytopenia, drug-induced thrombocytopenia, leukemia, and VWD. VWD is an autosomal dominant abnormality and, therefore, is seen with equal frequency in girls and boys.

14. What is one of the most important tests to perform in a sexually active adolescent who presents with excessive vaginal bleeding?

A **pregnancy test** should be obtained on all adolescents suspected of sexual activity who present with vaginal bleeding. The vaginal bleeding may be associated with a spontaneous or induced abortion, an ectopic pregnancy, or a hydatidiform mole. All of these diagnoses can be eliminated with a negative serum human chorionic gonadotropin (HCG) test.

15. What cervical abnormalities can present with abnormal vaginal bleeding?

Infections in the vagina, cervix, or endometrium can present with abnormal vaginal bleeding. If the vaginal bleeding is painful, pelvic inflammatory disease should be considered. Other relatively common cervical abnormalities include polyps and condylomata. Sarcoma botryoides and mixed mesodermal sarcoma are much less likely diagnoses.

16. What disorders of the vagina may be associated with abnormal vaginal bleeding?

Vaginitis may present with abnormal vaginal bleeding, as may the presence of a vaginal foreign body or a vaginal septum. Trauma to the vagina or hymen at the time of sexual intercourse or abuse also may present with excessive bleeding.

17. What is PMS and how do you diagnose it?

Premenstrual syndrome (PMS) is a combination of physical, emotional, and behavioral changes that occur after ovulation and before menstruation (i.e., during the luteal phase) and interfere with quality of life. Symptoms can be widely varied including bloating, food craving, breast tenderness, anger, anxiety, depression, fatigue, social isolation, and increased interpersonal conflict. Fundamental to the diagnosis of PMS is the prospective symptom calendar. Patients should record their symptoms prospectively for 3 months along with their menstrual cycle. With PMS, symptoms should be significantly worse the 5 days prior to menses with resolution of the symptoms after menstruation. Anovulation and irregular menstrual cycles are not compatible with the diagnosis of PMS, because there are no follicular and luteal phases in these conditions. If symptoms do not resolve after menses, or timing of symptoms appears to be random, the diagnosis of PMS is inappropriate. Other diagnostic possibilities include affective disorders, adjustment disorders, or normal adolescent behavior.

18. Are there any effective treatments for PMS?

Treatment of PMS should begin with educating the patient and her family that PMS is real and that certain feelings or behaviors may be due to PMS. For some patients, validating the experience of PMS can be helpful to improve self-confidence and emphasize coping mechanisms. Other self-help measures include adequate rest and sleep, stress management, aerobic exercise, and good nutrition. Other interventions are best focused on the patient's specific symptoms. For young women with mild complaints, over-the-counter medications containing a diuretic, analgesic, and antihistamine may be helpful. Therapies aimed to relieve specific complaints during the luteal phase include analgesics or antiprostaglandins for headache or low back pain, low doses of bromocriptine at bedtime for breast tenderness, and spironolactone (50–100 mg/day) for swelling. Agents shown as effective in treating PMS in controlled, double-blind studies include only fluoxetine, alprazolam, and gonadotropin-releasing hormone (GnRH). Fluoxetine can be used either daily or only during the symptomatic luteal phase. Alprazolam and GnRH have limited roles in the treatment of PMS in young women. Although some physicians have anecdotal success with other agents such as oral contraceptive pills (OCPs), progesterone, and vitamin B_6 in the treatment of PMS, these agents have not been demonstrated to be effective in controlled trials.

AMENORRHEA

19. What is the difference between primary and secondary amenorrhea?

Amenorrhea is the absence of menstrual flow for at least 6 months' duration. Primary amenorrhea is defined as the absence of any menses either by age 16, 3 years after the onset of secondary sexual differentiation, or within 1 year of developing Tanner V breasts and pubic hair. Patients with primary amenorrhea may or may not have other abnormalities in their growth and development. Patients with secondary amenorrhea experience the normal pubertal process culminating in menses, and then stop having menses.

20. How do you begin the evaluation of a patient with primary amenorrhea?

The initial evaluation begins with gathering information about the patient's growth and the development of her secondary sexual characteristics. The clinician should determine when and if pubertal landmarks such as breast bud development, axillary and pubic hair growth, and a linear growth spurt have occurred. It should be ascertained whether these changes were completed or interrupted during their development. It is important to ask about significant weight changes, and whether or not sexual activity has been initiated. The physical exam should begin with plotting the patient's height and weight on a growth chart and noting vital signs, particularly the blood pressure. Both short and tall statures are associated with specific syndromes involving primary amenorrhea. It is critical to assess the patient's growth history, because conditions such as Crohn's disease can cause primary amenorrhea as well as decreased growth velocity. The breast examination with Tanner staging can be very informative because estrogen production is necessary for breast development. The presence of axillary and pubic hair assures the clinician that the adrenal glands and ovaries are producing androgens (adrenarche) and that the body is having the appropriate physiologic response to their presence. Examination of the external and internal genitalia is of the utmost importance because primary amenorrhea is commonly due to a structural abnormality in the genital tract.

21. What kind of structural or anatomic abnormalities cause primary amenorrhea?

The most common anatomic abnormalities of the genital tract associated with primary amenorrhea are imperforate hymen and müllerian agenesis. These abnormalities occur with the failure of the canalization of the urogenital sinus (imperforate hymen) or failure of the formation, fusion, or canalization of the müllerian ducts (müllerian agenesis) during embryologic development. With both of these diagnoses, the ovaries are completely normal because they develop from a distinctly separate organ system.

22. What is imperforate hymen and how do you treat it?

Imperforate hymen occurs when the hymen covers the entire vagina and will not allow for egress of menstrual flow. These girls have normal ovaries and uteri and experience a normal pubertal process, but do not experience menarche because the menstrual flow cannot come through the vagina. If undetected prior to menarche, these girls often present with cyclic abdominal-pelvic pain as the menstrual flow is blocked behind the imperforate hymen. On physical examination, there is typically a bulging at the introitus, particularly with Valsalva maneuver. Treatment of imperforate hymen is a simple surgical procedure called hymenotomy whereby a cruciate incision is made in the hymen to allow menstrual egress.

23. What are the clinical findings of müllerian agenesis? Is it associated with any other abnormalities?

Müllerian agenesis (Rokitansky-Küster-Hauser syndrome) is the congenital absence of the uterus and vagina. On physical examination, height, weight, and secondary sexual characteristics are all normal, but the vagina is shortened, ending blindly with no evidence of a cervix. The midline uterus is absent on rectal examination. Up to 40% of patients with müllerian agenesis have a renal abnormality such as renal agenesis, malrotation, or ectopic kidney. Skeletal abnormalities include vertebral anomalies such as scoliosis; limb abnormalities can occur as well. Creation of a vagina for sexual activity can be accomplished either with the use of patient-directed vaginal dilators or by surgically creating a neovagina with split-thickness skin grafting. Rarely, patients may have a variant of müllerian agenesis with absence of a vagina but with the uterus and cervix present. Because these patients have a functional endometrium without a patent vagina for menstrual egress, they may present with cyclic abdominal or pelvic pain similar to patients with imperforate hymen.

24. What laboratory tests should you order for patients with primary amenorrhea? How do you interpret them?

The laboratory tests ordered should be tailored to the patient's history and physical findings. If you are unable to determine the cause of primary amenorrhea after the physical examination (i.e., you have verified a hymenal opening as well as the presence of a uterus), initial laboratory work-up commonly includes thyroid-stimulating hormone (TSH), prolactin, follicle-stimulating hormone (FSH), and luteinizing hormone (LH). Primary hypothyroidism is a rare cause of primary amenorrhea and can be associated with hyperprolactinemia. Hyperprolactinemia causes primary amenorrhea by suppressing LH and FSH, blocking the signal for stimulation of ovarian function. FSH and LH are in the low range when there is hypothalamic-pituitary dysfunction as the etiology of primary amenorrhea. When ovarian failure is the cause, FSH and LH will be elevated, as they are in menopausal women. As mentioned previously, patients with an anatomic cause of primary amenorrhea are eugonadal (normal FSH and LH) since their hypothalamic-pituitary axis and ovaries are functioning normally. If there is clinical evidence of androgen excess (hirsutism, acne, clitoromegaly), androstenedione, testosterone, and dehydroepiandrosterone sulfate (DHEAS) should also be measured. Finally, a CBC and erythrocyte sedimentation rate (ESR) should be considered to screen for occult inflammatory bowel disease.

25. Which patients presenting with primary amenorrhea need imaging studies of the head or chromosomal analyses?

If the patient has either hypothalamic hypogonadism (low FSH and LH) or hyperprolactinemia, magnetic resonance imaging (MRI) of the hypothalamic-pituitary area should be obtained to evaluate for lesions such as craniopharyngioma, hamartoma, and prolactin-secreting pituitary adenoma. Chromosomal studies should be ordered if the patient has ovarian failure (high FSH and LH) or if an intersex diagnosis is suspected.

26. What are the causes of primary amenorrhea due to hypothalamic-pituitary dysfunction (low FSH and LH)?

These include both primary and secondary causes of pituitary failure as well as neoplastic disorders. Kallmann's syndrome is a condition of hypoplasia of the olfactory tracts with coexisting dysfunction of the arcuate nucleus of the hypothalamus. The hypothalamus cannot secrete GnRH, leading to little or no secondary sexual development and amenorrhea; the sense of smell is also impaired. Isolated gonadotropin deficiency is a rare condition in which the hypothalamus cannot secrete GnRH and the patient has little or no secondary sexual differentiation and is amenorrheic. Sheehan's syndrome is uncommon in the adolescent; this syndrome occurs when the pituitary gland undergoes infarction and is no longer able to secrete tropic hormones. It is most commonly associated with post-partum hemorrhage and is therefore more likely to present as secondary amenorrhea. Neoplastic disorders associated with hypothalamic-pituitary dysfunction include craniopharyngioma and pituitary prolactinoma. These are diagnosed either by the presence of a visible abnormality on MRI or an elevated serum prolactin.

27. What causes ovarian failure (high FSH and LH) and primary amenorrhea?

Most cases of primary ovarian failure are due to aberrations of the X chromosome. Microdeletions in the long axis of the X chromosome or complete absence of the X chromosome results in accelerated atresia of the ovarian follicles and primary amenorrhea. The microdeletions are the most common abnormality, and affected patients will have a normal karyotype, 46XX. Absence of an X chromosome may be either complete (45,XO) or mosaic (46,XX/45,XO). Less common is ovarian failure due to alkylating chemotherapeutic agents or the very rare gonadotropin-resistant ovary syndrome (Savage syndrome).

28. What is the most common chromosomal abnormality associated with ovarian failure and primary amenorrhea?

Turner syndrome (45,XO) is the absence of one of the X chromosomes and is the most common chromosomal abnormality associated with primary amenorrhea due to ovarian failure. Patients with Turner syndrome undergo a more rapid atresia of their ovarian follicles due to the missing long arm of the X chromosome. Other characteristics of Turner syndrome include short stature, lack of development of secondary sexual characteristics, lymphedema, shield chest, webbed neck, and cubitus valgus (increased carrying angle of the arms). In mosaic Turner syndrome (45,XO/46,XX) some of the cell line has the normal chromosomal complement. Patients with mosaic Turner syndrome may undergo partial or full secondary sexual differentiation prior to ovarian failure.

29. What is Swyer's syndrome?

Swyer's syndrome (46,XY) is a variant of Turner syndrome. The testicles are dysgenetic during embryogenesis, resulting in failure to secrete müllerian duct inhibiting factor and testosterone. Therefore, patients are born with female external and internal genitalia. The patient is assigned female gender at birth, and the diagnosis is made at the time of puberty when there is no development of secondary sexual characteristics. The testicles need to be removed due to the high incidence (> 25%) of gonadoblastoma.

30. How do you treat a young woman with ovarian failure? Can she ever become pregnant?

Young women with ovarian failure may need to be given estrogen to complete the development of their breasts. After breast development is complete, they should be given estrogen and progestin therapy to facilitate sexual hair growth, stimulate uterine and endometrial growth, and initiate menses. If they are not given estrogen and progestin replacement therapy, they will develop significant osteoporosis due to hypoestrogenism. Young women are only able to become pregnant with the help of advanced reproductive technologies—specifically, oocyte donation or embryo transport.

31. How do you begin the evaluation of a patient with secondary amenorrhea?

Evaluation should begin by taking the patient's history with emphasis on weight changes, dietary habits, exercise patterns, sexual activity, life stressors, and previous menstrual history. Past surgical, gynecologic, and medical histories should also be obtained. A complete physical exam including pelvic examination should be performed.

32. What laboratory tests should be obtained in a patient with secondary amenorrhea?

The most important laboratory test to obtain in the patient who is sexually active is a pregnancy test. Pregnancy is a common diagnosis in sexually active adolescents who present with secondary amenorrhea. Other important laboratory tests include a TSH level to assess thyroid functioning and a prolactin level to rule out pituitary adenomas.

33. Why do clinicians give patients with secondary amenorrhea medroxyprogesterone acetate?

Medroxyprogesterone acetate, 10 mg daily for 10 days, is given once pregnancy has been ruled out to see if the patient responds with menses following progesterone withdrawal. This test is called the **progestin challenge**; if the patient begins menses, the test is positive. A positive test tells the clinician that the endometrium has been "primed" with estrogen from a functional hypothalamic-pituitary-ovarian axis and that the patient has a patent outflow track to allow menstrual egress.

34. If the pregnancy test, TSH, and prolactin are all normal, what is the most likely cause of the secondary amenorrhea?

If pregnancy has been ruled out and thyroid and prolactin values are normal, most cases of secondary amenorrhea are due to hypogonadotropic hypogonadism. Common factors in this syndrome include stress, strenuous exercise regimens, low weight, and low body fat. Typically these issues need to be addressed before the menses return to normal.

35. How would you counsel a 17-year-old track and field star who, after menarche at age 15, is now 66 inches tall and weighs 107 pounds, runs 20–40 miles per week, and has been amenorrheic (happily) for the last 9 months?

This is a typical presentation of the amenorrheic athlete who is exercising vigorously, is underweight with presumably a low body fat content, and has become amenorrheic. Even with her strenuous weight-bearing exercise, she is at increased risk for osteoporosis and stress-related injuries. She should be counseled to gain weight or reduce her weekly mileage and to take medications both to protect her bones from osteoporosis and to help her resume menstruation. Although OCPs have questionable benefit for prevention of osteoporosis in this clinical scenario, they are the treatment of choice if the patient is sexually active. If she is not sexually active, she could take hormone replacement therapy instead of OCPs. Calcium supplements should be taken if necessary, to ensure total calcium intake of 1200–1500 mg per day.

CERVICAL DYSPLASIA

36. How do you interpret Pap smear results? What is the Bethesda system?

Pap smears are tests developed to screen for cervical cancer. The National Cancer Institute met in Bethesda, Maryland, in 1988 to standardize cervical and vaginal cytology reports to facilitate peer review and quality assurance. From this workshop came a new system to report Pap smear results in three categories: adequacy of the specimen, general categorization, and descriptive diagnoses. **Adequacy** reflects whether the specimen was properly labeled and whether both the squamous and endocervical cells could be read without being obscured by blood or inflammation. Endocervical cells must be present for the Pap smear to be reported as "adequate." The **general categorization** is either "within normal limits," "benign cellular changes," or "epithelial cell abnormality." The **descriptive diagnosis** describes in greater detail the latter two categories.

37. What are some of the abnormalities that are reported as "benign cellular changes" on Pap smear?

Abnormalities associated with "benign cellular changes" are usually consistent with either infection or repair. Several infections such as trichomoniasis, yeast, and bacterial vaginosis can be identified cytologically with reasonable specificity. Of note, chlamydial infections cannot. The term *reactive changes* is used to report cellular findings that are consistent with a reactive reparative process.

38. How do you treat patients with benign cellular changes?

Treatment should be geared toward the specific result. If the Pap smear reports an infection, the patient should be treated with the appropriate antibiotics. Wet mount for various forms of vaginitis and cervical testing for gonorrhea and chlamydia may be indicated, particularly in patients who are sexually active. Reactive or reparative changes do not need further evaluation.

39. What are the "epithelial cell abnormalities" that are identified by Pap smear?

Epithelial cell abnormalities are divided into two groups: squamous and glandular. The squamous abnormalities include atypical squamous cells of undetermined significance (ASCUS), low-grade squamous intraepithelial lesion (LGSIL), high-grade intraepithelial lesion (HGSIL), and squamous cell carcinoma. The glandular abnormalities include the presence of endometrial cells, atypical glandular cells of undetermined significance, and adenocarcinoma.

40. What is colposcopy?

Colposcopy is a tool used to evaluate the cervix for dysplasia or cancer. It involves using a speculum to view the cervix, "staining" the cervix with dilute acetic acid, and examining the cervix through a large microscope called a colposcope. Dysplastic areas of the cervix stain white with the acetic acid, and different colored filters on the colposcope allow the clinician to see vascular changes also present with dysplasia. Both the ectocervix and endocervix are visualized and examined for abnormalities. If abnormalities are identified, they are biopsied and sent for pathologic evaluation. Clinicians may take one or more biopsies from the exocervix and may take a scraping, or endocervical curettage (ECC), of the endocervix. The clinician develops a treatment plan for the patient based on the Pap smear results, the visual appearance of the cervix on colposcopy, and the results of the cervical biopsies and ECC.

41. What is the appropriate follow-up for an ASCUS Pap smear result?

Several management options are available for patients with ASCUS. The incidence of dysplasia with ASCUS is reported to be from 10% to 40%, and the incidence of invasive cancer is very rare. The broad range of possible outcomes with ASCUS Pap smears forces the clinician to tailor the follow-up to the patient's history. Although the low incidence of cervical cancer in adolescents supports conservative follow-up, adolescents' notoriety with poor compliance suggests that under certain circumstances, aggressive evaluation may be indicated. One management option includes follow-up Pap smear in 3–6 months with colposcopy if the abnormality persists. Some clinicians move directly to colposcopy for all patients with one ASCUS Pap, whereas others move to colposcopy directly only for patients with a remote history of dysplasia or suspected poor compliance. Alternatively, some clinicians perform human papillomavirus (HPV) testing on patients with ASCUS Pap smears and perform colposcopy on patients who test positive for the more oncogenic HPV strains.

42. What evaluation is indicated for patients with LGSIL, HGSIL, or squamous carcinoma reported on Pap smear?

All patients with HGSIL or squamous cell carcinoma reported on Pap smear should undergo colposcopy. Because most LGSIL lesions (> 80%) will regress spontaneously in women younger than 34, some clinicians will repeat a LGSIL Pap smear and perform colposcopy only in patients with persistent lesions; however, most clinicians favor immediate colposcopy.

43. How should glandular abnormalities be evaluated?

The presence of endometrial cells is normal in menstruating women, regardless of when in the cycle the Pap smear was obtained and requires no further evaluation. Other glandular abnormalities are very rare in adolescents, but if reported should be evaluated with colposcopy and possible endometrial biopsy.

44. How do you define and treat cervical intraepithelial neoplasia (CIN)?

CIN, a pre-cancerous lesion (dysplasia), is limited to the squamous cells of the cervix superficial to the basement membrane. CIN I often will regress spontaneously and can be followed with Pap smears. If it does not regress within 1 year of diagnosis, it should be treated. Persistent CIN I and more aggressive lesions, CIN II or CIN III, often can be treated successfully with numerous methods including cryotherapy, laser vaporization, and loop electrosurgical excision (LEEP). The modality chosen depends on factors such as the size and shape of the lesion and the patient's cervix and should be tailored to the individual patient. All treatment modalities report a small chance of hemorrhage, cervical stenosis, and infertility. Treatment success depends on the modality used and the size and grade of the lesion but in general ranges from 77% to 96% cure rate.

45. What kind of follow-up do patients need after treatment for CIN?

Patients treated for CIN should undergo a repeat Pap smear 3 months after treatment; if normal continue Pap smears every 3 months for the first year. During the second year, they should have Pap smears every 6 months. If after 2 years of surveillance the Pap smears are normal, they may resume annual Pap smear screening.

VAGINITIS

46. How do you perform a microscopic examination of vaginal discharge?

A vaginal specimen is obtained by collecting the vaginal secretions from the posterior fornix of the vagina with a cotton-tipped swab. After collecting the specimen, the swab should be placed in a test tube with normal saline at room temperature. The pH of the sample is determined using pH indicator paper, and the sample is smeared on a slide. Normal saline is added to one part of the slide and potassium hydroxide (KOH) is added to another part of the slide; both parts are covered with cover slips. The slide can then be examined under the microscope. A "whiff test," or amine test, is performed when the KOH is added to detect any fishy odor. The examination under the microscope should include characterization of the epithelial cells, the predominant flora (i.e., bacilli or cocci), the presence of inflammatory cells, and the presence of any pathogens.

47. What is a normal vaginal discharge?

Normal vaginal discharge is white, homogeneous, and odorless. Its pH during the reproductive years is 3.5–4.2, but it may be more alkaline on exposure to semen or menstrual blood. Microscopically a normal discharge has superficial epithelial cells, flora composed of lactobacilli, and occasional leukocytes. Adding 10% KOH (the whiff test) does not change the odor.

48. What causes the physiologic leukorrhea of puberty?

During puberty adolescents may experience a copious clear-to-white colored vaginal discharge with a tenacious consistency and without odor. It may develop weeks to months prior to the onset of menarche and may persist for several years. It occurs in response to increased circulating levels of estrogens and is composed of desquamated vaginal cells, vaginal transudate, and endocervical mucus. The discharge is normal and requires no further intervention beyond reassuring the patient and her parents and ruling out other causes of vaginal discharge.

49. What are some of the common causes of abnormal vaginal discharge in adolescents?

Vaginitis in adolescents is usually due to a specific cause such as bacterial vaginosis, *Candida albicans*, or trichomoniasis. Diagnosis and treatment is based on vaginal pH and microscopic appearance of the discharge.

50. What is bacterial vaginosis? How do you diagnose and treat it?

Bacterial vaginosis is a mixed vaginal infection involving anaerobes with a relative loss of the normal vaginal lactobacillus. Patients may be asymptomatic or may complain of a thin discharge and fishy vaginal odor. Bacterial vaginosis is diagnosed with equal frequency in both sexually active and virginal adolescents. The exact cause of bacterial vaginosis is unknown. Diagnosis is made by elevation of vaginal pH above 4.5, positive whiff test, and the presence of greater than 20% clue cells on microscopy. Oral metronidazole, metronidazole vaginal gel, and clindamycin vaginal cream are all effective treatments for bacterial vaginosis. Treatment of the male sexual partner is not indicated.

51. How do you diagnosis and treat *Candida albicans*?

Patients with *Candida albicans* vaginitis typically experience vaginal itching and burning as well as a thick, yellowish vaginal discharge. Patients often will describe a discharge that looks like "cottage cheese." Diagnosis is confirmed by a vaginal pH < 4.5 and the presence of hyphae on microscopic examination. Treatment options include oral fluconazole (150 mg tablet given once) or various topical antifungal creams containing butoconazole, nystatom (Mycostatin), miconazole, tioconazole, terconazole, or clotrimazole.

52. How do you diagnose and treat *Trichomonas vaginalis*?

Trichomoniasis should be considered a sexually transmitted disease, and if the diagnosis is made, the patient should be screened for other STDs. Patients with trichomoniasis usually present with a copious yellow-gray or green, foamy vaginal discharge. Trichomoniasis is diagnosed by the presence of mobile flagellated organisms on a fresh wet-mount preparation. The pH level is usually greater than 4.5. The accepted treatment regimen for trichomoniasis is a single dose of metronidazole, 2 gm orally. Sexual partners need to be treated simultaneously for treatment to be effective. An alternative regimen is metronidazole, 500 mg orally twice daily for 7 days.

PELVIC PAIN

53. What is mittelschmerz?

Mittelschmerz is mid-cycle pain due to ovulation. Some patients experience a transient lower abdominal discomfort around the time of ovulation for 24–48 hours. The pain most likely is due to stretching of the ovarian capsule with ovulation or the release of follicular fluid causing irritation to the peritoneal lining. In most patients, this pain is relieved with the use of nonsteroidal anti-inflammatory drugs (NSAIDs) and does not interfere significantly with school, work, or other activities. In more severe cases, effective therapies include oral contraceptives and medroxyprogesterone acetate, which work by inhibiting ovulation.

54. What is primary dysmenorrhea and what causes it?

Dysmenorrhea includes a constellation of symptoms around the time of menses including cramping, lower abdominal pain, lower backache, nausea and vomiting, fatigue, diarrhea, and headache. The symptoms are usually worse during the first couple of days of the menses.

Primary dysmenorrhea occurs due to the increased production of prostaglandins E_2 (PGE_2) and prostaglandin $F_{2\alpha}$ ($PGF_{2\alpha}$) in a patient with an anatomically normal uterus. The increased prostaglandin production results in increased muscle tone both in the uterine muscle (the myometrium), leading to strong menstrual cramps, and in the wall of the intestine, leading to abdominal complaints. Primary dysmenorrhea is common in young women. It usually begins a couple of years after menarche, when the cycles are ovulatory, and usually resolves spontaneously in the late teens or early 20s.

55. What are effective treatments for primary dysmenorrhea?

For some patients, education, reassurance, and simple comfort measures are all that is necessary. If more intervention is required, NSAIDs can be very effective in the treatment of primary dysmenorrhea, because of their antiprostaglandin effect. It is important that patients take NSAIDs at their prescribed doses at the earliest onset of symptoms and continue to use them on a scheduled basis for the best symptom relief. If bothersome symptoms persist despite appropriately dosed NSAIDs, OCPs are an effective treatment with a > 90% response rate. The mechanism of action of OCPs is believed to include the thinning of the endometrial lining, resulting in decreased prostaglandin production. Some patients require OCPs and NSAIDs together for complete resolution of their symptoms. Medroxyprogesterone acetate can be used if the patient is unable to tolerate OCPs or if estrogen is contraindicated. The mechanism of action is similar to that of OCPs.

56. What is secondary dysmenorrhea?

Secondary dysmenorrhea is painful menstrual cycles due to significant pelvic pathology. The most common causes include endometriosis and obstructive müllerian anomalies. Endometriosis is defined as the presence of endometrial glands and stroma found outside of the uterine cavity. This tissue is responsive to hormonal changes in the menstrual cycle and can cause pain, painful periods, adhesion formation, and infertility. Young women with painful periods not resolving with the use of hormonal contraception and NSAIDs need to be evaluated for endometriosis with diagnostic laparoscopy. Mullerian anomalies that may cause dysmenorrhea include any anomaly of the vagina, cervix, or uterus preventing the egress of menstrual flow resulting in a collection of menstrual blood above the level of the obstruction, causing pain by distention. Symptoms usually begin with menarche and worsen progressively with each cycle until the obstruction is surgically corrected. Examples of müllerian anomalies include imperforate hymen, transverse vaginal septum, and bicornuate uterus with a noncommunicating horn. Other causes of secondary dysmenorrhea in adolescents include pelvic inflammatory disease, ovarian cysts, and cervical stenosis. Treatment for secondary dysmenorrhea focuses on treating the underlying pathology.

57. What are some of the causes of chronic pelvic pain in adolescents?

Chronic pelvic pain is defined as lower abdominal pain of at least 6 months' duration. The broad differential diagnosis for chronic pelvic pain in adolescents includes gastrointestinal (GI), musculoskeletal, urologic, psychosocial, and gynecologic causes. The etiology of the pain may be multifactorial.

58. How do you begin to evaluate a young woman with a complaint of chronic pelvic pain?

A variety of somatic, psychological, and social factors may, alone or in combination, play a role in the pain syndrome. All of these factors should be explored together from the onset of the evaluation. Like most aspects of medicine, the evaluation should begin with a complete and thorough history. The history should begin with the patient describing the nature, extent, and location of the pain as well as anything that causes exacerbation or brings relief. Medical and surgical evaluations and interventions to date should be reviewed. Past medical, surgical, gynecologic, and sexual histories also should be obtained. A pain calendar may be helpful to determine whether there is a cyclic component of the pain. Urologic, gastrointestinal, and musculoskeletal symptoms should be explored. Family history of endometriosis or other chronic pain syndromes or disabilities should be elicited. Psychosocial factors should be evaluated by asking about depression, eating disorders, substance abuse, sexual or physical abuse, number of school days missed, major life changes or stressors, and coping style.

59. After you have completed the history, what's next in the evaluation?

Physical examination comes next. The physical exam should be focused and directed to assess the various potential sources of pain elicited during the history. To screen for musculoskeletal causes of pain, examine the patient's posture for evidence of lordosis, one-legged standing, or leg-length discrepancy. Palpate the upper and lower back while the patient is sitting. When she is on her back, palpate her abdominal wall while she does leg flexion and head and leg raises. Ask her to point to the area where it hurts the most. With psychosomatic pain, the adolescent typically has difficulty isolating a small area where the pain originates. While performing a pelvic exam, consider urologic as well as gynecologic causes of pain. Palpate the urethra and bladder base, and note any specific tenderness. Also palpate the vaginal fornices for tenderness or masses. On bimanual exam, evaluate the uterus and palpate the adnexa. A rectal examination is essential, particularly if a GI source of pain is suspected.

60. What laboratories and imaging studies should be ordered for patients with chronic pelvic pain?

Laboratory tests should be tailored to the patient's initial evaluation but in general should include CBC with differential, urinalysis and culture, and ESR. Pelvic ultrasound should be reserved for patients with a suspected abnormality on pelvic exam or a compromised or incomplete pelvic examination.

61. What are the more common urologic causes of chronic pelvic pain?

Urinary tract infections and kidney stones are the more common urologic causes of chronic pelvic pain.

62. What are the more common gastroenterologic causes of chronic pelvic pain?

By far the most common GI cause of chronic pelvic pain is constipation, which is common in adolescents because of poor diet and bowel habits. Other less common causes include irritable bowel syndrome, inflammatory bowel disease, lactose intolerance, gastroenteritis, chronic appendicitis, and inguinal hernias.

63. What are some musculoskeletal causes of chronic pelvic pain?

Numerous musculoskeletal abnormalities can cause pelvic pain either directly or through referred pain. Most musculoskeletal abnormalities cause pain directly through increased muscle tone. Lumbar vertebrae, joint capsules, ligaments, discs, hip joints, and muscles such as the abdominals, iliopsoas, quadratus lumborum, piriformis, and obturator internus and externus are innervated from the T12–L4 region of the spine and can refer pain to the lower abdomen and the anterior thigh. This pain can change in character as progesterone and relaxin levels fluctuate during the menstrual cycle. Etiologies include postural abnormalities or leg length discrepancy, trigger points (areas of hyperirritability within a skeletal muscle), joint pain, inflammation, and spinal injury.

64. What type of psychosocial factors play a role in chronic pelvic pain?

Psychosocial factors may play a significant role in any chronic pain syndrome—either as a primary cause of the pain or as a modifier in the patient's response to painful stimuli. Patients should be evaluated for psychosocial abnormalities from the outset of their evaluation. Symptoms of depression, anxiety, sexual abuse, substance abuse, eating disorders, hypochondriasis, and school avoidance behavior should be appropriately evaluated. The patient's current life stresses as well as her ability to cope with problems also should be investigated.

65. What are the more common gynecologic disorders responsible for chronic pelvic pain in adolescents?

Endometriosis, pelvic inflammatory disease, pelvic adhesive disease, obstructive congenital anomalies, and ovarian masses are some of the more common causes of chronic pelvic pain in adolescents. Most of these conditions are diagnosed either by pelvic ultrasound or laparoscopy.

66. What is endometriosis, and how is it diagnosed?

Endometriosis is the presence of endometrial glands and stroma outside of the endometrial cavity. Symptoms of endometriosis include pelvic pain, dysmenorrhea, abnormal vaginal bleeding, and dyspareunia. Pelvic examination and ultrasound studies may be completely normal in patients with endometriosis. The diagnosis is made by laparoscopy, either by direct visualization of endometriotic implants on the peritoneum or by pathologic diagnosis of the peritoneum showing microscopic endometriosis.

67. What are the options for treating endometriosis?

Endometriosis is usually managed with a combination of surgical and medical therapies. Treatment typically begins at the time of laparoscopic diagnosis with surgical resection or ablation of the grossly visible lesions and resection of any adhesive disease. Postoperatively, patients are typically hormonally suppressed with continuous birth control pills, medroxyprogesterone acetate, or GnRH agonists. Patients with a family history of endometriosis are at increased risk for the same.

68. Which patients with chronic pelvic pain should undergo diagnostic laparoscopy? What are typical findings?

Laparoscopy can be extremely useful for both diagnosis and treatment in select cases. Patients with significant pain of unknown etiology after a comprehensive evaluation or patients with dysmenorrhea unresponsive to NSAIDs and OCPs are candidates for diagnostic laparoscopy. Patients with suspected pathology identified on physical examination or radiologic imaging such as adnexal masses or uterine abnormalities are also candidates for laparoscopy for both diagnostic and therapeutic purposes. The majority of appropriately selected adolescents undergoing diagnostic laparoscopy for chronic pelvic pain will have pathology at the time of surgery. The most common finding is endometriosis. Other potential causes of pain commonly identified at laparoscopy include pelvic adhesions, appendicitis, and evidence of pelvic inflammatory disease.

69. What kind of ovarian abnormalities can cause chronic pelvic pain?

The most common ovarian mass in the adolescent is the functional cyst, a simple, unilocular, fluid-filled mass that is a frequent ultrasound finding even in asymptomatic patients. Functional cysts are typically *not* a source of pelvic pain, do not require surgical intervention, and typically resolve spontaneously. They may be followed with repeat ultrasound evaluation. Clinicians should be careful not to attribute excessive pathology to functional cysts, thus failing to discover the true source(s) of the pain. Dermoids (mature cystic teratomas) are the most common ovarian neoplasms found in adolescents and can cause pain either by stretching the ovarian cortex, compressing adjacent structures, or leading to adnexal torsion. Ovarian cystectomy, with preservation of the remaining normal ovary, is the treatment of choice for dermoid tumors. Endometriomas are masses found on the ovary that represent an advanced stage of endometriosis and may be associated with pelvic pain. Endometriomas also require ovarian cystectomy for treatment. Tubo-ovarian abscesses (TOAs) or masses resulting from pelvic inflammatory disease may also present as chronic pelvic pain.

70. What types of uterine abnormalities can present with chronic pelvic pain?

The most common uterine abnormalities in adolescents with pelvic pain are the obstructive congenital müllerian anomalies. These include bicornuate uterus with a noncommunicating rudimentary horn and uterine didelphia with an obstructed hemi-vagina. These abnormalities typically present with lower abdominal pain worsening cyclically with menses. The abnormalities both have functional endometrium not connected to the vagina, and therefore menstrual egress is blocked. The menstrual blood accumulates in the obstructed organ causing pain due to distention. Retrograde menses from the obstructed organ increases the likelihood of endometriosis. Müllerian anomalies should be suspected when patients have other congenital anomalies, particularly renal or skeletal abnormalities. Diagnosis is usually made with pelvic ultrasound or pelvic MRI. Treatment involves surgical intervention with relief of the obstruction and preservation of fertility.

BIBLIOGRAPHY

1. American College of Obstetricians and Gynecologists: Amenorrhea. ACOG Technical Bulletin 128. Washington, DC, ACOG, 1989.
2. American College of Obstetricians and Gynecologists: Cervical Cytology: Evaluation and Management of Abnormalities. ACOG Technical Bulletin 183. Washington, DC, ACOG.
3. American College of Obstetricians and Gynecologists: Premenstrual Syndrome. ACOG Practice Bulletin 15. Washington, DC, ACOG, 2000.
4. American College of Obstetricians and Gynecologists: Vaginitis. ACOG Technical Bulletin 220. Washington, DC, ACOG, 1996.
5. American Fertility Society: Management of endometriosis in the presence of pelvic pain. Fertil Steril 60:952–955, 1993.
6. Claessens EA, Cowell CL: Acute adolescent menorrhagia. Am J Obstet Gynecol 139:277–280, 1981.
7. Falcone T, Desjardins C, Bourque J, et al: Dysfunctional uterine bleeding in the adolescents. J Repro Med 39:761–764, 1994.
8. Hertweck SP: Dysfunctional uterine bleeding. Obstet Gynecol Clin North Am 19:129–149, 1992.
9. Abnormal uterine bleeding. In Koehler SE, Carpenter J, Rock A (eds): Pediatric and Adolescent Gynecology. Philadelphia, Lippincott-Raven, 1996, pp 189–204.
10. Dysmenorrhea. In Koehler SE, Carpenter J, Rock A (eds): Pediatric and Adolescent Gynecology. Philadelphia, Lippincott-Raven, 1996, pp 205–221.
11. Ling Fu (ed): Contemporary Management of Chronic Pelvic Pain. Obstetrics and Gynecology Clinic of North America, volume 20. Philadelphia, W.B. Saunders, 1993.
12. National Cancer Institute Workshop: The 1988 Bethesda System for reporting cervical/vaginal cytological diagnoses. JAMA 262:931–934, 1989.

24. SEXUALLY TRANSMITTED INFECTIONS

Cynthia Holland-Hall, M.D., M.P.H.

TRENDS AND GENERAL INFORMATION

1. Who is more likely to be diagnosed with a sexually transmitted infection (STI)—a teenager or an adult?

Sexually active teens are more likely than adults to acquire an STI. An estimated 25% of teens develop an STI before graduating from high school. Although the incidence of many reported STIs has decreased during the past several years, adolescents and young adults continue to have higher age-specific rates of infection than any other age group. For example, in the U.S. in 1998, the rate of chlamydial infection among people 25–39 years of age was 201/100,000. For people 15–24 years of age, the rate was 1212/100,000.

2. Why do teenagers get more STIs than older adults?

Various factors contribute to this phenomenon. From a biologic standpoint, an adolescent girl is more likely than an adult woman to have exposed columnar epithelial cells on her ectocervix, referred to as the **ectropion**. As a woman ages, the transitional zone between the columnar and squamous cells on the cervix regresses into the endocervical canal. Because columnar cells are more susceptible to infection by certain sexually transmitted pathogens such as *Chlamydia* sp., teenage girls are more likely to acquire these infections if exposed. Furthermore, because they have been sexually active for a shorter time, teens are less likely than adults to have developed mucosal immunity to certain pathogens.

From a behavioral standpoint, teens are less likely than adults to be in long-term, monogamous relationships and more likely to have multiple sex partners. They may also be less experienced and less skilled at negotiating condom use with their partners and therefore more likely to have unprotected sex.

3. Why are females diagnosed with so many more infections than males?

The anatomy of the female genitalia, including the cervical ectropion, makes male-to-female transmission rates higher than female-to-male transmission rates for many organisms. In addition, asymptomatic females are frequently tested for STIs when they present for Pap smears, prescription contraceptives, or other gynecologic needs. Asymptomatic males are less likely to seek testing. Because females are more likely to be *tested* than males, they are also more likely to be *diagnosed* with STIs.

4. Do most people with STIs have symptoms?

No. Although most STIs can cause symptoms at times, infected persons are often asymptomatic and may not know they are infected. This is particularly true for chlamydial and viral STIs.

5. If a teen has one STI, how likely is it that he or she has others?

Having one STI is a strong risk factor for having another STI concurrently or developing another STI in the future. For example, in persons under 25 years old who are infected with *Neisseria gonorrhoeae*, 20–40% of women and 10–30% of men are coinfected with *Chlamydia trachomatis*. Teens who are diagnosed with one STI, therefore, should be screened for the presence of others.

6. Does condom use prevent STI transmission?

Rigorous studies of condom efficacy are difficult to perform, and solid data are lacking for many infections. Condoms clearly have been shown to reduce significantly the risk of human immunodeficiency virus (HIV) transmission when used consistently. Many studies also have demonstrated a protective effect against gonorrhea and, to a lesser extent, chlamydial infection. For ulcerative STIs, such as syphilis, herpes, and chancroid, condoms offer some protection, but protection is not complete. Condoms have *not* been shown to reduce the risk of human papillomavirus (HPV) acquisition, although some studies show a reduced risk of cervical changes and genital warts. Providers, therefore, must be careful when counseling teens about condom use. Teens should understand that using a condom does not eliminate the possibility of acquiring an STI but clearly reduces overall risk.

7. Which STIs are reportable to the local health department?
The following STIs are nationally reportable to the Centers for Disease Control and Prevention (CDC):

- Acquired immunodeficiency syndrome (AIDS)
- Chancroid
- *C. trachomatis*
- *N. gonorrhoeae*
- Hepatitis B
- HIV (pediatric)
- Syphilis (congenital or acquired)

However, reporting of these infections to the CDC by the states is voluntary. Because reporting can be mandated only by individual states, the above list may vary from state to state. Health care providers are responsible for notifying local, county, or state health departments when they diagnose a reportable infection. Clinical laboratories also may participate in the reporting process.

8. How can I predict which teens are most likely to have infections?
Certain behaviors place teens at particularly high risk of acquiring an STI (see table below). Nonetheless, infections are often diagnosed even in teens with single partners who report regular condom use. No constellation of demographic factors, sexual history, and clinical findings reliably predicts the presence of the majority of STIs. Therefore, routine screening of *all* sexually active teens is recommended.

Factors Placing Teens at High Risk of Acquiring an STI

Multiple sex partners	Signs or symptoms of STI
Young age at first intercourse	No/inconsistent condom use
New sex partner	Exchanging sex for drugs, money, food
Partner with an STI	Men who have sex with men
Prior STI	

9. How often should sexually active teenagers be tested for STIs?
Sexually active teenage girls should receive annual pelvic examinations, including the following components: visual inspection of the genitalia for evidence of herpetic lesions or genital warts; a Papanicolaou smear for evidence of cervical dysplasia caused by HPV; microscopy or culture of vaginal fluids to detect *Trichomonas vaginalis*; and endocervical testing for *N. gonorrhoeae* and *C. trachomatis*. Most adolescent health experts recommend semiannual screening for *C. trachomatis* because of its high prevalence and the asymptomatic nature of most infections. More frequent testing for all treatable infections should be considered in teens with multiple partners, teens who engage in unprotected sex, and those teens with history of a prior STI. Asymptomatic teenage boys should be screened for gonococcal and chlamydial urethritis, although recommendations for the timing of routine screening of males are less clear. Serologic screening for HIV and syphilis should be routinely performed where these infections are endemic and strongly considered in any sexually active teen.

10. What types of tests are available for diagnosing *N. gonorrhoeae* and *C. trachomatis*?
Bacterial culture is the traditional gold standard for identifying both organisms. Because of the high specificity of culture, it is the only diagnostic test admissible as evidence of infection

in the legal setting. Culture is sensitive for *N. gonorrhoeae*, but poor (about 70%) for *C. trachomatis*. In either case, sensitivity decreases when specimens are not quickly transported to a laboratory and processed under appropriate conditions.

Antigen detection techniques, such as enzyme immunosorbent assays (EIA), are generally less expensive and easily processed. They offer increased sensitivity over culture for *C. trachomatis* but not for *N. gonorrhoeae*.

Nonamplified DNA probes are widely used because of the ease of specimen handling, reasonable cost, and 80–85% sensitivity.

Nucleic acid amplification (NAA) techniques, such as polymerase chain reaction (PCR) and ligase chain reaction (LCR), are extremely sensitive and quite specific for both organisms, although false positives may occur. Although they are among the more expensive diagnostic tests for gonococcal and chlamydial infections, the increased rate of detection, particularly for chlamydial infections, makes them cost-effective in high-prevalence settings.

11. Does the provider have to do a pelvic exam and/or urethral swab to diagnose gonococcal and chlamydial infection?

It depends on the diagnostic technique. Cultures require viable organisms for successful diagnosis. Therefore, endocervical and/or urethral specimens must be obtained. NAA requires only tiny amounts of genetic material, which remains stable even in a nonviable organism. PCR and LCR, therefore, may be used on first-void urine samples and vaginal introital swabs, although at present only urine testing is approved by the Food and Drug Administration.

12. If a physician diagnoses an STI, may he or she prescribe antibiotics for the patient's partner as well as for the patient?

Partner treatment is one of the greatest challenges in STI management, and it is critical for the prevention of reinfection. It may be tempting to write an additional prescription for the patient's partner rather than trusting that he or she will be evaluated and appropriately treated elsewhere. Before considering this option, make sure that you are familiar with prescribing laws in your state (e.g., the legality of prescribing to a patient whom you have not examined in person), and do not forget to take into account the possibility of the partner's underlying medical conditions, medication allergies, and ability to adhere properly to the prescribed regimen. It is always preferable for partners to be evaluated and treated individually, by you or another provider.

ORGANISMS THAT CAUSE CERVICITIS AND URETHRITIS

13. What organisms cause nongonococcal urethritis (NGU) in males?

C. trachomatis causes 25–55% of cases overall. *Mycoplasma genitalium* and *Ureaplasma urealyticum* are implicated in up to one-third of cases. These three organisms are generally susceptible to the same antibiotics. *T. vaginalis* and herpes simplex virus may cause NGU as well. Empiric treatment should be considered when treatment for the former organisms fails to relieve symptoms.

14. What organisms are most likely to be isolated in women with mucopurulent cervicitis (MPC)?

N. gonorrhoeae and *C. trachomatis*. However, in many women with MPC, which is characterized by a purulent endocervical discharge or exudate and possibly friability of the cervix, tests for both organisms are negative. Conversely, most women infected with these organisms do not have MPC.

15. Are gonococcal infections increasing or decreasing in the U.S.?

After years of declining rates, gonorrhea has slowly been increasing since the late 1990s. Rates of infection are highest in females 15–19 years of age and males 20–24 years of age. In recent years, about 75% of all reported cases of gonorrhea occurred in persons 15–29 years old. Over 75% of all reported cases occurred in African Americans.

16. What are the symptoms of gonococcal genital infection?

Males with gonococcal urethritis usually experience dysuria and a purulent penile discharge. Ascending infection may lead to epididymitis. Females with genital infections may develop a purulent vaginal discharge and have milder, nonspecific signs of infection such as dysuria—or they may be completely asymptomatic. Untreated infection may progress to pelvic inflammatory disease. Rectal infections may present with anal itching, discharge, pain, or bleeding.

17. What is the most common cause of infectious arthritis in teens?

Staphylococcus aureus is the most common organism in teens, just as it is in other age groups. *N. gonorrhoeae*, however, is the second most common organism isolated in adolescents with septic joints.

18. How does gonococcal pharyngitis differ clinically from group A streptocccocal pharyngitis?

Pharyngeal infection with *N. gonorrhoeae* is usually asymptomatic. Parenteral treatment with ceftriaxone may be necessary to eradicate the organism from the pharynx.

19. What are symptoms of disseminated gonococcal infection (DGI)?

DGI may occur after gonococcal bacteremia (gonococcemia). Symptoms include arthritis or migratory arthralgias, skin lesions, tenosynovitis, fever, and mild hepatitis. Meningitis, endocarditis, and glomerulonephritis occur rarely. Several studies indicate that DGI is more likely to occur in the presence of pharyngeal gonorrhea; therefore, pharyngeal as well as genital cultures should be performed if DGI or gonococcal arthritis is suspected.

20. Which cultures are most likely to be positive for *N. gonorrhoeae* in a patient with DGI?

Genital and pharyngeal cultures are most likely to be positive. Cultures of the blood, skin lesions, or synovial fluid are much less likely to result in isolation of the organism.

21. What is appropriate treatment for gonococcal infection?

A number of single-dose treatments are available to treat uncomplicated cervicitis or urethritis. Parenteral treatment and more prolonged courses of antibiotics are required for pelvic inflammatory disease, pharyngitis, arthritis, or DGI. Because of the high coinfection rate with *C. trachomatis*, cotreatment for this organism is recommended.

Single-Dose Treatment for Gonococcal Cervicitis and Urethritis

Cefixime, 400 mg orally, *or*
Ceftriaxone, 125 mg intramuscularly, *or*
Ciprofloxacin, 500 mg orally, *or*
Ofloxacin, 400 mg orally

22. What is the most common bacterial sexually transmitted infection?

C. trachomatis is not only the most common bacterial STI; it is the most commonly reported infectious disease in the United States. Because of increased screening and treatment efforts throughout the country, it is believed that chlamydial infection may be declining. Nonetheless, it is perhaps the most serious STI epidemic facing teens today. In many parts of the country, prevalence of infection is 5–10% or more among sexually active teens.

23. What are symptoms of chlamydial infection?

Women with chlamydial infections may present with mucopurulent cervicitis, urethritis, or symptoms of pelvic inflammatory disease. Men may present with urethritis or epididymitis. Both males and females with chlamydial infections, however, are most likely to have no symptoms at all; for this reason, routine screening is necessary. It is estimated that as many as 80–90% of chlamydial infections in women are asymptomatic.

24. How are chlamydial infections treated?

Uncomplicated urethritis or cervicitis can be treated with a single dose of azithromycin, 1 gm orally. This regimen has become popular because of its simplicity and high efficacy. Doxycycline, 100 mg twice daily for 7 days, is equally efficacious if taken correctly, but adherence can be a problem in teens. This regimen is significantly less expensive—an important factor for teens who are paying for their own medications. Pelvic inflammatory disease and epididymitis require additional therapy.

25. What is Reiter's syndrome?

Reiter's syndrome consists of the triad of arthritis, urethritis, and conjunctivitis or other ocular manifestations. Additional mucocutaneous manifestations are often present as well. It often follows infection with *C. trachomatis*, although it may occur after a gonococcal infection or an enteric bacterial infection as well. Reiter's syndrome after an STI typically affects men more than women.

26. Is a "test of cure" necessary after treating a gonococcal or chlamydial infection?

Given the highly efficacious single-dose treatment regimens now available, test of cure is no longer routinely recommended. Test of cure may be considered if a multidose regimen is used and adherence is questionable. In this case, however, testing should not be performed until 3 weeks after treatment is completed, because highly sensitive diagnostic techniques may identify remnants of nonviable organisms for several days after successful treatment. Because of the challenges of ensuring partner treatment, many experts recommend performing "test of reinfection" several weeks after initial diagnosis and treatment.

TRICHOMONIASIS

27. What are the classic features of *T. vaginalis* infections?

T. vaginalis, a single-celled, flagellated protozoan, is one of the most common treatable STIs. Women with trichomoniasis may present with vulvovaginal signs and symptoms, including a frothy, malodorous vaginal discharge, dysuria, and vulvar itching and irritation. The classic "strawberry cervix" is seen in a minority of patients. Women may have asymptomatic infections as well. Men with trichomonal infections are usually asymptomatic but may report mild dysuria or a penile discharge.

28. How is trichomoniasis diagnosed?

Microscopy of vaginal or urethral secretions is the most common means of diagnosis and has the advantage of providing immediate information. Motile trichomonads may be seen under light microscopy, often in the presence of significant inflammation. The sensitivity of this technique, however, is poor. Even a skilled microscopist may miss up to 30% of infections. Culture is much more sensitive but may take 5–7 days to complete.

29. Why is treatment of trichomonas important?

Treatment provides symptomatic relief and prevents further transmission of the infection to sexual partners. Because trichomoniasis is often associated with significant genital inflammation, it may increase a woman's risk of acquiring HIV infection if she is exposed. Pregnant women with *T. vaginalis* may be at increased risk of preterm delivery or premature rupture of the membranes.

30. How is trichomoniasis treated?

Oral metronidazole is the only approved treatment available in the U.S. It may be given in a single 2-gm dose or as 500 mg twice daily for 7 days. The single 2-gm dose may be used during pregnancy. Both regimens result in cure in 90–95% of cases. Test of cure is not necessary if symptoms resolve. Sexual partners must be treated as well, and patients should abstain from intercourse until both partners are treated and symptom-free. If both partners are treated and the infection persists, retreat with metronidazole, 500 mg twice daily for 7 days. Because metronidazole causes a disulfiram-like reaction, counsel patients not to drink alcohol until at least 48 hours after completing treatment.

31. Why is topical (i.e., vaginal) metronidazole not used to treat this infection?

T. vaginalis may invade the urethra and perivaginal glands. Topical metronidazole is unlikely to achieve therapeutic levels in these sites and therefore is not recommended.

INFECTIONS CAUSING GENITAL ULCERS

32. Which organisms cause genital ulcers?

Herpes simplex virus (genital herpes), *Treponema pallidum* (syphilis), *Hemophilus ducreyi* (chancroid), *Calymmatobacterium granulomatis* (granuloma inguinale or donovanosis), and *C. trachomatis* serovars L1, L2, or L3 (lymphogranuloma venereum). The latter two are rarely seen in the United States. Herpes simplex virus (HSV) is the most common cause of genital ulcers in the U.S.

33. Which herpesvirus is more likely to cause genital ulcers, HSV-1 or HSV-2?

HSV-2 is more strongly associated with genital ulcers, particularly with recurrent genital outbreaks. HSV-1 causes oral infections ("cold sores" and "fever blisters") and can cause genital lesions after oral-genital contact.

34. How many teens are infected with HSV-2?

Because most infected persons are asymptomatic and no screening test is widely used for asymptomatic infection, the precise prevalence of herpesvirus infection in teens is unknown. However, serologic studies suggest that by the time they reach adulthood, 15–20% of young people are infected with HSV-2. This is a 5-fold increase over the estimated prevalence 20 years ago.

35. What is the best way to test for HSV?

Viral culture is the gold standard for diagnosis. The highest yield is from an early vesicular lesion that is unroofed at the time of specimen collection. Virus also may be isolated by scraping the base of an ulcer. The sensitivity of culture is inversely related to the time since onset of symptoms. Type-specific antibody assays for HSV-2 are now available and may be used to identify asymptomatic carriers of the virus. Widespread use for routine screening of asymptomatic people is controversial.

36. How do primary and secondary herpes outbreaks differ clinically?

Primary outbreaks classically are characterized by painful vesicular genital lesions accompanied by inguinal lymphadenopathy, fever, malaise, and myalgia. The vesicles break, leaving tender ulcers that may coalesce into larger lesions that may take 2–4 weeks to heal. The virus then goes into a subclinical or latent state in the spinal cord ganglia. Secondary genital outbreaks may appear weeks or months later and are usually less severe and shorter in duration than the primary outbreak. They have fewer associated systemic symptoms.

37. Can genital herpes ever look like anything else?

Absolutely. In fact, most cases probably do not present with the "classic" findings of vesicles and/or ulcerative lesions. Patients may present with genital pruritus, excoriations, fissures, or skin irritations that test positive for HSV. The patient or clinician may mistake the lesions for a fungal infection ("jock itch" or "yeast infection"), folliculitis, contact dermatitis, latex allergy, or another cause of vulvitis. Failure to recognize these "atypical" symptoms may lead to increased HSV transmission.

38. How does treatment differ for primary and secondary outbreaks?

Primary outbreaks are treated with higher doses of antiviral therapy, and the duration of treatment is longer. In either case, treatment should be initiated as soon as possible (within 24–48 hours of the onset of symptoms) in order to minimize the severity and duration of symptoms.

Treatment Regimens for Genital Herpes Infections (All Oral)

FIRST CLINICAL EPISODE	RECURRENT OUTBREAKS	DAILY SUPPRESSIVE THERAPY
Acyclovir, 400 mg 3 times/day × 7–10 days	Acyclovir, 800 mg 2 times/day × 5 days	Acyclovir, 400 mg 2 times/day
Acyclovir, 200 mg 5 times/day × 7–10 days	Acyclovir, 400 mg 3 times/day × 5 days	Famciclovir, 250 mg 2 times/day
Famciclovir, 250 mg 3 times/day × 7–10 days	Famciclovir, 125 mg 2 times/day × 5 days	Valacyclovir, 500 mg/day
Valacyclovir, 1 gm 2 times/day × 7–10 days	Valacyclovir, 500 mg 2 times/day × 3–5 days	Valacyclovir, 1 gm/day

39. When should suppressive therapy be considered?

Suppressive therapy may be considered in any patient but is most appropriate for patients with at least 4–6 outbreaks per year. It has been shown to decrease the frequency of recurrent outbreaks by over 75% in patients with frequent outbreaks. Several possible regimens are included in question 38. Keep in mind, however, that the natural history of HSV includes decreasing frequency of recurrent outbreaks as time passes. Therefore, suppressive therapy should not be continued indefinitely.

40. What important elements should be included in counseling a patient with herpes?

Patients must inform future sexual partners of their diagnosis. Teens may benefit from role-playing to practice this difficult conversation. Although the risk of transmitting the virus is highest during an outbreak, subclinical shedding (and therefore transmission) may occur at any time. Condoms do not effectively prevent transmission but should be used to reduce risk. Women who become pregnant must inform their obstetricians that they are infected so that the risk of transmission to the infant during delivery is minimized. Herpes infection carries substantial social stigma. Remind the patient that it is a common infection and offer any necessary emotional support while the patient learns to live with the diagnosis.

41. Which sexually transmitted disease is known as "the great imitator"?

Syphilis. The protean signs and symptoms may be difficult to differentiate from other diseases.

42. Is syphilis increasing or decreasing in the U.S.?

The reported rate of syphilis in the U.S. is currently the lowest since reporting began in 1941. Most cases occur in just 20% of U.S. counties. The Centers for Disease Control and Prevention launched the National Plan to Eliminate Syphilis in the United States in 1999.

43. What populations are at highest risk for syphilis?

African Americans have much higher rates of infection that non-Hispanic whites, reflecting the significant racial disparity in health status in the U.S. Young adults (20–35 years old) have higher rates than teens. Recent increases have been seen in men who have sex with men and in the Hispanic population. The highest rates of infection are found in the southeastern United States and in large urban areas.

44. What are the stages of syphilis infection?

Primary infection: an ulcer (chancre) at the site of infection with the organism *T. pallidum*. The chancre is typically a single, firm, painless lesion that occurs 10–90 days after exposure to *T. pallidum* and resolves in 3–6 weeks.

Secondary infection: a nonpruritic rash that often appears on the palms and soles and resolves spontaneously. Lymphadenopathy, alopecia, condyloma lata, and constitutional symptoms such as fever, malaise, weight loss, and fatigue also may be present.

Latent infection: may be either early (infection acquired within the past year) or late/unknown duration and persist for years without symptoms.

Tertiary infection: may include degenerative neurologic changes, blindness, cardiac, auditory, or gummatous lesions.

45. Can transmission occur during any stage of syphilis infection?

Transmission of *T. pallidum* can occur only when mucocutaneous lesions are present. It is therefore unlikely after the first year of infection. Nonetheless, persons reporting sexual contact with a partner with known syphilis in any stage should be tested, and treatment should be considered on a case-by-case basis.

46. How does treatment differ according to stage of infection?

Parenteral penicillin G is the treatment of choice for all stages. A single intramuscular (IM) dose of benzathine penicillin G is adequate treatment for primary and secondary syphilis as well as early latent syphilis. Late latent syphilis, latent syphilis of unknown duration, and tertiary syphilis (without evidence of neurosyphilis) is treated with 3 consecutive weekly IM doses of penicillin G. Patients with neurosyphilis or syphilitic eye disease require intravenous treatment or daily IM injections in conjunction with oral probenecid for 10–14 days.

47. How do I test for syphilis infection?

In early syphilis, exudate or tissue from the chancre may be examined using darkfield microscopy or direct fluorescent antibody testing. Serologic studies include nontreponemal tests (Venereal Disease Research Laboratory [VDRL] and rapid plasma reagin [RPR]) and treponemal tests (fluorescent treponemal antibody absorbed [FTA-ABS] as well as microhemagglutinin assay for antibody to *T. pallidum* [MTA-TP]). All serologic tests have significant false-negative rates during primary syphilis but excellent sensitivity during secondary syphilis. Nontreponemal tests alone are inadequate because of potential false positives, but they may be used for screening in asymptomatic patients. Treponemal antibody tests alone correlate poorly with disease activity and tend to stay positive despite adequate treatment. Treponemal and nontreponemal tests, therefore, are best used in combination for diagnosis and disease monitoring. The VDRL-CFS may be used to diagnose neurosyphilis, although false negatives may occur.

48. What may cause a false-positive RPR or VDRL?

Twenty to forty percent of all positive nontreponemal tests are false positives. Possible causes include:

Rheumatologic disease	Acute infection
HIV infection	Cirrhosis
Hashimoto's thyroiditis	Narcotic addiction
Lymphoma	Older age

49. Describe the clinical features of chancroid.

One or more painful genital ulcers may be accompanied by tender inguinal lymphadenopathy. Suppurative adenopathy is highly suggestive of chancroid. Testing for HSV and *T. pallidum* should be performed, and results should be negative. Because culture for *H. ducreyi* is not widely available, chancroid is often a clinical diagnosis.

VIRAL SEXUALLY TRANSMITTED INFECTIONS

50. What is the most common viral STI?
Human papillomavirus (HPV). As many as 25–50% of women under the age of 25 are infected with HPV, and an estimated 50–75% of all sexually active men and women are infected with HPV at some point in their lives. Most remain asymptomatic and undiagnosed.

51. Which HPV serotypes are most often associated with genital warts?
There are over 30 serotypes of HPV. HPV types 6 and 11 are most likely to cause external genital warts and also may cause warts on the cervix, vaginal walls, and urethral and perianal areas.

52. Which HPV serotypes are the most strongly associated with cervical dysplasia and cancer?
HPV types 16, 18, 31, 33, and 35, which occasionally are found in visible genital warts as well. These serotypes have been associated with squamous intraepithelial neoplasia of the external genitalia and perianal area as well as the cervix.

53. Why should external genital warts be treated?
Primarily for cosmetic reasons and to relieve symptoms. Although most warts are asymptomatic, some may be itchy, painful, or friable. It has never been shown that removal of warts decreases the likelihood of transmitting HPV to a sexual partner or alters the natural history of HPV infection in any way. Untreated warts often resolve spontaneously; alternatively, they may spread.

54. What options are available for treating external genital warts?
There are several possible treatments for the destruction of genital warts. As is often the case in medicine, this variety reflects the fact that no single treatment has been shown clearly to be superior to the others in every case. Treatment regimens include:
Patient-applied therapies
• Podofilox, 0.5% solution or gel   • Imiquimod, 5% cream
Clinician-applied therapies
• Trichloroacetic acid (TCA), 85%   • Surgical removal
• Podophyllin resin, 10–25%   • Intralesional interferon
• Cryotherapy (liquid nitrogen)   • Laser surgery
Patients with relatively few warts (< 10–12) in the anogenital area generally respond well to most therapies, including patient-applied therapies. Patients with extensive lesions may benefit most from surgical therapies.

55. Are cervical, deep vaginal, urethral, and anal lesions treated the same as external genital and perianal lesion?
These lesions, particularly cervical lesions, should be treated only by an experienced clinician. Cryotherapy, TCA, and podophyllin may be appropriate choices. Overly aggressive treatment may result in fistula formation or other complications. Patient-applied therapies are not appropriate for treatment of these lesions.

56. Once infected with HPV, does a person remain infected for life?
Although the virus may be present for several months or even years after symptoms are resolved, most people ultimately clear HPV infections. HPV types associated with cervical dysplasia may be more likely to persist.

57. Which STI is preventable by a vaccine?

Hepatitis B. Sexual transmission is responsible for up to 60% of all new cases of hepatitis B. All adolescents, therefore, should receive this very safe vaccination series.

58. How do you treat the sexual contact of a person known to have acute or chronic hepatitis B?

Sexual contacts of persons with acute hepatitis B should receive hepatitis B immune globulin (HBIG) and receive the hepatitis B vaccination series, initiated within 14 days of the sexual contact. Partners of persons with chronic hepatitis B should receive the vaccination, which is highly effective in preventing acquisition of the virus.

59. What is pediculosis pubis? How is it treated?

Pediculosis pubis (pubic lice or "crabs") is generally acquired through sex with an infected partner, although it may be acquired by sharing infested clothing or bedding. Patients may present with intense pruritus in the pubic area. Although the actual louse may be seen on exam, it is more common to see the oblong eggs ("nits") attached to the pubic hair. Treatment options include permethrin cream rinse, pyrethrins, or lindane shampoo. Lice and nits should be combed out with a fine-tooth comb after treatment. Patients should be reevaluated in 1 week if symptoms persist; repeat treatment may be necessary. Clothing and bedding should be washed in hot water, dry cleaned, or sealed in a plastic bag for 1 week. Lice and nits in the eyebrows or eyelashes may be suffocated by applying petroleum jelly.

PELVIC INFLAMMATORY DISEASE

60. What is pelvic inflammatory disease (PID)?

PID is an infection of the upper female genital tract, including any combination of salpingitis, endometritis, and pelvic peritonitis. Salpingitis (infection and inflammation of the fallopian tubes) is the most typical presentation, with or without the development of a tubo-ovarian abscess. The infection is caused by ascension of sexually transmitted pathogens from the lower to the upper genital tract, which may occur when the mechanical and immunologic barrier of the cervix is breached. In some cases, organisms may be transported through the cervical canal via sperm, trichomonads, instrumentation during a surgical procedure, along an IUD string, or during menses.

61. What are the typical presenting symptoms?

Teens with PID typically present with lower abdominal/pelvic pain that is continuous and bilateral, although one side may be more painful than the other. Pain with movement and intercourse is common. About one-half of patients with PID complain of a vaginal discharge, and one-third report abnormal vaginal bleeding. Up to 40% have fever. Patients occasionally experience right upper quadrant pain as well. Other gastrointestinal symptoms, such as nausea, vomiting, and diarrhea, may occur, but their prominence should prompt the search for an alternative diagnosis.

62. What is the "PID shuffle"?

This irreverent phrase describes the stooped over, shuffling gait displayed by patients in whom normal, upright posture with ambulation is impossible because of pain. Its presence suggests peritoneal irritation.

63. What is the relationship of PID to age in sexually active females?

The risk of infection increases with decreasing age. Of the one million cases of PID diagnosed per year, up to 20% occur in teens. A sexually active teen is up to 10 times more likely to be diagnosed with PID than a 25–29-year-old woman.

64. What organisms most commonly cause PID?

N. gonorrhoeae and *C. trachomatis* are the sexually transmitted bacteria most commonly implicated in PID. Most infections, however, are polymicrobial, including anaerobic bacteria (such as *Bacteroides fragilis*, *Peptococcus* species, and *Peptostreptococcus* species) as well as facultative bacteria (such as *Gardnerella vaginalis* and *Streptococcus* species). These anaerobic and facultative bacteria typically are not isolated from the endocervix but have been identified in specimens obtained via laparoscopy or culdocentesis. The mycoplasmas, such as *Mycoplasma hominis*, *Ureaplasma urealyticum*, and *Mycoplasma genitalium*, may be cultured from the cervix of some patients with PID, although their role in infection remains unclear. *Actinomyces* sp. is a rare cause of PID.

65. How many cases of untreated gonococcal or chlamydial infections develop into PID?

15–40% of chlamydial and 9–15% of gonococcal infections of the lower genital tract, if left untreated, progress to clinically symptomatic PID. Infection is more likely to progress in a young teen than in an older woman.

66. What are the minimal clinical criteria for diagnosing PID?

• Lower abdominal tenderness,
• Cervical motion tenderness, and
• Adnexal tenderness.

The presence of these three findings in a sexually active female with no other explanation for her symptoms should prompt empiric treatment for PID.

67. What additional criteria provide further support to the diagnosis of PID?

• Oral temperature > 101°F (> 38.3°C)
• Cervical or vaginal discharge
• Elevated erythrocyte sedimentation rate (> 15 mm/hr) or C-reactive protein
• Laboratory documentation of cervical infection with *N. gonorrhoeae* or *C. trachomatis*
• Clinical evidence of cervicitis, such as a friable cervix, mucopurulent discharge from the cervical os, and evidence of inflammation on microscopic evaluation of cervical secretions
• Abnormal or postcoital vaginal bleeding
• Sexual contact with a partner with known infection

68. What is the gold standard for the diagnosis of PID?

Laparoscopy. Findings may include hyperemia, ischemia, edema, or necrosis of the fallopian tubes. Involvement of the ovary and/or abscess formation also may be seen. The sensitivity of this technique is as high as 95% for diagnosing PID. Laparoscopy may miss more subtle findings, however, such as mild inflammation of the tubes, or endometritis. Histologic evidence of endometritis on endometrial biopsy is also considered a definitive diagnostic criterion. The invasive nature of these procedures limits their widespread use, but they should be considered when the diagnosis is in question.

69. How accurate is the clinical exam in the diagnosis of PID?

The minimal criteria of lower abdominal tenderness, cervical motion tenderness, and adnexal tenderness are present in up to 90% of laparoscopically confirmed cases of PID. The predictive value of the clinical exam, however, is relatively poor. Only 60–70% of clinically diagnosed PID is confirmed laparoscopically in studies evaluating the accuracy of clinical diagnosis. Alternative findings explaining the symptoms may include ovarian cysts, ectopic pregnancy, endometriosis, or appendicitis; a significant proportion have no abnormal findings on laparoscopy. In fact, no constellation of standardized clinical and/or laboratory criteria has been found to be highly sensitive and specific for PID. It is generally accepted that it is better to overtreat than undertreat adolescent patients because of the potential long-term morbidity associated with an untreated infection.

70. What laboratory studies should be obtained in evaluation?

Aside from endocervical testing for *N. gonorrhoeae* and *C. trachomatis*, laboratory studies are rarely helpful in confirming a diagnosis of PID. The white blood cell count is elevated in only about 50% of cases. Sedimentation rate and C-reactive protein are generally mildly elevated, but these findings are also nonspecific. Urine pregnancy testing is essential to rule out pregnancy and its complications as the cause of pelvic pain. Syphilis and HIV screening may be appropriate, but they are not useful in diagnosis or management of PID per se.

71. What is the relationship between PID and menstruation?

Up to 75% of cases of PID occur within the first 7 days of the menstrual cycle. The vast majority of infections with onset in the perimenstrual period are caused by gonococcal or chlamydial infection. Conversely, most cases with onset of symptoms after day 14 of the menstrual cycle involve nongonococcal, nonchlamydial organisms. It is postulated that the mucus plug in the endocervical canal serves as a barrier, protecting the upper genital tract from vaginal bacteria. The disruption of this plug during menses may predispose to ascending infection. Menstrual blood is an outstanding culture medium, particularly for *N. gonorrhoeae*. Bacteria may be carried upward toward the tubes via retrograde menstruation. The shedding of the endometrium itself also may facilitate infection by removing another protective barrier.

72. What is Fitz-Hugh-Curtis syndrome?

Inflammation of the hepatic capsule and adjacent peritoneum ("perihepatitis"), which occurs in conjunction with PID in 5–20% of cases. Patients present with right upper quadrant pain in addition to the pelvic symptoms. In some cases Fitz-Hugh-Curtis syndrome may occur in the absence of the clinical findings of PID; such patients present with abdominal or right upper quadrant pain and may have positive cervical or laparoscopic cultures for *C. trachomatis* or *N. gonorrhoeae*. Because the liver parenchyma is not involved, liver function tests are normal or only mildly elevated. It is not known whether perihepatic involvement results from direct peritoneal spread or lymphatic or hematologic spread.

73. What is the role of ultrasonography in the evaluation of PID?

Ultrasound (particularly transvaginal ultrasound) is superior to the bimanual exam in identifying adnexal masses and is the most common diagnostic procedure for identifying a tubo-ovarian abscess. The exam may demonstrate thickened, fluid-filled fallopian tubes or more complex cystic structures. Ultrasonography can easily miss the subtle findings seen on laparoscopy. Nonetheless, it should be used liberally in the evaluation of PID, particularly when guarding or obesity limit the quality of the bimanual exam or response to appropriate therapy is inadequate.

74. Why is tubo-ovarian abscess a misnomer?

Tubo-ovarian abscess (TOA) occurs in 15–20% of teens with PID and is the most severe acute complication of this infection. In most cases a TOA is not a true abscess; rather, it is a complex mass involving a thickened, tortuous, fluid-filled tube that may contain cystic elements as well. TOA is typically a polymicrobial infection with anaerobes present; it is uncommon to isolate *N. gonorrhoeae* or *C. trachomatis*.

75. If the endocervical cultures are negative, does that mean the diagnosis of PID was incorrect?

Not necessarily. The longer the duration of symptoms before cultures are obtained, the less likely one is to recover a pathogen from the cervix, particularly in the case of PID caused by gonorrhea. Also consider the type of testing used for diagnosis; some, such as culture for *C. trachomatis*, have significant false-negative rates. Lastly, it is possible for the patient to clear a lower genital tract infection but still have upper tract disease. The absence of any findings of lower genital tract infection, however, should call into question the diagnosis of PID.

76. Can PID caused by gonococcal vs. chlamydial infection be distinguished clinically?

Gonococcal PID typically has an acute onset of severe symptoms, a fulminant course if untreated, and a rapid, dramatic response to antibiotics. Onset is most likely to be within the first week of the menstrual cycle, with a short clinical course before presentation to a medical provider. Temperature and white blood cell count are more consistently elevated than in chlamydial disease.

PID caused by chlamydial infection may have a more indolent onset with milder symptoms, and response to treatment may be slower. Onset is more likely to occur in the week after menses, with a longer duration of symptoms before presentation. However, there is no known difference in the development of long-term sequelae caused by these two infections. In addition, the rate of comcomitant infection by both organisms is as high as 40%.

77. Is there an association between choice of contraceptive and development of PID?

Barrier methods of contraception reduce the risk of PID by reducing bacterial STI transmission. Spermicides containing nonoxynol-9 have been shown to cause cell wall destruction in some bacterial pathogens. Oral contraceptive pills are associated with a decreased risk of symptomatic PID, possibly because their effect on the quality of the cervical mucus impedes the transport of ascending pathogens.

The intrauterine device (IUD) is rarely used in adolescents, in part because of its association with increased risk of PID. A nulliparous female with an IUD is 7–9 times more likely to be diagnosed with PID than the general female population. The greatest risk seems to be in the weeks immediately after IUD insertion; the insertion process may be a greater predisposing factor than simply having the IUD in place. The new levonorgestrel IUDs may have a less marked effect on the development of PID.

78. Describe the appropriate outpatient management of PID.

The goal of treatment is to relieve symptoms and prevent the long-term sequelae of the infection. Antibiotics should be chosen to cover not only *N. gonorrhoeae* and *C. trachomatis* but also must be effective against anaerobes and gram-negative facultative bacteria, particularly when symptoms have been present for several days. Two appropriate regimens are listed in question 80. A follow-up visit within 72 hours is essential. Counseling about the potential sequelae of PID and the importance of partner treatment are also critical components of therapy. Partners should be treated for gonococcal and chlamydial infection regardless of their culture results.

79. What are the indications for admitting a patient with PID to the hospital?

- Severe illness at presentation
- Uncertain diagnosis
- Inadequate response to outpatient therapy at follow-up visit
- Pregnancy
- HIV or other immunodeficiency
- TOA or other significant adnexal mass
- Patient inability to adhere to the outpatient treatment regimen (e.g., patients who are vomiting and cannot tolerate oral medications, patients who are unlikely to fill their prescriptions, and patients who cannot return for a follow-up appointment within 72 hours)

The last criterion may be relevant to teens, who cannot always see long-term consequences of their actions (i.e., failure to take medications). In fact, many adolescent medicine providers believe that all teens should be admitted to the hospital for the initiation of therapy, although this approach is not always feasible.

80. What antibiotics should be used in hospitalized patients?

Treatment goals are the same as for outpatient therapy. Two appropriate parenteral regimens are listed below. Doxycycline may be given orally in patients who are not vomiting; it may be preferred because intravenous infusion of this antibiotic can be painful. Patients may be changed to oral antibiotics 24–48 hours after significant clinical improvement to complete a total of 14 days of therapy. They should be reevaluated within 72 hours of discharge from the hospital.

Suggested Regimens for Treatment of Pelvic Inflammatory Disease

INPATIENT THERAPIES	OUTPATIENT THERAPIES
Cefoxitin, 2 gm IV every 6 hr *and* Doxycycline, 100 mg orally twice daily × 14 days	Ceftriaxone, 250 mg IM, single dose *and* Doxycycline, 100 mg orally twice daily × 14 days
Clindamycin, 900 mg IV every 8 hr *and* Gentamicin, loading dose (2 mg/kg) followed by maintenance dose (1.5 mg/kg) every 8 hr	Ofloxacin, 400 mg orally twice daily × 14 days *and* Metronidazole, 500 mg orally twice daily × 14 days

81. How does management change if TOA is present?

A patient with TOA must be managed in the hospital with broad-spectrum intravenous antibiotics. Some studies suggest 7 days of parenteral therapy before changing to oral antibiotics. In addition to treating for *N. gonorrhoeae* and *C. trachomatis*, good anaerobic coverage with clindamycin or metronidazole is essential throughout the course of treatment. Medical management of TOA is usually successful. However, if the patient has persistent fevers or worsening pain or fails to respond to antibiotics within 72 hours, surgical intervention may be necessary. Bilateral abscesses or abscesses > 8 cm are more likely to require surgical treatment. A ruptured TOA is a medical emergency with a 7% mortality rate. Surgery may include abscess drainage and, in some cases, removal of the adnexal structures on the affected side.

82. What are the potential long-term sequelae of PID?

Chronic pelvic pain is common after PID, including severe dysmenorrhea and/or dyspareunia. Nearly 20% of women with PID have a subsequent episode of pelvic pain lasting longer than 6 months. The pain may be related to pelvic adhesions that form after resolution of the acute inflammation. **Ectopic pregnancy** is 5–10 times more likely to occur in women with a history of PID than in women with no history of infection. PID is the most common predisposing factor to ectopic pregnancy in young women. About 10% of women with PID who subsequently conceive develop this life-threatening complication. PID is also believed to be responsible for 30–40% of female **infertility**, again due to adhesions and scarring of the fallopian tubes. The **recurrence** rate of PID is 12–33% and higher in younger women. The severity of symptoms on presentation correlates poorly with development of long-term sequelae and damage to the tubes—even "mild" infections can cause significant tubal scarring.

83. How does the risk of tubal infertility increase with multiple episodes of PID?

The risk of tubal infertility is roughly 10% after the first episode of PID, 20–30% after the second episode, and 50% after three or more episodes of PID. Delay in seeking care for symptoms is also associated with an increased risk of impaired fertility.

84. What is meant by "silent PID"?

Many episodes of PID are asymptomatic or minimally symptomatic and never diagnosed or treated. Indeed, the acute signs and symptoms of infection eventually resolve in up to 85% of untreated women. Women with infertility secondary to tubal obstruction often have no history of STIs or clinical PID, but many (up to 70%) have positive titers indicating prior infection with *C. trachomatis* or *N. gonorrhoeae*.

BIBLIOGRAPHY

1. Buchan H, Vessey M, Goldacre M, Fairweather J: Morbidity following pelvic inflammatory disease. Br J Obstst Gynaecol 100:558–562, 1993.
2. Centers for Disease Control and Prevention: 1998 Guidelines for treatment of sexually transmitted diseases. MMWR 47(No. RR-1), 1998.
3. Centers for Disease Control and Prevention: Tracking the Hidden Epidemics. Trends in STDs in the United States, 2000. Atlanta, Department of Health and Human Services, Centers for Disease Control and Prevention, 2001.
4. Emans SJ, Laufer M, Goldstein D: Pediatric and Adolescent Gynecology, 4th ed. Philadelphia, Lippincott-Raven, 1998.
5. Eng TR, Butler WT (eds): The Hidden Epidemic: Confronting Sexually Transmitted Diseases. Washington, D.C., National Academy Press, 1997.
6. Holmes KK, Sparling PF, Mårdh P, et al (eds): Sexually Transmitted Diseases, 3rd ed. New York, McGraw-Hill, 1999.
7. Jacobson L, Westrom L: Objective diagnosis of acute pelvic inflammatory disease: Diagnostic and prognostic value of routine laparoscopy. Am J Obstet Gynecol 105:1088–1098, 1969.
8. Lawson MA, Blythe MJ: Pelvic inflammatory disease in adolescents. Pediatr Clin North Am 46:767–782, 1999.
9. Pickering LK (ed): 2000 Red Book: Report of the Committee on Infectious Diseases, 25th ed. Elk Grove Village, IL, American Academy of Pediatrics, 2000.
10. Westrom L: Incidence, prevalence, and trends of acute pelvic inflammatory disease and its consequences in industrialized countries. Am J Obstet Gynecol 138:880, 1980.

25. CONTRACEPTION

Melanie A. Gold, D.O., and Kym A. Smith, B.S.

1. What is the newest combination injectable contraceptive? Is it appropriate for adolescents?

In October 2000, the Food and Drug Administration approved Lunelle, a combination estrogen-progesterone injectable contraceptive that is composed of 5 mg of estradiol cypionate and 25 mg of depot medroxyprogesterone acetate (DMPA). Lunelle is a highly effective contraceptive with a 0.3% failure rate. The first injection is best administered within the first 5 days of menses and should be administered every 28 days for highest effectiveness. This contraceptive method may be best suited to adolescents who like the menstrual regularity of the pill but have difficulty remembering to take it on a regular basis. Like other hormonal contraceptive methods, Lunelle provides no protection against sexually transmitted diseases (STDs), including HIV; therefore, condom use should be recommended.

2. How do oral contraceptive pills (OCPs), Lunelle, and Depo-Provera compare in terms of efficacy, safety, and side effects?

CHARACTERISTIC	OCPS	LUNELLE*	DEPO-PROVERA
Failure rate			
Theoretical	1%	0.3%	0.3%
Typical	5%	0.3%	0.3%
Duration of action	24 hr	28 days	12 wks
Safety window for missed dose	48 hr	± 5 days	± 14 days
% menstrual irregularity in first 3 months of use	30%	30%	80%
% with amenorrhea at 1 year of use	6%	4%	50%
Weight gain	+	++	+++
Time to resume fertility after discontinuing	1–2 mo	2–3 mo	6–18 mo

OCPs = oral contraceptive pills.
* Reported patterns are based on studies of adult women. Less is known about Lunelle's effects (especially menstrual and weight changes) on adolescent girls.

3. How should you counsel a patient who complains of irritation when using condoms from "an allergy to latex"?

First, make sure that the irritation is really an allergy. True latex allergy is not common; however, irritation from the spermicidal lubricant (e.g., nonoxonyl 9) on condoms occurs frequently. Initially suggest switching to a latex condom that is lubricated (but not with a spermicide), or suggest using a nonlubricated latex condom together with a separate water-based lubricant. Patient populations such as those with spina bifida or multiple surgical or medical exposures to latex are more apt to have true allergies.

4. For patients with true latex allergy, what types of condoms can be recommended?

For patients with latex allergy, you can recommend a male polyurethane condom such as Avanti (made by Durex) or Supra (made by Trojan). However, polyurethane condoms have been shown to be less effective at preventing pregnancies and STDs and have higher breakage and slippage rates compared with condoms made of latex. Thus, polyurethane condoms should be reserved for true latex allergy. Condoms made of lambskin also can be used for pregnancy prevention by latex-allergic patients, but they do not afford adequate protection against STDs and thus should be reserved for adolescents who are at low risk of exposure to STDs.

5. Is the female condom a good choice for adolescents?

The female condom is made of polyurethane and may be another alternative method of barrier protection for adolescents with true latex allergy. However, use of the female condom requires a high degree of comfort with insertion and removal from the vagina—a level of comfort that many adolescents do not possess. Latex male condoms are the preferred method for barrier protection. The female condom may be an appropriate choice of barrier protection when true latex allergy is present or when a female adolescent wants barrier protection and her partner will not wear a male condom.

6. Which lubricants are safe to use with latex condoms?

Water-based lubricants, such as KY-Jelly, AstroGlide, or Slippery Stuff, are safe to use with latex condoms and prevent breakage or slippage from friction. Oil-based lubricants, (e.g., mineral oil, hand lotion, massage oil, vegetable oil, vegetable shortening, coconut oil, butter, whipped cream) are unsafe because they weaken latex and increase the likelihood of condom breakage or leakage. Saliva is a water-based lubricant but in rare instances can transmit sexually transmitted infections and is best avoided. Oil-based lubricants do not weaken polyurethane and can be safely used with polyurethane male and female condoms.

7. What is new on the horizon for male condoms?

The baggy latex condom is a latex condom that is loose-fitting with a ballooned distal end. In clinical trials with adult men, there was less slippage compared with standard latex condoms, but slightly more breakage. Male users preferred the baggy condoms and reported that they felt more natural, were easier to keep on, caused less disruption, and made sex more enjoyable.

The tactylon condom is made of a synthetic thermoplastic elastomer called styrene ethylene butylene styrene (SBES). This material is already used in medical gloves and resists decomposition. Tactylon condoms were compared to latex, baggy, and low-molecule condoms (low resistance to stretch and high elasticity). Men using the tactylon condoms reported more slippage and breakage compared with latex condoms. However, both males and females preferred tactylon condoms over the other condoms because they were easy to put on and had no odor. The aesthetic improvements in condoms (e.g., feel and smell) should be weighed against slippage and breakage rates. However, such improvement may lead to increased usage among male adolescents and result in lower STD rates.

8. Do spermicides increase the risk of contracting human immunodeficiency virus (HIV)?

Spermicides such as nonoxynol 9 can cause vaginal irritation, leading to vaginal mucosal breakdown and increased susceptibility to HIV acquisition. One study found that sex workers who used frequent applications of vaginal spermicide (e.g., 7 times or more a day) had higher rates of HIV seroconversion than sex workers who did not use vaginal spermicide. However, no current data indicate that use of vaginal spermicide under usual conditions (e.g., less than 7 times a day with a single partner) is correlated with higher HIV acquisition rates. Likewise, no evidence indicates that latex condoms which are merely lubricated with spermicide increase the risk of HIV with typical use. However, because condoms lubricated with spermicide do not provide substantially better protection against pregnancy than condoms lubricated without spermicide, it is reasonable to recommend that adolescents use lubricated condoms without spermicide. If additional nonhormonal pregnancy prevention is desired, a separate vaginal spermicide can be used with the condom.

9. What are the two main progestin families? How do they differ from each other?

Estranes: norethindrone, norethindrone acetate, and ethinodiol diacetate.

Gonanes: norgestrel, levonorgestel, norgestimate, desogestrel, and gestodene (not available in pill preparation in the U.S.).

Estrane-family progestins have a shorter half-life than gonane-family progestins.

10. What is the best combination oral contraceptive pill for an adolescent who has never taken pills before?

Although all oral contraceptive pills (OCPs) can effectively prevent pregnancy, for a first-time user some health care providers prefer a 20–25 μg estrogen pill (an ultra-low-dose pill) to a 30–35 μg pill (a low-dose pill). A high-dose 50 μg estrogen pill should not be prescribed for routine contraception in first-time pill users. Prescribing a lower-dose pill lessens the incidence of nausea and vomiting but may increase the likelihood of breakthrough bleeding (BTB), particularly within the first three cycles of use. Pills that contain the progestins in the gonane family are less likely to result in BTB than pills containing progestins in the estrane family, which have a shorter half-life. One study found that 20-μg pills containing desogestrel cause less initial BTB than 20-μg pills containing levonorgestrel. These data should be weighed against the potentially higher risk of thromboembolism among women taking pills with desogestrel compared with those taking pills with levonorgestrel, as demonstrated in European epidemiologic studies.

11. Is there any advantage to choosing a triphasic pill over a monophasic pill?

Monophasic pill preparations contain the same dose of estrogen and progestin for each day of the pill pack with the exception of the placebo pills. Triphasic preparations vary in the dose of estrogen, progestin, or both over the course of the pack. In a monophasic preparation every hormonally active pill is the same color, whereas in triphasic preparations pills of differing doses are different colors or shapes. Monophasic and triphasic pills are equally effective at preventing pregnancy. Monophasic preparations may be preferable to triphasic preparations because adolescents may become confused when they miss a pill and need to double up on pills that are different colors or shapes.

12. When counseling a first-time pill user, which combination OCP side effects are most important to discuss?

It is critical to counsel first-time pill users that nausea, breast tenderness, breakthrough bleeding, headaches, and mood changes are the most common side effects. However, it is important to stress that these nuisance side effects usually disappear within three cycles of starting the pills. Although thromboembolism is a rare complication, it is important to review signs of thromboembolism with the acronym **ACHES**:

A = **A**bdominal pain
C = **C**hest pain or shortness of breath
H = **H**eadache (severe, crushing)
E = **E**ye or visual disturbance
S = **S**evere leg pain or swelling

13. What are the most common side effects associated with the estrogen and progestin components of combination oral contraceptive pills?

Estrogen-related adverse effects
- Nausea, vomiting
- Breast tenderness
- Telangiectasia, chloasma
- Vascular type headache
- Thromboembolism
- Cholestasis
- Benign liver tumor (hepatoma)

Progestin-related adverse effects
- Mood changes, fatigue
- Decrease libido
- Breast enlargement
- Increased appetite
- Acne
- Abnormal carbohydrate and lipid metabolism

14. When an adolescent is starting pills, when should she start taking them?

OCPs can be initiated in one of three ways: (1) visit start, (2) menses start, or (3) Sunday start.

With the **visit start**, the adolescent takes the first pill on the "visit" day that she is prescribed the pills, regardless of where she is in her menstrual cycle.

- Advantage. Patient benefits from starting the method while she is highly motivated.
- Disadvantage. Pills will not effectively suppress ovulation for 14 days. Counsel her that her next menses may be delayed from the time when it was expected or that breakthrough bleeding may occur.

With the **menses start**, the adolescent takes the first pill of the pack on the first day of her next menses.

- Advantages. Menses are often a good reminder of when to start taking the pill, pregnancy is adequately ruled out, and the pill is immediately effective because the patient is at a time in her cycle when she is unlikely to ovulate.
- Disadvantages. Many adolescents have irregular cycles and may accidentally get pregnant while waiting for menses to start the pills.

With the **Sunday start**, the adolescent starts taking the pill on the Sunday after the first day of her next menses (unless the menses starts on a Sunday, in which case the pills are started that day).

- Advantage. Future menses usually occur during the week, leaving the weekends (when adolescents may be more likely to have sex) menses-free.
- Disadvantages. An adolescent who starts her menses on a Monday may not remember to start the pill the following Sunday when she is no longer menstruating. Pills will not effectively suppress ovulation for 14 days if the Sunday start day is more than 5 days after menses began. When the next menses begins on a Sunday, adolescents become confused and do not remember that they should start taking the pills that day (they often wait until the following Sunday).

In general, the visit start is preferred unless an adolescent has a strong preference to avoid menses on the weekend or if she expects menses to start within a day or two, her menses are regular, and she prefers to wait.

15. What are the noncontraceptive benefits of combination OCPs?

- Decrease menstrual flow
- Regulate periods
- Decrease menstrual cramps
- Decrease anemia
- Decrease risk of ovarian cysts
- Decrease risk of ovarian cancer
- Decrease risk of uterine cancer
- Reduce symptoms of endometriosis
- May reduce symptoms of premenstrual syndrome
- Decrease risk of pelvic inflammatory disease
- Decrease risk of fibrocystic breast changes and benign breast disease

16. What is the best instruction to give an adolescent about missed or late pills?

1. Ideally OCPs are most effective when taken every 24 hours. A pill is not considered "late" unless it is taken more than 4–6 hours after the time it was supposed to be taken. Adolescent and adult women frequently take pills late or miss them, thus compromising their efficacy.

2. If she is late taking a pill, tell her to take it as soon as she remembers.

3. If she does not realize that she has missed the pill until the next day's dose is due, tell her to take the forgotten pill and that day's pill together ("doubling up").

4. If she misses pills two days in a row, tell her to double up two days in a row.

5. If she misses pills three days in a row, tell her to throw the pack out and immediately start a brand new pack of pills. Counsel her that she is not protected against pregnancy from the new pack of pills until she completes 14 days of pills and that breakthrough bleeding may occur.

6. The only pills in the pack that can be safely missed or taken late are the placebo pills; placebo pills do not need to be doubled up.

7. Counsel her that whenever a pill is missed or late (even if she catches up by doubling up), she may have breakthrough bleeding.

8. Tell her that anytime two or more pills in a row are missed, especially during the first or third week of the pack, she is not protected against pregnancy. If unprotected intercourse occurs under these circumstances, emergency contraceptive pills (ECPs) should be offered. Some clinicians offer ECPs if unprotected intercourse occurs when only one pill is missed. Whenever the pill-free or placebo interval is prolonged beyond 9 days, there is significant risk of ovulation. The next worst time to miss pills is in the first and third weeks of the pill pack.

9. Some clinicians advocate shortening the pill-free interval from 7 days to only 3 or 4 days (or even eliminating the pill-free interval altogether) so that when pills are missed, contraceptive efficacy will not be compromised as much.

17. What is "continuous" or "extended cycling" with OCPs?

Usually, combination OCP regimens consist of 21 days of hormonally active pills followed by a 7-day interval of hormone-free or placebo pills to allow a withdrawal bleed. For continuous cycling, one hormonally active low-dose OCP is taken every day and the usual hormone-free interval (or 7 days of placebo pills) is skipped. The length of cycling (i.e., the number of days hormonally active pills are taken continuously) can vary:
- Two cycles or 42 days continuously ("bi-cycling")
- Three cycles or 63 days continuously ("tri-cycling")
- Four cycles or 84 days continuously ("quad-cycling")

These regimens usually are followed by a scheduled 7-day hormone-free or placebo interval to allow a controlled withdrawal bleed. The Food and Drug Administration is currently evaluating an application for a 30-µg estrogen and progestin monophasic pill called Seasonale for continuous cycling with an 84-day cycle and a 7-day placebo interval.

18. How does a clinician know how many days to extend the continuous cycling?

Some family planning experts advocate starting with a 42-day cycle and then extending each cycle (by 21 days) until an 84-day cycle is reached. Others advocate prescribing continuous hormonally active pills with no prescheduled pill-free interval. In this case, when a woman experiences breakthrough bleeding that lasts more than 3–5 days while taking the hormonally active pills, she can be advised to discontinue the pills for 3–7 days. After the withdrawal bleed and hormone-free interval, hormonally active pills can be resumed continuously until the next breakthrough bleeding episode. Although traditionally the hormone-free or placebo interval has been 7 days, some family planning experts suggest that a 3- or 4-day hormone-free interval is sufficient to allow a controlled withdrawal bleed.

19. For which medical conditions may continuously cycled pills be most beneficial?
- Endometriosis
- Coagulopathies, such as von Willibrand's disease
- Severe dysmenorrhea
- Premenstrual syndrome
- Estrogen withdrawal headaches during hormone-free interval
- Anemia
- Women who frequently are late or miss pills
- Women who prefer amenorrhea on an OCP

20. What are the major health benefits of continuously cycling combination pills?

1. Women who continuously cycle on OCPs bleed less frequently, and when they do bleed, they do so lightly. Thus they are less likely to develop or exacerbate preexisting anemia.

2. Because pills are not 100% effective at preventing pregnancy and missed pills compromise efficacy, some clinicians advocate continuous cycling for all adolescents relying on combination pills for contraception if they desire and are comfortable with amenorrhea.

21. Are any health risks associated with continuous cycling of OCPs?

There has been concern that continuous cycling may cause endometrial hyperplasia and subsequent endometrial cancer. No evidence supports this concern. In fact, an endometrium exposed to continuous low doses of estrogen and progesterone becomes thin (not hypertrophic), and this exerts a protective effect. However, no long-term studies have evaluated the safety of extended or continuous cycling.

22. How do you prescribe combination OCPs for continuous cycling?

1. Only monophasic pills are appropriate for continuous cycling. When triphasic or biphasic pills are used, breakthrough bleeding may occur when a new pack is started because of the drop in estrogen and/or progestin dose.

2. To avoid patient confusion or accidental ingestion of placebo pills, it may be less confusing to prescribe 21-day pill packs rather than 28-day packs of a monophasic OCP.

3. One important consideration before prescribing OCPs for continuous use is whether the patient's insurance plan limits the number of pill packs that can be filled to 13 packs per year (1 pack every 28 days). As many as 4 additional packs per year may be needed for continuous cycling and may require preauthorization and/or extra expense.

23. For the most common pill-related side effects, what changes should be made?

First, determine whether the side effect is related to estrogen or progestin.

- Nausea or vomiting: take pill at night and with food; decrease estrogen content in pill.
- Breast tenderness: decrease estrogen content in pill.
- Migraine headache: decrease estrogen content in pill.
- Headaches during pill-free interval: shorten pill-free interval or prescribe continuous pill cycling.
- Moodiness: change progestin family (e.g., if patient is using a pill with an estrane-family progestin, change to a gonane-family pill) or lower progestin dose.
- Weight gain: counsel about diet and exercise; change progestin family or lower progestin dose.
- Spotting or irregular bleeding in third week: change to gonane family progestin or increase progestin dose; consider change from monophasic to triphasic.
- Spotting or irregular bleeding in first or second week: increase estrogen content in pill.
- Amenorrhea: exclude pregnancy with a urine pregnancy test and reassure that this is not a problem; if pregnancy is excluded and patient wishes menses, increase estrogen content in pill.

24. What are the newest OCPs on the market?

In the spring of 2001, the FDA approved two new oral contraceptive pills, Cyclessa and Yasmin.

Cyclessa is a triphasic pill formulation with 25 µg ethinyl estradiol and increasing dosages of desogestrel (100 mg in week 1, 125 mg in week 2, and 150 mg in week 3). In a 6-month trial, Cyclessa was compared with Ortho Novum 7/7/7, which contains 35 µg of ethinyl estradiol and increasing dosages of norethindrone (0.5 mg in week 1, 0.75 mg in week 2, and 1.0 mg in week 3). Cyclessa provided superior cycle control at every point in time over the 6-month study period; fewer Cyclessa users reported amenorrhea and breakthrough bleeding than Ortho Novum 7/7/7 users. However, those who took Cyclessa reported slightly higher rates of nausea and emotional lability.

Yasmin is a monophasic pill containing 30 μg of ethinyl estradiol and 3 mg of drospirenone. Drospirenone is a new category of progestin that binds competitively to androgen receptors and has a spironolactone-like effect. In addition to suppressing ovarian function, this progestin also suppresses adrenal production of mineralocorticoids. Overall, it has been shown to decrease average diastolic blood pressure. Some weight loss has been documented within the first 6 months of use. Adolescents who have weight concerns may find Yasmin particularly attractive. Pills containing drospirenone may be particularly useful for adolescents with ovarian hyperandrogenism, hirsutism, and excessive acne, but comparative studies with other pill formulations have not yet been published. Pills containing drospirenone are contraindicated in conditions that predispose to hyperkalemia, such as kidney, liver, and adrenal disease, and in women taking nonsteroidal anti-inflammatory drugs chronically or women who use potassium-sparing diuretics, angiotensin-converting enzyme inhibitors, or heparin.

25. For the adolescent starting depot medroxyprogesterone acetate (Depo-Provera), when is the best time to administer the first injection?

Depo-Provera can be initiated in one of two ways: (1) the menses start or (2) the visit start.

With the **menses start**, the adolescent gets her first Depo-Provera injection within the first 5 days of menses.
  • Advantages. Pregnancy is adequately ruled out (although a urine pregnancy test is still recommended before administering the injection, and the injection is immediately effective because the adolescent is at a time in her cycle when she is unlikely to ovulate.
  • Disadvantages. Many adolescents have irregular cycles and may accidentally get pregnant while waiting for the menses to get the first injection.

With the **visit start**, the adolescent gets her first injection on the day of her office visit, regardless of where she may be in her menstrual cycle. The injection can be given as long as the last time the adolescent had unprotected intercourse was at least 14 days earlier and her urine pregnancy test is negative on the day of the visit.
  • Advantage. She starts the method when she is highly motivated.
  • Disadvantage. She may not be protected from pregnancy until 14 days after she gets the first injection.

In general, the visit start is preferred unless an adolescent has had unprotected intercourse within the past 14 days and pregnancy cannot adequately be ruled out by a urine pregnancy test. Depo-Provera is not teratogenic if accidentally given early in the first trimester of pregnancy, but its use has been associated with small-for-gestational-age growth of the fetus.

26. What are the most important side effects to discuss when counseling an adolescent about Depo-Provera?
  • Irregular menses: intermittent spotting, irregular bleeding, prolonged bleeding, and/or amenorrhea; 25–50% will have amenorrhea after 1 year of use, 80% by 5 years of use.
  • Weight gain, averaging 5.4 pounds during the first year of use, 8.1 pounds after 2 years of use, and 13.8 pounds after 4 years of use.
  • Delay in return to fertility (6–12-month delay starting from 3 months after the last injection).
  • Mood changes (associated with depression).
  • Bitemporal thinning of hair or alopecia occurs rarely.

27. What effect does Depo-Provera have on bone mineral density in adolescents?

A number of studies in adult women have shown a decrease in bone mineral density following Depo-Provera use. However, these studies suffer from small sample size, lack of control for confounding factors (e.g., dietary calcium, exercise, cigarette use) and rarely include adolescent subjects. A multicenter study investigating the impact of Depo-Provera on adolescents' bone mineral density is under way; preliminary results may be available in 2002. To date, no evidence-based studies support providing estrogen supplementation to preserve bone mineral density in adolescent Depo-Provera users. All adolescents, but particularly those on Depo-Provera, should be counseled to optimize calcium intake to 1200–1500 mg/day, do regular weight-bearing exercise, and avoid tobacco as well as beverages containing caffeine or alcohol, which may compromise calcium absorption or maintenance in bones.

28. How should breakthrough bleeding on Depo-Provera be evaluated?

1. Rule out pregnancy (ectopic, placenta previa, implantation bleeding) with a urine human chorionic gonadotropin test.

2. Rule out trauma, foreign body, and cervical polyps with a thorough history and an external genital examination plus a speculum examination.

3. Rule out cervicitis (from gonorrhea, chlamydia, or trichomonas) with cultures and vaginal microscopy.

4. Rule out anemia by measuring a hemoglobin and checking orthostatic blood pressure (blood pressure with pulse in supine and standing positions).

29. Once other causes of bleeding have been ruled out, how should breakthrough bleeding be managed?

1. Ibuprofen, 800 mg orally 3 times/day for 5 days (if no response go to next step).

2. Either Estrace, 1 mg/day orally for 7–14 days, or Premarin, 0.625 mg/day orally for 7–14 days (may either increase Estrace to 2 mg/day or Premarin to 1.25 mg/day if no response within 7 days).

3. If you need to repeat estrogen supplementation several times, consider cycling with combination OCPs.

4. Give daily iron supplementation if hemoglobin is less than 12.0.

30. How do emergency contraceptive pills (ECPs) work to prevent pregnancy?

ECPs prevent pregnancy primarily by preventing ovulation and implantation. ECPs also may prevent fertilization. Alteration of cervical mucus thickness and changes in tubal transport of sperm or ova have been determined to be mechanisms of action in animal models, but these findings have not been confirmed in human studies. ECPs will not dislodge implanted fertilized ova (i.e., they are not abortifacients).

31. What are the indications for prescribing ECPs?

Whenever unprotected sexual intercourse has occurred within the past 72 hours. Common examples include:

- Condom broke or slipped off
- No contraception use
- Rape or sexual assault
- Patient missed 2 pills in a row or was late in starting next pack by 2 days or more
- More than 14 weeks from last Depo-Provera injection
- More than 33 days from last Lunelle injection
- Slipped or dislodged diaphragm, sponge, or cervical cap

32. What are the contraindications to prescribing ECPs?

Pregnancy is the only contraindication, not because ECPs are teratogenic but because they are ineffective after implantation and will not disrupt a pregnancy. The contraindications for ECPs are not the same as contraindications for ongoing combination OCP use. For patients with a history of thromboembolism, current migraine headache with neurologic deficits, or a history of myocardial infarction, breast cancer, or stroke, ECPs can be prescribed; however, the progestin-only regimen is preferred over the combination pill regimen (Yuzpe).

33. Which pills can be used for emergency contraception (EC)?

1. **Yuzpe (or combination pill) regimen**: 200 µg ethinyl estradiol plus either 1 mg of levonorgestrel or 2 mg of norgestrel (divided into two doses and given 12 hours apart)
   - **Preven (prepackaged EC)**: 2 tablets initially, repeated in 12 hours; includes home pregnancy test.
   - **Ovral, Ogestrel**: 2 tablets initially, repeated in 12 hours
   - **Lo/Ovral, Low Ogestrel, Nordette, Levora, Levlen**: 4 tablets initially, repeated in 12 hours.
   - **Trivora, Triphasil (yellow tablets only)**: 4 tablets initially, repeated in 12 hours.
   - **Alesse, Levlite, Aviane**: 5 tablets initially, repeated in 12 hours
2. **Progestin-only regimen**: 3.0 mg of norgestel or 1.5 mg of levonorgestrel (divided into 2 doses and given 12 hours apart)
   - **Plan B (prepackaged EC)**: 1 tablet initially, repeated in 12 hours.
   - **Ovrette**: 20 tablets initially and repeat in 12 hours.

The progestin-only method is preferred over the Yuzpe regimen because of its higher efficacy and fewer side effects, particularly nausea and vomiting. If the Yuzpe regimen is used, provide an antiemetic (e.g., meclizine, 50 mg) 1 hour before administering the first dose.

34. How long after unprotected intercourse are ECPs effective?

Both prepackaged ECP methods (Plan B and Preven) are FDA-approved for use up to 72 hours after unprotected intercourse. However, data support prescribing EC up to 120 hours (5 days) after unprotected intercourse. The Yuzpe method was found to be 87% effective in 169 women who used it 72–120 hours after intercourse. ECP efficacy decreases as time increases after an episode of unprotected intercourse.

Pregnancy Rate for Yuzpe and Progestin-only ECPs by Timing from Intercourse

TIMING AFTER COITUS (HR)	YUZPE (%)	PROGESTIN-ONLY (%)
≤ 24	2.0	0.4
25–48	4.1	1.2
49–72	4.7	2.7
73–120	1.1	—
Overall	3.2	1.1

35. Should ECPs be prescribed to adolescent patients in advance? What effect will prophylactically prescribing ECPs have on contraceptive behavior?

Three studies have assessed the effect of providing prophylactic ECPs on women's contraceptive behaviors. Two demonstrated no change in ongoing contraceptive use after giving ECPs to women in advance of need. One study showed that women who received ECPs in advance were more likely to have switched to a less effective birth control method. The first two studies had a 1-year follow-up interval (the third only a 4-month follow-up interval), and none of the studies assessed effect on a predominantly adolescent population. The different outcome of the three studies illustrates the need for additional research involving larger numbers of adolescents with longer follow-up to understand more clearly the behavioral and biologic outcomes of advance provision of ECPs. Prescribing prophylactic ECPs to adolescents is supported by most family planning experts because it is difficult for adolescents to obtain ECPs in a timely manner, and ECPs are more effective the sooner they are taken after unprotected intercourse.

36. What is Norplant? How does it work?

Norplant is a reversible, 5-year, low-dose, progestin-only subdermal implant. It consists of six soft flexible capsules that are placed under the skin of the upper arm during an in-office procedure. Norplant continuously releases a progestin (levonorgestrel) to prevent pregnancy in two ways: it inhibits ovulation and thickens cervical mucus, making it more difficult for the sperm to ascend the reproductive tract.

37. Is Norplant a good contraceptive option for adolescents?

Norplant was initially a popular method of long-acting contraception, especially among postpartum adolescents. However, at present Norplant is no longer produced by the Wyeth-Ayerst pharmaceutical company because of an FDA concern that some lots currently available in the U.S. were providing inadequate serum levels of levonorgestrel (LN) and thus increasing the risk of pregnancy. To date, the FDA has not allowed the use of these previous lots, and new Norplant is not being distributed. Norplant probably will be replaced by the introduction of a new single-rod subdermal implant called Implanon (see below).

38. What is Mirena? How does it work?

In December 2000, the FDA approved Mirena, a new levonorgestrel-releasing intrauterine device (IUD). The Mirena IUD releases the same amount of levonorgestrel as one or two Ovrette minipills (0.075 mg norgestrel) per day. The levonorgestrel causes the cervical mucus to thicken so that sperm cannot reach the egg. The Mirena IUD has been found to be safe and cost-effective and provides extremely effective long-term contraception among adult women.

39. What are the advantages and disadvantages of Mirena?

The Mirena IUD is as effective as tubal ligation (> 99% effective at preventing pregnancy) and works for 5 years or until it is removed. It prevents ectopic pregnancies, decreases menstrual cramping, and dramatically decreases menstrual blood loss. In Europe the Mirena IUD has been used as a treatment for menorrhagia in adult women. Another advantage is that return to fertility is immediate once Mirena is removed. After removal, 80% of women desiring pregnancy will become pregnant in the first year. Disadvantages include the high initial cost of insertion, lack of protection against sexually transmitted diseases, and menstrual cycle alterations, such as irregularity or amenorrhea.

40. Is a levonorgestrel IUD an appropriate method of contraception for adolescents?

Currently, many clinicians feel that an IUD is not a good contraceptive choice for a nulliparous adolescent. Adolescents often engage in high-risk sexual behaviors, such as multiple sexual partners and inconsistent use of condoms. There is controversy over whether the high effectiveness of the levonorgestrel IUD outweighs the potential risk of pelvic inflammatory disease (PID) among adolescents who are nulliparous and may have high-risk sexual practices.

41. Do IUDs increase the risk of PID?

Higher rates of PID were noted in early studies of IUD users compared with women who used condoms or OCPs. More recent studies show that the increased risk of PID with the IUD seems restricted to women at high risk for STDs. Most episodes of PID associated with IUDs are infections that result from the insertion of the device through a cervix previously infected with gonorrhea or chlamydia. The previous use of a copper IUD is not associated with an increased incidence of tubal infertility among never-pregnant women.

42. What is the newest contraceptive method available to adolescents?

NuvaRing contraceptive vaginal ring is a flexible, transparent ring (54 mm in diameter) that continuously releases a new progestin (etonogestrel) and an estrogen (ethinyl estradiol). The FDA approved the ring for contraceptive use in October 2001. The ring is placed inside the vagina for 3 weeks and then removed for 1 week to allow a withdrawal bleed. It is left in place during intercourse.

43. How well does NuvaRing prevent pregnancy?
The overall failure rate is 0.6–1.8 pregnancies per 100 woman years. There were significantly higher failure rates among U.S. ring users (1.8 pregnancies/100 woman-years) compared with European ring-users (0.6/100 woman-years). However, these differences were believed to be due to user failure rather than method failure; in the U.S., women temporarily removed the device before intercourse and failed to replace the ring after intercourse.

44. How appropriate is the NuvaRing for adolescent contraception?
Adult users seem to find NuvaRing to be an acceptable method of contraception with a 60–70% continuation rate. However, the contraceptive ring may not be an acceptable method among adolescents who often feel uncomfortable touching their vaginas to put the ring in place or among those who are not able to keep of track of when it should be removed.

45. What new contraceptive methods are on the horizon? Are they appropriate for adolescents?
The **EVRA Contraceptive Patch** is a 20-cm^2 adhesive transdermal patch that contains a new progestin (17-deacetylnorgestimate) and an estrogen (ethinyl estradiol). The patch is placed on the trunk, buttock, or arm once a week and changed each week for 3 weeks. On the fourth week the patch is left off to allow a withdrawal bleed. Failure rates have not been published at this time, but efficacy and side effects are described as similar to those of combination OCPs. Among adult users in study trials, acceptability was high, and compliance was perfect. This new method has the greatest potential for acceptability and effective use among adolescents that may translate into high contraceptive efficacy. Some adolescents may not like the patch because it is visible when wearing a bathing suit and may be perceived as less private than other methods of birth control.

Implanon is a 3-year subdermal implant made of one ethylene vinyl acetate rod that contains a new progestin (etonogestrel). The rod is 4 cm × 2 mm and is inserted under the skin during an in-office procedure, much the way Norplant was inserted. The method appears to be highly effective; no pregnancies were observed among 13 trials of 70,000 cycles of use. Ovulation is completely suppressed in the first two years of use, and in the third year the rate of ovulation is 3%. Return to fertility is rapid when Implanon is removed; 94% of women ovulated within 3 weeks after the device was removed. Side effects are also similar to those seen with other progestin-only methods and include irregular menstrual bleeding, weight increases, and acne. Implanon may be a good method of contraception for adolescents who are able to make a commitment to three years of effective contraception and who are comfortable with the requirement for surgical insertion and removal of the method. Given the current lack of availability of Norplant, Implanon may be the best choice for postpartum adolescents who wish for longer-acting hormonal contraception.

BIBLIOGRAPHY

1. Burkman RT, Kaunitz AM, Shulman LP, Sulak PJ: Oral contraceptives and noncontraceptive benefits: Summary and application of data. Int J Fertil 45:143–147, 2000.
2. Ellertson C, Ambardekar S, Hedley A, et al: Emergency contraception: Randomized comparison of advance provision and information only. Obstet Gynecol 98:570–575, 2001.
3. Glasier A, Baird D: The effects of self-administering emergency contraception. N Engl J Med 339:1–4, 1998.
4. Gold MA: Emergency contraception: Another opportunity to prevent adolescent pregnancy. Adv Pediatr 47:309–334, 2000.
5. Gold MA: Prescribing and managing oral contraceptive pills and emergency contraception. Pediatr Clin North Am 46:695–718, 1999.
6. Hall PE: New once-a-month injectable contraceptives, with particular reference to Cyclofem/Cyclo-Provera. Int J Gynaecol Obstet 62(Suppl 1):S43–S56, 1998.
7. Hatcher RA, Trussell J, Stewart F, et al: Contraceptive Technology, 16th ed. New York, Ardent Media, 1998.

8. Hubacher D, Lara-Ricalde R, Taylor DJ, et al: Use of copper intrauterine devices and the risk of tubal infertility among nulligravid women. N Engl J Med 345:561–567, 2001.

9. Kaunitz AM: Menstruation: Choosing whether . . . and when. Contraception 62(6):277–284, 2000.

10. Piaggio G, von Hertzen H, Grimes DA, Van Look PF: Timing of emergency contraception with levonorgestrel or the Yuzpe regimen. Task Force on Postovulatory Methods of Fertility Regulation. Lancet 353:721, 1999.

11. Raine T, Harper C, Leon K, Darney P: Emergency contraception: Advance provision in a young, high-risk clinic population. Obstet Gynecol 96:1–7, 2000.

12. Rodrigues I, Grou F, Joly J: Effectiveness of emergency contraceptive pills between 72 and 120 hours after unprotected sexual intercourse. Am J Obstet Gynecol 184:531–537, 2001.

13. Task Force on Postovulatory Methods of Fertility Regulation (WHO): Randomised controlled trial of levonorgestrel versus the Yuzpe regimen of combined oral contraceptives for emergency contraception. Lancet 352:428, 1998.

Websites

www.managingcontraception.com : includes R.A. Hatcher's *A Pocket Guide to Managing Contraception*.

www.arhp.org : Association of Reproductive Health Professionals

www.not-2-late.com: Emergency Contraception Website

www.ppfa.org: Planned Parenthood Federation of America

www.cdc.gov : Centers for Disease Control and Prevention

26. THE PREGNANT TEEN

Tahniat S. Syed, M.D., and Melanie A. Gold, D.O.

1. How many adolescents become pregnant and give birth annually in the United States?

The U.S. adolescent birth rate, the highest of any industrialized country, has declined steadily from its peak in 1991. By 1997, the birth rate had decreased by 16% for women 15–17 years of age and by 11% for women 18–19 years of age. The decrease occurred in all racial and ethnic groups. The largest decline was in African-American adolescents, especially those aged 15–17 years.

In 1997, there were 94.3 pregnancies/1,000 women 15–19 years of age (19% lower than 1991) and 52.9 live births/1,000 women 15–19 years of age. In 1996, 14% of pregnancies in adolescents aged 15–19 years resulted in miscarriage, 35% in induced abortion, and 51% in live births. In 1999, the total birth rate among adolescents aged 15–17 years was 28.7 births/1,000 women, resulting in 63,588 total births. For adolescents aged 18–19 years, there were 80.3 births/1,000 women, or 312,462 total births. Despite a decrease in the adolescent birth rate every year since 1992, the rate in 1999 was still higher than the rate in 1980.

2. List the indications for a pregnancy test in adolescents.

- History of unprotected sexual intercourse at least 10–14 days previously
- Amenorrhea (no menses for longer than one of patient's usual menstrual cycles)
- Breast tenderness/fullness
- Nausea and/or vomiting
- Weight gain
- Fatigue/dizziness
- Pelvic pain, abdominal pain
- Vaginal spotting or irregular menses

3. How do you decide whether to do a urine or serum pregnancy test?

Approximately 1 week after fertilization, the blastocyst implants into the endometrium to form the syncytiotrophoblast, which produces rising levels of human chorionic gonadotropin (hCG). The hCG concentration peaks at 10 weeks' gestation. Pregnancy tests measure the amount of the beta subunit of hCG in a patient's urine or serum. Urine hCG concentrations approximate serum hCG concentrations; thus, urine hCG measurement is an easy, accurate, valid and cost-effective way to detect most pregnancies. Most urine pregnancy tests are based on monoclonal antibodies to beta-hCG and detect levels as low as 25–50 mIU/mL. Thus urine testing can accurately diagnose pregnancy in an adolescent whose last sexual intercourse occurred at least 10–14 days previously. Serum hCG can be measured qualitatively or quantitatively. Quantitative serum hCG testing is used to diagnose suspected cases of ectopic pregnancy or other abnormalities (e.g., molar pregnancies, blighted ovum). In a normal pregnancy, the hCG should double every 48–72 hours; failure to double suggests an abnormality such as an ectopic pregnancy. There is no significant advantage to serum qualitative hCG for routine pregnancy testing; urine testing is adequate in most circumstances.

4. What are the signs and symptoms of an ectopic pregnancy?

An ectopic pregnancy is a life-threatening surgical emergency. An ectopic pregnancy must be ruled out in any adolescent with a positive hCG who also has pelvic or abdominal pain, vaginal bleeding, cervical motion tenderness, a palpable adnexal mass, or hemodynamic shock.

5. What components of options counseling should be provided to an adolescent with a positive pregnancy test?

An adolescent with a positive pregnancy test should be counseled that she has the following three options:

1. Carry the pregnancy to delivery and raise the baby
2. Carry the pregnancy to delivery and place the baby in adoption or foster care
3. Terminate the pregnancy

Clinicians should identify convenient referral locations as well as local funding resources to assist adolescents in pregnancy outcome choices. If the adolescent decides to continue the pregnancy, refer her for prenatal care and start her on prenatal vitamins. If the patient chooses adoption, refer her for medical, legal, social service, and counseling resources. If the adolescent decides to terminate the pregnancy, refer her for medical or surgical services. All patients considering termination of pregnancy should have a pelvic examination to test for sexually transmitted infections (STIs) and to screen for bacterial vaginosis and a bimanual exam to estimate gestational age. Ensure that a successful referral took place by phone or office visit follow-up. Counseling should include discussions about future plans for preventing unintended pregnancies as well as for continuing education.

6. What psychosocial issues should be considered in counseling an adolescent with a positive pregnancy test?

Be aware of family, social, religious, and cultural issues, and ask how they affect the adolescent's decision about the pregnancy. Provide a supportive environment so that she feels secure enough to examine her own feelings about pregnancy. Reinforce that the decision about the outcome of the pregnancy is hers, and encourage involvement of her parents, a trusted adult, and/or her male partner, all of whom may be helpful and supportive in her decision-making. Be a supportive listener; explain pregnancy options in a nonjudgmental, nondirective way. In addition to options counseling, the pregnant adolescent should be screened for tobacco use and other substance abuse and counseled about the effects of substance use on her unborn child.

7. What consent and confidentiality laws apply to an adolescent with a positive pregnancy test?

Inform the adolescent of the results of her pregnancy test alone in a confidential manner; minors have legal rights that protect their privacy about the diagnosis and treatment of pregnancy. Unless she is suicidal or homicidal or the pregnancy is the result of sexual abuse or rape, consent should be obtained from the patient before disclosing the diagnosis of pregnancy to parents or others. Knowledge of state laws about confidentiality and reporting of suspected abuse, statutory rape, and impaired mental competence is critical to providing appropriate care.

8. How many adolescents receive abortions in the United States?

In 1996, approximately 274,000 abortions were performed in adolescents. Since 1991, the abortion rate has declined 16% among adolescents aged 15–19 years.

9. List common barriers to accessing abortion.

- Delays in recognizing pregnancy, resulting in less time for decision-making
- Distance from an abortion provider
- Inadequate means of transportation to a provider
- Lack of abortion providers
- Lack of available timely appointment
- Cost of procedure and travel
- Harassment and violence by antiabortion protesters
- Perceived stigma of getting an abortion

- Fear of effect on future fertility
- Fear of pain and uncertainty about what to expect from procedure
- State-mandated 24-hour waiting periods, which vary from state to state
- State-mandated parental consent, notification, or judicial court bypass for minors, which vary from state to state

10. What should be included in a preabortion evaluation?

Before having an abortion procedure, an adolescent should be counseled to reduce anxiety, to provide information about the procedure, to screen for underlying psychopathology (e.g., depression, suicidality, ambivalence or coercion to have the abortion, physical or sexual abuse), and to identify how she plans to prevent future unintended pregnancies.

Review her current state of health and medical history. Assess the stability of chronic health problems, such as anemia, diabetes, chronic steroid use, and bleeding disorders. Ask about current respiratory illness, medications, allergies, substance use, history of STIs, previous surgeries, and prior reaction to anesthetics. Perform a complete general physical exam, including a bimanual pelvic exam to assess uterine size, position, and estimation of gestational age.

Preabortion laboratory testing should include screening for STIs and bacterial vaginosis, collecting an annual Papanicolaou smear (if due), checking hemoglobin and/or hematocrit, and determining the patient's Rho(D) antigen status and giving immunoglobulin (RhoGAM), when indicated. The site performing the abortion procedure usually determines the Rh status. An ultrasound to confirm gestational age is indicated if the date of the patient's last menstrual period is unclear or if uterine size is difficult to assess during the bimanual exam because of obesity, anxiety, or uterine retroversion.

11. What are the medical methods of abortion?

	MIFEPRISTONE (MFP) + MISOPROSTOL (MSP)	METHOTREXATE (MTX) + MISOPROSTOL (MSP)
Action	MFP: antiprogesterone, softens and opens the cervix, thins uterine lining MSP: prostaglandin that induces contractions	MTX: cytotoxic folic acid antagonist that impairs rapidly dividing cells MSP: prostaglandin that induces contractions
Administration	MFP: 600 mg orally MSP: 800 µg given 2 days later vaginally or orally	MTX: 50 mg/m^2 given as intramuscular injection or 50 mg orally MSP: 800 µg given 5–7 days later orally or vaginally
Number of visits	Three	Two to three
Efficacy	95–97% at 14 days	90–95% at 14 days
Side effects	MFP: vaginally bleeding (8 ± 4 days) MSP: cramping, nausea, vomiting, diarrhea	MTX: vaginal bleeding (14 ± 7 days) MSP: cramping, nausea, vomiting, diarrhea
Gestational limits:	Up to 49 days' gestation	Up to 49 days' gestation
FDA-approved?	Yes	No, but standard of care allows "off label" use

12. What are the surgical methods of abortion?

Manual vacuum aspiration (MVA), previously known as menstrual extraction
- Gestational limits: 4–10 weeks' gestational age.
- Procedure: a soft, small-bore catheter is inserted through the cervical os, and uterine contents are manually aspirated using a 60-ml syringe.

Dilation and curettage (D&C), also known as dilation and aspiration (D&A); approximately 99% of abortions are performed by this method

- Gestational limits: usually up to 12 weeks, although D&C may be performed up to 18 weeks in some cases.
- Procedure: after administration of local anesthesia (cervical block) or IV sedation, dilator rods of progressively larger diameters are inserted and removed to dilate the cervix. After cervical dilation, a cannula attached to a suction aspiration machine is inserted through the os. The uterine contents are then removed by the mild suction over 10 minutes. Menstrual cramping can occur during the procedure, and bleeding may last for several days afterwards.

Dilation and evacuation (D&E)
- Gestational limits: from 12 to 26 weeks.
- Procedure: the cervix is dilated for a few hours to two days using osmotic dilators. After dilation, a large-bore cannula is used to suction the uterine contents, and tissue forceps are used to grasp and remove parts too large to be suctioned. This procedure takes about 30 minutes and is usually performed under general anesthesia.

13. What is a "partial birth abortion"?

Partial birth abortion is an inaccurate and inflammatory term used to argue against abortions. It is used to describe the abortion procedure dilation and extraction (D&X), which is performed after 19 weeks' gestation but may be indicated at any time after 16 weeks. The D&X is a variation of the D&E in which the cervix is dilated completely to allow the removal of an intact fetus by breech delivery after partial evacuation of intracranial contents to facilitate delivery of the head.

14. What is the average cost of an abortion?

According to the Alan Guttmacher Institute, the average cost of a nonhospital abortion in 1997 was $316 when performed up to 12 weeks, $618 at 16 weeks, and $1,109 at 20 weeks. Few states have medical assistance coverage for elective abortions.

15. How safe are medical and surgical abortion procedures?

Abortion is one the most common and safest surgical procedures performed in the U.S. The risk of death from pregnancy and childbirth is 16 times greater than the risk of death from abortion. The greatest medical risks are usually those associated with general anesthesia or IV sedation rather than with the procedure itself.

16. What are the most common complications associated with surgical abortion?

COMPLICATIONS	INCIDENCE (% OF CASES)
Vasovagal symptoms (diaphoresis, bradycardia, hypotension)	Exact incidence unknown; most commonly occurs during or immediately after completion of the procedure
Missed abortions (retention of viable fetus)	< 0.5%; more common when abortion procedure is done < 6 weeks from LMP without ultrasound confirmation
Incomplete abortion (retention of tissue	< 0.5%
Retention of blood clots	< 1%
Infections (usually from preexisting gonococcal or chlamydial infection)	< 3%
Cervical tears or lacerations	< 1%
Uterine perforation with associated bowel injury	< 0.5%
Uterine hypotonia	< 1%

17. What are the common signs of postabortion complications?

- Severe abdominal or pelvic pain
- Chills
- Fever
- Heavy vaginal bleeding
- Passage of large clots (size of a quarter or larger)
- Foul-smelling vaginal discharge
- Continuing symptoms of pregnancy

18. When should a postabortion check-up be done? What should it include?

The postabortion check up is scheduled within 2–3 weeks after the procedure and can be performed by the patient's primary care provider. The practitioner should ensure that the patient has recovered both emotionally and physically from the procedure and that she has chosen a contraceptive plan for the future. Severe psychological or psychiatric disturbances after an abortion occur in a small percentage of women and usually consist of depression and/or anxiety. The most common emotional response reported after an abortion is relief. Psychological distress is usually greater before the procedure is done and is higher among patients who are scheduled to receive general anesthesia.

The practitioner should assess the severity and duration of pain, need for analgesia, bleeding severity (clot size), duration and history of fever, and sexual intercourse since the procedure. The physical exam should include a breast exam, looking for nipple discharge, masses, and tenderness; a speculum exam to visualize closure of the external cervical os and abnormal discharge; and a bimanual exam to confirm that the uterus is small, firm, and nontender and has involuted to its usual intrapelvic position. A wet mount should be done to evaluate for bacterial vaginosis or other infections.

19. What characteristics of adolescents are associated with a high risk for postabortion adjustment problems?

- Single status
- Nulliparity
- History of serious emotional problems
- Conflictual relationships with sexual partners
- Lack of social support for her decision
- Ambivalence about abortion
- Negative religious or cultural attitudes toward abortion

20. What is the role of hCG testing in the postabortion period?

Levels of hCG usually decrease at least 66% within 48 hours of a successful abortion. A less sensitive pregnancy test that detects 1,000 mIU or more of hCG can confirm successful termination of pregnancy at the postabortion check-up, or the patient can return in another 2–3 weeks for a standard urine pregnancy test that detects 25–50 mIU of hCG.

21. Discuss the legal aspects of abortion in adolescents.

Physicians must provide care that is consistent with state laws. Many states restrict access of a minor (adolescents under age 18) to abortion by requiring single or dual parent notification and/or consent. Over one-half of states mandate some degree of parental involvement in a minor's decision. Only Connecticut, Maine, and the District of Columbia have laws that specifically permit a minor to obtain an abortion by her own consent. Parental notification laws require medical personnel to notify a minor's parents of her intention to obtain an abortion, whereas parental consent laws require medical personnel to obtain written permission from one or both parents before the abortion can be performed. All states with parental notification or consent laws must provide an alternative court bypass system in which a judge can authorize the abortion if he or she determines that the minor is mature enough to make the decision by herself or deems that it is in her best interest. Some states allow a physician to waive parental involvement, and some allow professional counseling instead of parental involvement. Restrictive laws vary greatly from state to state and change frequently. See www.guttmacherinstitute.net for up-to-date information about current state laws regarding minors' consent for abortion.

BIBLIOGRAPHY

1. American Academy of Pediatrics, Committee on Adolescence: Counseling the adolescent about pregnancy options. Pediatrics 101:938–940, 1998.
2. American Academy of Pediatrics, Committee on Adolescence: The adolescent's right to confidential care when considering abortion. Pediatrics 1996;97:746–751, 1996.
3. Cates W, Schulz K, Grimes D: The risks associated with teenage abortion. N Engl J Med 309:621–624, 1983.
4. Creinin M: Medical abortion regimens: Historical context and overview. Am J Obstet Gynecol 183:S3–S9, 2000.
5. Gold M: Abortion. In Coupey SM (ed): Primary Care of Adolescent Girls. Philadelphia, Hanley & Belfus, 2000, pp 319–334.
6. Henshaw S: Factors hindering access to abortion services. Fam Plann Perspect 27:54–59, 87, 1995.
7. Henshaw R, Naji S, Russell I, Templeton A: Psychological responses following medical abortion (using mifepristone and gemeprost) and surgical vacuum aspiration. Acta Obstet Gynecol Scand 73:812–818, 1994.
8. Major B, Cozzarelli C, Cooper M, et al: Psychological responses of women after first-trimester abortion. Arch Gen Psychol 57:777–784, 2000.
9. Paul M, Lichtenberg E, Borgatta L, et al: A Clinician's Guide to Medical and Surgical Abortion. New York, Churchill Livingstone, 1999.
10. Paul M, Schaff E, Nichols M: The roles of clinical assessment, human chorionic gonadotropin assays, and ultrasonography in medical abortion practice. Am J Obstet Gynecol 183:S34–S43, 2000.
11. Ventura S, Mosher W, Curtin S, Abma J: Trends in pregnancy rates for the United States, 1976–97: An update. National Vital Statistics Reports 49:1–10, 2001.

27. SEXUAL ASSAULT

Cynthia Holland-Hall, M.D., M.P.H.

BACKGROUND

1. How many adolescents experience forced and/or unwanted sexual contact?

Rape and other sexual assault rates are higher for adolescents than for any other age group. In an anonymous survey of high school students, about one in five stated that they had experienced some form of unwanted sexual contact. About 10% of eighth- and tenth-grade students stated they had experienced forced intercourse. Young women in the twelfth grade or in their freshman year of college report particularly high rates of acquaintance rape.

2. Are most assaults reported to the police?

Assault episodes frequently are not reported to law enforcement agencies or even to friends or parents. According to the National Crime Victimization Survey, only 30% of all rapes are reported to the police. Adolescents may be less likely to report than adults. Fear, guilt, embarrassment, confusion, and lack of knowledge of their rights are reasons that adolescents may not disclose sexual victimization.

3. How many adolescent sexual assault victims are males?

Female adolescent sexual assault victims outnumber male victims by a ratio of 13.5 to 1. Because male victims are less likely to report sexual assault than female victims, the actual prevalence of sexual assault against males may be higher than realized.

4. What percentage of adolescent rapes and sexual assaults are committed by people known to the victim?

Over 75% of sexual assaults are committed by relatives or acquaintances of the victim. Among older adolescents, the assailant is likely to be a date or social acquaintance; among younger victims, the assailant is likely to be an extended family member. Ninety percent of rapes that are committed on college campuses are committed by someone known to the victim.

5. Where do most of these assaults take place?

A study of adolescents presenting to an emergency department for care after sexual assault revealed that nearly 80% of incidents took place inside homes or vehicles. Far fewer took place on the streets or in woods or parks.

6. What do adolescents think about forced sexual intercourse?

A study of adolescents' perceptions toward violence revealed the following troublesome perceptions about forced sexual intercourse in a dating couple:
- One-third of young women believed that forced intercourse was acceptable if the couple had been dating a long time.
- One-third of young women believed that forced intercourse was acceptable if the woman had initially agreed to have sex but then changed her mind.
- Over one-fourth of young women believed that forced intercourse was acceptable if the woman "led the man on."
- Over one-half of young men believed that forced intercourse was acceptable if the woman initially agreed to have sex but then changed her mind.
- Forty percent of young men believed that forced intercourse was acceptable if the man spent a lot of money on the date.

7. Define statutory rape.

Statutory rape is sexual intercourse with a person under a specified age, which may vary from state to state. Laws in most states are based on the severity of the crime, the age of the victim, and the age difference between victim and assailant. Many states require physicians to report statutory rape.

8. When should a provider suspect that an adolescent has been the victim of sexual assault?

A victim of sexual assault may not immediately disclose what has happened. A girl may present for pregnancy testing or concerns about sexually transmitted infections (STIs). The provider must gently inquire as to why she has these concerns. Victims may alternatively present with chronic somatic complaints unrelated to reproductive health. Very early onset of sexual activity should also raise suspicion of prior sexual abuse or assault; one study showed that nearly three-fourths of adolescents who had sex before 14 years of age had sex involuntarily at an earlier point in their lives. Although the following physical and behavioral symptoms are not necessarily indicative of prior sexual assault, they should lead the provider to consider this possibility.

Physical symptoms	Behavioral/psychological symptoms
Chronic pelvic or abdominal pain	Risky sexual behaviors
Chronic gastrointestinal symptoms	Substance use
Pain with intercourse	Depression
Breast pain	Somatization
Sexually transmitted infections	Problems with interpersonal relations
Chronic headache	Eating disorders/obesity
Musculoskeletal complaints	Insomnia/nightmares
Pregnancy	Depression or suicidality
	Anxiety or posttraumatic stress disorder
	School failure

9. What is the "date-rape" drug?

Flunitrazepam (Rohypnol) and gamma-hydroxybutyrate (GHB) are illicit drugs whose recent increased availability has been temporally associated with increased rates of date and acquaintance rape. Effects of these drugs include sedation, muscle relaxation, and amnesia. They are essentially colorless and odorless substances that can be added to the victim's drink, and they are particularly potent when combined with alcohol. Because they may be undetectable in a routine urine drug test, notify the toxicology laboratory that you are suspicious of their use. Many labs can then test specifically for these drugs.

10. After sexual assault, how likely is it that a patient will acquire a sexually transmitted infection (STI)?

The Centers for Disease Control and Prevention estimates the following risks for STI acquisition after sexual assault:

• *Neisseria gonorrhoeae*: 6–12%
• *Chlamydia trachomatis*: 4–17%
• Syphilis: 0.5–3%
• Human immunodeficiency virus (HIV): < 1%

11. What is rape survivor syndrome?

Also known as rape trauma syndrome, rape survivor syndrome includes mood swings and feelings of disbelief, anxiety, fear, and guilt in the weeks after the assault. This reaction is followed by an adjustment/reorganization phase that may last from months to years until the victim finally recovers. Some form of posttraumatic stress disorder occurs in up to 80% of rape survivors. Depression is also a common sequela.

EVALUATION OF THE SEXUAL ASSAULT VICTIM

12. What special measures should be taken during the evaluation of the adolescent assault victim?

Sexual assault evaluations can be particularly traumatic for young victims. Perform the evaluation in a quiet, private room if possible. Female victims should have a female chaperone or family member with them during the evaluation if they so desire. Proceed with the physical evaluation and forensic evidence collection only with the patient's consent.

13. What are the goals of the initial sexual assault evaluation?
- Evaluate and treat traumatic injuries.
- Provide prophylaxis against sexually transmitted infections.
- Provide prophylaxis against pregnancy.
- Collect forensic evidence.
- Ensure social and psychological support.
- Arrange medical and mental health follow-up.
- Provide the above in a safe, private environment.

If the evaluation takes place more than 72 hours after the assault, certain elements, such as collecting forensic evidence and providing prophylaxis against pregnancy, may no longer be possible.

14. What is a "rape kit"?

These forensic evidence kits are usually available in emergency departments and other places where sexual assault victims present for care. One can also obtain a kit from the local law enforcement agency. If the assault took place within the previous 72 hours and the patient has not bathed, physical evidence may be collected that can be used if the victim chooses to pursue prosecution of the assailant. Whenever possible, specially trained personnel should be involved in the collection and processing of the forensic evidence kit. If the protocol for collecting evidence is not strictly followed or if the chain of custody of the evidence (i.e., appropriate handling and protection of the evidence by designated personnel) is broken, the evidence may not be admissible in a court of law.

15. What kind of forensic evidence is collected?

In addition to collecting specimens for STI identification and specimens to assist in distinguishing the victim's secretions from the assailant's, potential evidence includes:
- The victim's underwear and other clothing, which may contain debris to aid in the identification of the assailant
- Swabs of the assailant's saliva, semen, or blood from the victim's skin and/or the genital area
- Scrapings/debris from under the victim's fingernails or from the pubic hair
- Blood for baseline HIV and syphilis testing

16. What are the most pertinent historical elements of a sexual assault evaluation?

The following should be obtained in a sensitive, nonjudgmental manner and should be clearly documented in the medical record. Use the victim's own words whenever possible.
- Use of physical force/violence
- Particular sexual acts performed (e.g., vaginal, anal, oral penetration)
- Ejaculation
- Condom use (recall that many assaults occur on dates and with known assailants)
- Previous consensual sex with assailant
- Alcohol or drug use at time of assault (by victim or perpetrator)
- Actions taken after the assault
- Last menstrual period/possibility of preexisting pregnancy

17. What should be documented from the physical exam?
Careful description of both genital trauma and nongenital injuries (e.g., bruises, bite marks), including drawings or photographs. Include documentation of the presence of sperm on microscopic evaluation of vaginal/rectal secretions.

18. What laboratory studies should be obtained?
Victims should be tested for gonococcal and chlamydial infection at all sites of genital contact. Although nonculture tests such as nucleic acid amplification tests are most sensitive, they are not approved for all testing sites (e.g., anal and pharyngeal specimens) and may lead to false-positive results. Because of its high specificity, culture is the only test admissible as evidence in most courts. Microscopic evaluation and/or culture of vaginal secretions for trichomoniasis should be performed. Baseline serologies for syphilis, hepatitis B virus, and HIV may be obtained to document the absence of these infections at the time of initial assessment. A pregnancy test can evaluate for preexisting pregnancy.

TREATMENT

19. What is appropriate prophylactic antibiotic treatment for a sexual assault victim?
The victim should be treated empirically for gonococcal, chlamydial, and trichomonal infections. The following regimen may be used:
• Ceftriaxone, 125 mg intramuscularly, single dose
• Azithromycin, 1 gm orally, single dose
• Metronidazole, 2 gm orally, single dose
Azithromycin and metronidazole may be taken at separate times to avoid excessive gastrointestinal upset. Prophylaxis against HIV infection is not routinely recommended because of the low risk of acquiring this infection.

20. When should you consider offering HIV prophylaxis?
The risks and benefits of HIV prophylaxis should be discussed with the victim. Consider any information known about the assailant's HIV risk behaviors, such as intravenous drug use and sexual practices, and the epidemiology of HIV infection in your geographic area. The victim must understand the potential side effects of antiretroviral therapy, the need to adhere strictly to the prescribed regimen, and the importance of close follow-up. The decision should then be made on a case-by-case basis. Choose the medication regimen according to current guidelines for occupational mucous membrane exposure.

21. Should any other STI prophylaxis be offered?
Adolescents who have not previously been immunized against hepatitis B virus (HBV) should receive the first dose of the vaccination. Follow-up doses should be administered 1–2 months and 4–6 months after the first dose. The vaccine should adequately protect against HBV acquisition. Routine use of hepatitis B immunoglobulin is not recommended.

22. Should you protect against anything else?
Pregnancy prophylaxis should be offered if the patient presents within 72–120 hours of sexual assault involving vaginal penetration. Ideally, pregnancy prophylaxis should be available at the time of evaluation, because emergency contraception is most efficacious when given as soon as possible after unprotected intercourse. Several regimens for emergency contraception are described in Chapter 25.

23. When should follow-up be arranged?
A follow-up visit should occur 2–3 weeks after the assault. When possible, it should be arranged before the patient leaves the initial visit. Follow-up STI screening should be considered at this visit, particularly if the victim did not receive prophylactic antibiotics. A pregnancy

test should be performed if the patient has not had her menses. Syphilis testing should be performed 4–6 weeks after the assault, and HIV testing should be performed 3–6 months after the assault. The patient's psychological state should be assessed during the follow-up visit, and referrals for mental health services may be made if this step has not already been taken.

PREVENTION

24. How should adolescents be screened for a history of sexual assault?
Adolescents should be directly interviewed about this issue in private during routine exams or when they present with reproductive health concerns or other vague or chronic symptoms. Questions you may use include the following:
- How old were you the first time you had sex?
- Did you ever have sex when you really did not want to do so?
- Has anyone ever forced you to participate in a sexual act against your will?

Pay attention not only to verbal answers but also to nonverbal communication cues that may indicate the need to probe further.

25. What advice can a clinician give an adolescent or young woman to help her prevent becoming a victim of sexual assault?
- You make the ultimate decisions about your body—no one else.
- You have the right to refuse any unwanted touching at any time by saying "No" or "Stop."
- You have the right to decide the limits of sexual involvement with your partner and to insist that he respect them, even if you have been dating for a long time.
- You are allowed to change your mind about whether you want to have sex with someone.
- Avoid being alone or in an isolated place with anyone whom you do not know very well.
- At a party or bar, get your drinks yourself and keep them in your sight at all times.
- Avoid using alcohol or drugs.
- If a situation makes you feel unsafe or uncomfortable, even if you are not sure why, leave.
- On a date, make sure that you are able to get home on your own if necessary. Have money to make a phone call or to pay bus or cab fare.

BIBLIOGRAPHY

1. American Academy of Pediatrics, Committee on Adolescence: Care of the adolescent sexual assault victim. Pediatrics 107:1476, 2001.
2. American College of Emergency Physicians: Evaluation and Management of the Sexually Assaulted or Sexually Abused Patient. Dallas, American College of Emergency Physicians, 1999. Available at www.acep.org/library/index.cfm/id/2101.
3. American College of Obstetricians and Gynecologists, Committee on Adolescent Health Care: Adolescent Victims of Sexual Assault. ACOG Educational Bulletin No. 252, 1998.
4. American Medical Association: Strategies for the Treatment and Prevention of Sexual Assault. Chicago, AMA, 1995.
5. Bechtel K, Podrazik M: Evaluation of the adolescent rape victim. Pediatr Clin North Am 46:809, 1999.
6. Centers for Disease Control and Prevention: 1998 Guidelines for treatment of sexually transmitted diseases. MMWR 47(RR-1):108–116, 1998.
7. Elstein SG, Davis N: Sexual Relationships between Adult Males and Young Teen Girls: Exploring the Legal and Social Responses. Chicago, American Bar Association, 1997.
8. Newell AR, Richardson C, et al: Treatment of the adolescent survivor of sexual assault. Clin Fam Pract 2:883, 2000.
9. Parrot A: Acquaintance rape among adolescents: Identifying risk groups and intervention strategies. J Soc Work Hum Sex 8:47, 1989.
10. Peipert JF, Domagalski LR: Epidemiology of adolescent sexual assault. Obstet Gynecol 84:867, 1994.

28. GENITAL DISORDERS IN MALES

Cynthia Holland-Hall, M.D., M.P.H.

1. What are the common causes of painless testicular swelling or masses?
- Hydrocele
- Varicocele
- Spermatocele
- Hernia (not incarcerated)
- Testicular tumor
- Idiopathic scrotal edema (more common in prepubertal boys)

2. What is a varicocele?
The venous drainage system of the testis is complex, and varies among individuals. The pampiniform plexus is a branching, interconnected system of veins that surround the testicular artery, perhaps serving as a cooling mechanism for blood flowing to the testis. The pampiniform plexus originates at the testis and extends into the spermatic cord. A varicocele forms when these vessels become dilated.

3. How many teens have a varicocele?
Up to 15% of male adolescents have a varicocele. This is about the same as the prevalence in older men.

4. How is a varicocele diagnosed?
Although most varicoceles are asymptomatic, the patient may complain of a fullness or dragging sensation. Varicoceles are typically found during routine physical exams. The clinician may palpate a "bag of worms" or soft tubular structures above the testis when the patient is standing. In the supine position, this gravity-dependent lesion decreases or disappears entirely. If it is still palpable, consider alternative diagnoses or the possibility of an intra-abdominal structure impeding venous return.

5. How are varicoceles classified?
- Grade I: Varicocele is detectable only when the patient performs a Valsalva maneuver
- Grade II: Varicocele is palpable but not visible
- Grade III: Varicocele is visible on inspection

6. On which side is a varicocele typically found? Why?
About 85% of young men with varicoceles have the lesion on the left side only. Of the remaining 15%, most have bilateral varicoceles. This is likely due to the anatomic differences in venous return between the two testicles. The right testicular (or internal spermatic) vein drains directly into the inferior vena cava, a very low-pressure system, at an oblique angle. The left testicular vein drains into the left renal vein, a smaller vein with higher pressures, at a right angle. This higher pressure is transmitted to the pampiniform plexus, and venous dilatation occurs. An isolated right-sided varicocele is unusual and should be referred to a urologist for further evaluation.

7. What kind of problems can a varicocele cause?
Varicoceles are clearly associated with time-dependent decline in testicular function. They are the most common cause of adult male factor infertility, although only 15–20% of men with a varicocele ever seek treatment for infertility. Testicular atrophy (relative to the unaffected side) is an indicator of decreasing testicular function and is more commonly found when the varicocele is large. The precise mechanism of decreased testicular function is unclear.

8. When should a patient with a varicocele be referred for possible correction?

Testicular size should be assessed with an orchidometer or with ultrasound. Patients with a difference in testicular volume of more than 2–3 ml should be evaluated by a urologist. Following surgical repair or embolization, "catch up" testicular growth occurs in 80% of patients. Patients who are symptomatic or who have very large varicoceles, bilateral varicoceles, or right-sided varicoceles may be considered for treatment as well. Semen analysis or gonadotropin-releasing hormone (GnRH) stimulation testing may be useful in selected patients to guide therapy.

9. What is the recurrence rate following surgical repair?

Adolescents have a 9–16% recurrence rate for varicocele following surgical repair. This is significantly higher than the recurrence rate for adults.

10. How do you counsel a patient with a varicocele who does not need referral to a urologist?

Reassure the patient that this is a common lesion among young men, and it is generally benign. Remind him that although there is an increased risk of infertility, most young men with varicoceles are fertile, and he must still practice contraception with his partner(s). Most varicoceles can simply be followed by the primary care provider during annual exams. Teach testicular self-examination (TSE), and instruct the patient to note testicular size and watch for evidence of atrophy. As an adult, he may see a urologist for semen analysis to assess fertility. Be aware of the potential psychological impact of telling a young man that he has a genital lesion, encourage him to ask questions, and provide reassurance that his sexual performance should not be impaired.

11. How do you counsel a patient with an inguinal hernia?

An asymptomatic patient with an inguinal hernia should be referred for elective surgical correction in the near future. The adolescent should be taught how to reduce the hernia and the signs and symptoms of incarceration (scrotal pain and swelling, abdominal pain, nausea and vomiting) and to seek medical attention immediately should he experience these symptoms.

12. How does a patient with hydrocele typically present?

Hydroceles are painless, soft, cystic masses that typically are found anterior to the testis. They may increase in size over the course of the day. Although hydroceles are generally painless, patients occasionally may complain of a heaviness or mild aching sensation. On physical exam, the testis should be palpable and discrete from the hydrocele. The hydrocele itself will transilluminate when a light source is placed behind it. In the presence of scrotal pathology, a reactive hydrocele may develop. The examiner must therefore be certain that the underlying testis is normal when a hydrocele is noted.

13. Should a hydrocele be surgically corrected?

No intervention is required for most hydroceles. If the patient experiences discomfort or dislikes the cosmetic appearance of the hydrocele, surgical correction may be undertaken.

14. How can you tell the difference between a hydrocele and a spermatocele?

Spermatoceles are painless, pea-sized cystic lesions that contain sperm. Spermatoceles are smaller than most hydroceles, and they are located at the upper portion of the epididymis, superior and posterior to the testis. Like hydroceles, they may transilluminate.

15. Should a spermatocele be surgically corrected?

Spermatoceles are typically benign, painless lesions, although rarely they may undergo torsion. Surgical correction is not necessary and is relatively contraindicated because removing a spermatocele may actually compromise fertility by damaging the vas deferens.

16. How common is testicular cancer in teens?

Testicular cancer is the most common solid tumor in males 15–34 years old, with an incidence of 1 in 10,000 in this age group. Most testicular tumors in adolescents are seminomas. The cure rate is excellent when the primary lesion is identified early. Teaching TSE to young men is, therefore, critical.

17. What are risk factors for testicular cancer?

Caucasians have a fourfold higher incidence of testicular cancer than non-caucasians. Young men who have a history of an undescended testicle have a 20–40-fold increased risk of cancer as well, even after surgical fixation of the testis in the scrotum. Orchipexy is still recommended, however, because it allows earlier detection of a testicular mass. Patients with a history of an undescended testicle should have regular follow-up with a urologist throughout adulthood.

18. How should male adolescents be counseled regarding testicular cancer?

Male adolescents should be taught TSE when their genital development reaches Sexual Maturity Rating III or when they are cognitively mature enough to understand the teaching. Begin by asking the teen what he knows about testicular cancer. Correct any misinformation, such as the belief that testicular cancer generally affects elderly men. Adolescents and young men should perform TSE monthly, preferably in the shower. Instruct your patient to roll each testicle between his thumb and fingers until the entire surface is felt, noting any lumps, hard pieces, changes in size, or painful areas and informing a doctor of any changes found. Review TSE technique with the patient at subsequent visits.

19. What is the differential diagnosis of testicular pain?

Testicular torsion	Hematoma secondary to trauma
Torsion of the appendix testis	Incarcerated hernia
Epididymitis	Henoch-Schönlein syndrome
Orchitis	

The first three diagnoses on this list account for the vast majority of cases of acute testicular pain.

20. Why is orchitis less common today than it used to be?

Because most children in the United States are now immunized against mumps virus. Previously, up to 1 in 3 adolescents infected with mumps developed orchitis.

21. What are risk factors for testicular torsion?

The peak incidence of testicular torsion is in male adolescents 12–18 years old. Incidence is about 1 in 4000 in males younger than 25 years. When the testis is undescended, the incidence increases tenfold. Once the testis is surgically fixed in the scrotum, however, the risk of torsion is low. Young men with the "bell clapper deformity" of the testis are predisposed to developing torsion as well.

22. What is the "bell clapper deformity"?

Embryologically, when the testis descends into the scrotum, it pulls the tunica vaginalis fascial layer with it. The tunica vaginalis remnant typically is primarily anterior to the testis. When it more completely surrounds the testis, the testis moves more freely in the scrotum, like the clapper of a bell.

23. How does a patient with testicular torsion typically present?

When the testis twists on the spermatic cord, blood flow to the testis is compromised and infarction begins. The onset of unilateral scrotal pain typically is abrupt. Pain often begins while the patient is at rest, but it may begin with activity. Abdominal pain, nausea, and vomiting may be present. About 50% of men with torsion retrospectively report prior similar episodes of pain that were self-limited.

24. What is the physical exam like in a patient with torsion?

On physical exam, the patient clearly is in a great deal of discomfort. Unilateral scrotal swelling and tenderness are present. The affected testis often is higher in the scrotum than the unaffected testis, and the testis may lay in a transverse orientation. The torsed testis may appear larger than the contralateral testis because of venous congestion and edema. The thickened spermatic cord may be palpable in the inguinal canal. The cremasteric reflex is absent on the affected side.

25. What laboratory studies are useful for diagnosing testicular torsion?

No serum or urine abnormalities are typically found in the presence of torsion. Although laboratory studies may be obtained to evaluate for epididymitis, which may be on the differential, do not wait for laboratory results to proceed with the evaluation of torsion.

26. What imaging studies may be used to aid in the diagnosis of testicular torsion?

Radionucleotide scintigraphy or Doppler flow studies may confirm the clinical diagnosis of torsion. These tests should be used only when the diagnosis of torsion is in question; it is not necessary to prove that the patient has torsion with an imaging study if the clinical presentation is consistent with this diagnosis.

27. What are the advantages and disadvantages of radionucleotide scintigraphy scans in the diagnosis of torsion?

Nuclear medicine scans have 95% diagnostic accuracy in diagnosing torsion. The impeded blood flow to the torsed testicle shows up as a "cold" spot on the scan. Epididymitis and other acute inflammatory lesions often show up as "hot" spots. Because of the time required to perform the exam, the need for intravenous access, and the more limited availability, this study is used less frequently than ultrasound to diagnose torsion.

28. What are the advantages and disadvantages of ultrasound in the diagnosis of torsion?

Color Doppler flow studies assess blood flow to the testis. They are quick, noninvasive, and inexpensive. They are, however, highly operator dependent and give higher rates of indeterminate and false-negative exams than radionucleotide scintigraphy. They may be useful for diagnosing other scrotal pathology, such as a hydrocele or hematoma.

29. How is suspected testicular torsion managed?

Testicular torsion is a surgical emergency, and the treating clinician must proceed quickly with diagnosis and management. Notify the urologist as soon as possible when seriously considering this diagnosis, and begin preparing the patient for probable surgery (e.g., keep the patient NPO, start an IV). The diagnosis is often clinical, and there may be little utility in waiting for test results. In the operating room, detorsion is performed. If the testis is viable when blood flow is restored, orchipexy is performed to fix the testis in the scrotum. If it is not viable, orchiectomy is performed. Fixation of the contralateral testis is performed as well, since up to 40% of patients may develop contralateral torsion.

30. Why is it so important to diagnose testicular torsion quickly?

If surgery is undertaken within 6 hours of the onset of symptoms, the prognosis is excellent. However, the success rate (i.e., the ability to save a viable testis) drops to 20% when surgery is delayed to 12 hours after the onset of symptoms. Testicular salvage is highly unlikely after 24 hours. Torsion is the most common cause of testicular loss in young men.

31. What if surgery has to be delayed? Is there anything you can do for your patient in the meantime?

If a significant delay in surgery is anticipated, manual detorsion may be attempted as a temporizing measure to prevent further testicular ischemia. In most cases of torsion, the anterior aspect of the testis rotates medially. Detorsion therefore is performed by gently externally rotating the testis. As a mnemonic, when standing at the supine patient's feet, the detorsion movement is similar to opening a book.

32. How is torsion of the appendix testis diagnosed?

The appendix testis, a small, often pedunculated müllerian duct remnant on the anterior aspect of the testis, may undergo torsion. This typically occurs in young adolescents and is rare after 20 years of age. Onset of pain is more gradual and less severe than for testicular torsion. The classic "blue dot sign" may be present when the infarcting appendix testis can be seen through the scrotal skin. Torsion of the appendix epididymis, an appendage at the head of the epididymis, may cause similar symptoms.

33. What is the treatment for torsion of the appendix testis?

This condition is self-limited. The appendix testis undergoes auto-infarction, and the pain gradually resolves. Bed rest, analgesia, and scrotal elevation using an athletic supporter may reduce the inflammation and associated edema. Pain and swelling should resolve within 1 week.

34. What organisms are usually responsible for causing epididymitis?

Chlamydia trachomatis and *Neisseria gonorrhoeae* are the most common causative organisms. It should, therefore, come as no surprise that epididymitis occurs primarily in sexually active adolescents. If other organisms such as gram-negative enteric pathogens are isolated, the patient may have an anatomic genitourinary anomaly, may engage in anal intercourse, or may have inserted a foreign body into the urethra thereby introducing unusual pathogens.

35. How does the presentation of epididymitis differ from the presentation of torsion?

The onset of pain is usually subacute with epididymitis, compared to the abrupt onset of pain with torsion. Patients with epididymitis often have had pain for 24 hours or more before presentation. Urethral discharge, dysuria, and fever are helpful diagnostic findings suggesting epididymitis, but they are not reliably present. It may be possible to localize the tenderness to the epididymis at the superior posterior aspect of the testis. The cremasteric reflex may be present or absent.

36. What is Prehn's sign?

A patient with epididymitis may have some alleviation of his pain when the scrotum is elevated manually. This is Prehn's sign.

37. Are laboratory studies useful for diagnosing epididymitis?

Although laboratory studies may all be normal, some can be useful if positive. Gram stain of a urethral swab may show white blood cells (WBCs) and gram-negative diplococci if *N. gonorrhoeae* is the pathogen. Urinalysis may be positive for leukocytes. Of course urethral culture or nonculture testing for *N. gonorrhoeae* and *C. trachomatis* are useful, but these results are not generally available for immediate clinical decision-making. Serum WBC count is not useful in distinguishing epididymitis from torsion.

38. How is epididymitis treated?

To cover the suspected pathogens, a single dose of ceftriaxone, 250 mg, may be given intramuscularly, followed by doxycycline, 100 mg orally twice a day for 10 days. Patients over

18 years old may be treated with oral ofloxacin, 300 mg twice a day for 10 days. If sexually acquired epididymitis is suspected, sexual partners should be notified and treated. The infection should improve quickly and resolve within 2 weeks of initiating treatment. If epididymitis was not sexually acquired, or if it does not respond as anticipated to antibiotic treatment, consider further anatomic investigation of the urinary tract.

39. What is an approach to the acute presentation of an adolescent with a painful scrotum?

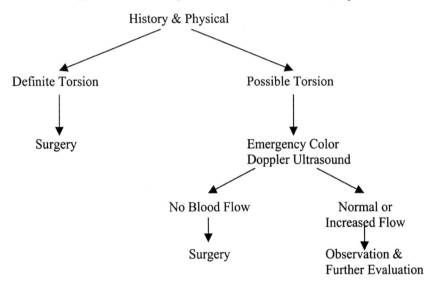

BIBLIOGRAPHY

1. Goldenring JM: A lifesaving exam for young men. Contemp Pediatr (Apr):63, 1992.
2. Kass EJ: Adolescent varicocele. Pediatr Clin North Am 48:1559–1569, 2001.
3. Luzzi GA, O'Brien TS: Acute epididymitis. BJU Int 87:747–755, 2001.
4. Marcozzi D, Suner S: The nontraumatic, acute scrotum. Emerg Med Clin North Am 19:547–568, 2001.
5. Pillai SB, Besner GE: Pediatric testicular problems. Pediatr Clin North Am 45:813–830, 1998.
6. Skoog S, Roberts K, Goldstein M, Pryor JL: The adolescent varicocele: What's new with an old problem in young patients? Pediatrics 100:112–121, 1997.
7. Thomas R: Testicular tumors. Adoles Med State Art Rev 7:149–156, 1996.

IV. Mental Health and Psychosocial Concerns

29. SUBSTANCE ABUSE

Peter Rogers, M.D., M.P.H.

1. List early conduct problems that have been associated with a later substance abuse disorder among adolescents.

Aggressiveness, emotional lability, negativity, sulkiness, and blaming others at age 3 years have been associated with a substance abuse disorder at age 14 years.

2. What family factors may influence the development of an adolescent substance abuse disorder?

Parental separation/divorce; parental attitudes about use of drugs and alcohol; a father with a substance abuse disorder; history of physical or sexual abuse; lack of parental closeness; lack of family activities; inconsistent discipline.

3. Comment on the percentages of high school students who use illicit drugs other than marijuana since 1990.

The lifetime prevalence of use of illicit drugs other than marijuana has increased among 12th graders and 10th graders but decreased for 8th graders since 1990. Approximately 25% of 12th graders, 22% of 10th graders, and 18% of 8th grade students in the year 2000 had used illicit drugs other than marijuana.

MARIJUANA

4. What is the most common illicit drug of abuse among 8th, 10th, and 12th grade students?

Marijuana. According to the Monitoring the Future Study conducted in 2000, 9% of 8th graders, 20% of 10th graders, and 21.6% of 12th graders state that they have smoked marijuana in the previous 30 days.

5. What percent of 12th-grade students state that they smoke marijuana daily?

Six percent of 12th-grade students in the 2000 Monitoring the Future Study stated that they smoke marijuana daily. This percent is virtually unchanged from 1998 data.

6. According to the Monitoring the Future Study, what three factors contribute to the continued increased use of marijuana?

1. Marijuana is universally available; 90% of high school seniors say that they know where to get the drug if they want to use it.

2. The perceived risk of marijuana as a harmful drug continues to decline.

3. The personal disapproval rating for marijuana use is low compared with other illicit drug use.

7. In what two areas of the brain are most of the receptor sites for delta-9-tetrahydrocannabinol (THC)?

1. The hippocampus, which is involved in short-term memory formation.

2. The cerebellum, which is involved in balance. A chronic user of marijuana may have poor short-term memory and often has a positive Romberg test.

8. How has the potency of marijuana changed in the past 25 years?
The potency of marijuana is defined as the percent of delta-9-THC in the dried sample. Since 1973, the Marijuana Potency Project at the University of Mississippi has determined the potency of street samples of marijuana submitted by the U.S. Drug Enforcement Agency. In 1973, the average potency of street samples of marijuana was approximately 2%. The current potency of selected grades of sensimilla is about 12%. Some believe that the increase in potency has increased addiction liability. In 1964, John Lennon made the comment that "Marijuana is nothing more than a harmless giggle." It is not a "harmless giggle" anymore.

9. Is cannabis withdrawal a recognized clinical entity?
Cannabis withdrawal is not recognized in the *Diagnostic and Statistical Manual of Mental Disorders* (DSM-IV). Because delta-9-THC is lipophilic, it is slowly released from fat stores. When use is discontinued, THC continues to be released slowly; therefore, withdrawal is not as dramatic as, for example, with alcohol. Although no toxic syndrome is associated with cannabis withdrawal, abrupt cessation after chronic, heavy use is associated with insomnia, irritability, restlessness, depression, drug craving, and nervousness.

10. What is amotivational syndrome?
This expression describes the apathy, loss of energy, and decreased goal-directed activity that may be seen in frequent users of marijuana.

ALCOHOL

11. What percent of 12th grade students state that they had five or more drinks on one occasion in the past two weeks?
Thirty percent of 12th-grade students have had five or more drinks at one time in the past two weeks, according to the Monitoring the Future study. This percentage has remained virtually unchanged over the past 15 years, reflecting the problem of binge drinking among adolescents and young adults.

12. What percent of parents know that their high school senior drinks every 2 weeks?
According to a Johnson Institute study, only 3% of parents believe that their high school senior son or daughter drinks every 2 weeks.

13. What other adolescent risk-taking behaviors are associated with alcohol abuse?
Alcohol use contributes significantly to adolescent accidents, homicide, and suicide, the top three causes of death in people aged 15–24 years. Furthermore, alcohol use is associated with acts of violence (intentional and unintentional), motor vehicle accidents (fatal and nonfatal), sexual assault, and more frequent sexual intercourse with more partners.

14. Do many adolescents drink and drive?
In an anonymous survey of high school students, one-third stated that within the past month they had ridden in a car with a driver who had been drinking alcohol, and 17% had driven after drinking alcohol.

15. Is there a genetic predisposition to alcohol abuse?
Sons of alcoholic fathers have 1 in 4 risk of becoming alcoholics. Daughters of alcoholic fathers also are at an increased risk of becoming alcoholics and marrying an alcoholic.

16. Children of alcoholics are at an increased risk for what problems?
Children of alcohol abusers are at increased risk for delinquent behavior, learning disorders, attention deficit–hyperactivity disorder, psychosomatic complaints, and problem drinking and alcoholism as adults.

17. What effect has raising the minimum legal drinking age (MLDA) to 21 years had on traffic fatalities?

Based on multiple studies, the National Highway Traffic Safety Administration estimates that raising the MLDA has reduced traffic fatalities among 18- to 20-year-old drivers by 13%. Twenty of 29 studies conducted between 1981 and 1992 reported significant reduction in traffic crashes and fatalities since the MLDA was raised.

18. What effect have "zero tolerance" laws had on traffic fatalities?

Zero tolerance laws state that the blood alcohol concentration for drivers under the age of 21 years must be less than 0.02. These laws have resulted in a 20% decline in the proportion of drinking drivers involved in fatal crashes who were younger than 21 as well as a significant decline in single-vehicle, nighttime fatal crashes among drivers under 21 years old.

19. How do parental attitudes affect adolescent drinking behavior?

Parents' favorable attitudes about alcohol use and parents' drinking behavior have been positively associated with adolescents' initiating and continuing to drink. Early initiation of drinking has been identified as an important risk factor for later alcohol-related problems. Lack of parental support, monitoring, and communication have been significantly related to frequency of drinking, heavy drinking, and drunkenness among adolescents. In addition, harsh and inconsistent discipline and hostility and rejection toward children have been shown to predict adolescent drinking and alcohol-related problems. Children who report being warned about alcohol use by their parents and who report being close to their parents are less likely to start drinking during adolescence.

"CLUB" DRUGS

20. Name the six drugs that the National Institute of Drug Abuse refers to as "club drugs."
- Ecstasy (3,4-methylenedioxymethamphetamine)
- Gamma-hydroxybutyrate (GHB)
- Ketamine
- Rohypnol (flunitrazepam)
- Methamphetamine
- Lysergic acid diethylamide (LSD)

21. Use of what illicit drug has increased most dramatically among 12th-grade students between 1995 and 2000?

Ecstasy. In the year 2000, 11% of high school seniors had tried ecstasy, approximately double the percent of 12th graders who had used the drug in 1995.

22. What makes Ecstasy chemically unique?

Ecstasy, or 3,4-methylenedioxymethamphetamine (MDMA), is unique because it is both a hallucinogen and an amphetamine stimulant.

23. What two drugs are commonly referred to as "date rape" drugs?

Flunitrazepam (Rohypnol), a benzodiazepine, and gamma-hydroxybutyrate (GHB) are the two drugs most commonly reported to be used in "date rapes." Both drugs are short-acting. Rohypnol is commonly given to the victim with alcohol. GHB can have its effects if given alone; it is tasteless and odorless.

24. Is the use of LSD within the past 30 days increasing or decreasing among 8th, 10th, and 12th graders?

LSD use is decreasing in all three grade levels. In the year 2000, 1% of 8th graders, 1.6 % of 10th graders, and 1.6% of 12th graders reported use in the previous month. The use of LSD by 12th graders has hovered around 2% for the past 10 years. The adolescent who uses LSD is probably past the experimental stage of drug and alcohol use and should be considered a candidate for substance abuse treatment. Because the tolerance to LSD increases dramatically, most adolescents who use the drug rarely use it more than 2–3 times per week.

25. What were the rates of ketamine use and GHB use among 8th, 10th, and 12th graders in the year 2000?

	8TH GRADE	10TH GRADE	12TH GRADE
Ketamine	1.2%	1%	2%
GHB	1.6%	2.1%	2.5%

INHALANTS

26. The greatest prevalence of inhalant abuse occurs among which racial/ethnic group?
Non-Hispanic white adolescents have the highest prevalence of inhalant abuse. Non-Hispanic black adolescents have the lowest prevalence of inhalant abuse among all age groups.

27. What are the gender differences in inhalant abuse?
Boys report a slightly increased lifetime usage rate compared with girls (17.6% vs. 14%, respectively). Girls, however, report beginning use of inhalants at a younger age, often at age 12 or 13 years.

28. What methods do adolescents use to get the psychoactive effect of inhalants?
Inhalation is achieved through several methods: "sniffing" involves inhaling the vapors directly from an open container or heated pan; "bagging" refers to inhalation of vapors from a plastic or paper bag containing the substance; "huffing" refers to the oral or nasal inhalation of vapors by holding a piece of cloth that has been soaked in the volatile substance against the nose and/or mouth.

29. What types of inhaled substances are used by adolescents?
The most common types of abused inhalants fall into 5 groups:
1. Aliphatic hydrocarbons (e.g., gasoline, propane, butane).
2. Alkylhalides, which are found in dry cleaning fluids, paint stripper, and spot removers. They contain trichloroethane and trichloroethylene.
3. Aromatic hydrocarbons (e.g., toluene, benzene), which are contained in spray paint, paint thinner, and glues and varnishes.
4. Nitrites, which are contained in room air fresheners and vasodilators.
5. Ketones (e.g., acetone, butanone), which are contained in nail polish removers and spray paints.

30. How do inhalants affect the brain?
Most solvents are absorbed rapidly into neurons (from the blood) because of their high lipid content. Most volatile agents act as central nervous system (CNS) depressants due to generalized alteration of neuronal function. Toluene is probably the most damaging to the CNS, causing an acute encephalopathic syndrome characterized by euphoria, hallucinations, seizures, and coma. Chronic toluene exposure has been shown to cause cortical atrophy and cerebellar damage.

31. Describe the sudden sniffing death syndrome.
Hydrocarbons contained in inhalants appear to sensitize the myocardium to epinephrine. Anything that can cause a sudden release of endogenous catecholamines while a person is using a hydrocarbon-containing inhalant may lead to ventricular fibrillation and death.

32. How do inhalants affect the lungs?

The most common effects of inhalants on the lungs include asphyxiation and direct damage to pulmonary tissue. Volatile substances may displace oxygen, leading to signs and symptoms of hypoxia and loss of consciousness. Hydrocarbons may cause a chemical pneumonitis.

33. What is "huffer's rash"?

Repeated use of volatiles may cause desiccation and cracking of the skin. Secondary bacterial infections of cracked skin in the perioral/perinasal area is often referred to as "huffer's rash." It may be seen in frequent users of inhalants.

STIMULANTS

34. How many high school seniors have used cocaine?

Cocaine use peaked in the 1980s, before its dangerous and highly addictive nature was widely recognized. Although it has decreased significantly since that time, cocaine use has been slowly increasing again since the early 1990s. Nearly 9% of high school seniors have tried it.

35. What is "ice"?

"Ice," also known as "crystal meth," is the smokable form of the potent D-methamphetamine. Some adolescents use methamphetamine and other stimulants to increase alertness or promote weight loss; others use it for its euphoric and hypomanic effect. Ice is generally used for the latter.

ASSESSMENT AND INTERVENTION

36. How can a provider screen an adolescent for substance use or abuse?

Interview the patient alone after reviewing your confidentiality policy. Inquire directly about what drugs the adolescent has used, how much and how often, and the settings in which they are used. Determine the extent to which the adolescent's home, school, and social functioning are impaired by substance use. Sample questions to initiate a discussion of substance abuse include the following:

- Do any of the kids in your school/neighborhood use drugs?
- What drugs have your friends tried in the past?
- Do any of your friends use drugs regularly?
- Have you tried drugs yourself? Which ones?
- Have you ever inhaled anything to get high?

37. When is treatment at an inpatient or residential treatment facility indicated?

The American Academy of Pediatrics recommends inpatient treatment in the following situations:

1. The patient is unable to discontinue use despite a trial of appropriate outpatient management.

2. The patient is no longer in control and demonstrates abusive or dangerous behavior toward self or others.

3. The patient demonstrates runaway behavior or suicidality.

4. The patient's physical and emotional condition has deteriorated to a level that threatens his or her life.

38. What are important characteristics of drug treatment programs for adolescents?

Programs should demand total abstinence; any substance use is considered abuse. The staff should be knowledgeable about adolescent development and chemical dependency.

Family therapy and support groups should be integrated into treatment whenever possible. Follow-up and continuing outpatient therapy are critical for success.

39. What substances are most strongly associated with relapse following treatment?

Alcohol and marijuana. Continuing outpatient therapy after discharge from a treatment program is strongly correlated with ongoing success.

DRUG TESTING

40. Should an adolescent who is suspected of using drugs have a urine drug screen without his or her consent?

According to an American Academy of Pediatrics Policy Statement, the answer is "no" as long as the adolescent is competent to make the choice. If the patient is obtunded or otherwise incapable of making the choice, a physician needs to decide whether drug testing is indicated for diagnosis and treatment. A 1995 Supreme Court decision states that random urine drug screening is legal in the United States.

41. Do most urine drug screens test for alcohol?

No. Urine drug screens do not routinely screen for alcohol. If alcohol use is suspected, it is best to measure blood alcohol level.

42. Does a negative urine drug screen effectively rule out a substance abuse problem?

No. A negative urine drug screen means only that the screened-for drugs were not present above the arbitrary cut-off level at the time the test was performed. A negative urine drug screen means little in terms of patient assessment and management. This concept is important for providers to convey to parents who request drug screens of their children in hope of determining whether they are using drugs.

43. What drugs of abuse used by teenagers are not routinely included in a drug screen?

LSD, Ecstasy, alcohol, GHB, dextromethorphan, ephedrine, and ketamine.

44. If you suspect that urine submitted for a drug screen has been adulterated, what tests can be done by you or by the lab to screen for adulteration?

- Temperature should be between 90.5 and 98.6°F.
- pH should be between 4.6 and 8.0.
- Urine creatinine should not be less than 0.2 mg/ml.
- Urine specific gravity should be > 1.003.
- Urine nitrites should be negative. (Some commercially available adulterants dramatically increase the concentration of nitrites in urine and interfere with screening for drugs of abuse.)

45. Can second-hand inhalation of marijuana cause a positive urine drug screen for delta-9-THC?

It depends on the cut-off level that the lab uses for its marijuana screen. If the cut-off level for delta-9-THC is 20 ng/ml, second-hand marijuana inhalation may have caused the positive urine drug screen. Many labs use 50 ng/ml as the cut-off level; this level precludes second-hand inhalation as a cause of the positive screen.

ADDICTION AND DEPENDENCY

46. What is considered the hallmark of addiction?

Continued use of a psychoactive substance despite harmful consequences. These consequences may include school failure, strained interpersonal relationships, motor vehicle or other accidents, or time spent in the juvenile justice system.

47. What does CRAFFT stand for?

CRAFFT is a brief screening test for adolescent substance abuse:

C = Have you ever ridden in a **car** driven by someone who was high or had been drinking or using drugs?

R = Do you ever use alcohol or drugs to **relax**, feel better about yourself, or fit in?

A = Do you ever use alcohol or drugs while you are **alone**?

F = Do your family or **friends** ever tell you that you should cut down on your drinking or drug use?

F = Do you ever **forget** things that you did while using alcohol or drugs?

T = Have you gotten into **trouble** while you were using alcohol or drugs?

BIBLIOGRAPHY

1. Catalano RF, Hawkins JD, et al: Evaluation of the effectiveness of adolescent drug abuse treatment, assessment of risks for relapse, and promising approaches for relapse prevention. Int J Addict 25:1085, 1991.
2. Friedman LS, Johnson B, et al: Evaluation of substance-abusing adolescents by primary care physicians. J Adolesc Health Care 11:227, 1990.
3. Fuller PG, Cavanaugh RM: Basic assessment and screening for substance abuse in the pediatrician's office. Pediatr Clin North Am 42:295, 1995.
4. Johnston L, O'Malley P, Bachman J: Monitoring the Future—National Survey Results on Drug Use, Vol. 1: Secondary School Students. Washington, DC, National Institute on Drug Abuse, 2001.
5. Miller N, Gold M, Smith D: Manual of Therapeutics for Addictions. New York, Wiley-Liss, 1997.
6. Provisional Committee on Substance Abuse, American Academy of Pediatrics: Selection of substance abuse treatment programs. Pediatrics 86:139, 1990.
7. Rogers P, Heyman R: Addiction medicine: Adolescent substance abuse. Pediatr Clin North Am 49:245–246, 2002.
8. Substance Abuse and Mental Health Services Administration: Screening and Assessing Adolescents for Substance Use Disorders. Treatment Improvement Protocol Series, No. 31. Washington, DC, DHHS Publication. No. 99.3344, 1999.
9. Strasburger V, Greydanus D (eds): At-risk Adolescents: An Update for the New Century. Adolescent Medicine: State of the Art Reviews, volume 11, no. 1. Philadelphia, Hanley & Belfus, 2000.

30. TOBACCO USE

Maurice S. Clifton, M.D.

1. Why should physicians learn about smoking tobacco?

Smoking tobacco is the leading cause of preventable death in the United States. Over 430,000 Americans die each year of smoking-related causes (the equivalent of three jumbo jets crashing each day). More Americans die from smoking than AIDS, alcohol, motor vehicle accidents, homicide, suicide, and illegal drugs combined.

2. But those deaths are in adults. Why is adolescent smoking important in pediatrics and adolescent medicine?

• Most smokers start smoking as adolescents.
• Most adolescents want to stop smoking.
• Cigarette use has been linked with other risky behaviors in teens.
• Exposure to second hand tobacco smoke increases the prevalence of many pediatric conditions including otitis media, asthma exacerbations, and sudden infant death syndrome.
• The more a person smokes as an adolescent, the more he or she will smoke as an adult and the more health problems he or she will experience as an adult.
• Counseling teens about how to stop smoking is effective and can be fun.

3. How many adolescents smoke cigarettes?

Over 3 million adolescents smoke in the U.S. From 1991 to 1996, there was a marked increase in the smoking rate reported by adolescents. During that time the percentage of 8th graders that reported smoking at least one cigarette in the past 30 days (the definition of current smoker) rose from 14% to 21%. From 1992 to 1997, the rate of current smoking in 12th graders increased from 28% to 36%. The rates have been decreasing since that time, with 21% of eighth graders and 31% of twelfth graders reporting current smoking in 2000.

4. What are the causes of the recent trends?

Although it is difficult to find the exact cause of trends in populations, many factors probably contributed to the recent decrease. More adolescents perceive smoking to be detrimental to their health. In addition, there have been anti-smoking ad campaigns, restrictions on tobacco industry advertisements, an increase in the price of cigarettes, and increased limitations on the access to cigarettes by teens.

5. When do teens start smoking?

Each day 6,000 children and adolescents try smoking for the first time, and 3,000 become daily smokers. Children begin to try cigarettes between the ages of 11 and 13 and progress to daily use an average of 2 years later. Of current adult smokers, 89% tried their first cigarette and 71% became daily smokers by the time they were age 18. Despite decreases in the smoking rates, teens who smoke are trying their first cigarette and becoming daily smokers at a younger age.

6. Why do teens start smoking?

Teens start smoking for various reasons, and it is hard to determine cause and effect. Individual attributes associated with initiation of smoking include positive attitudes toward smoking, concerns with body weight, perception of accessibility, parental smoking and approval, and number of smoking friends.

7. Do teenagers want to stop smoking?

The common misperception is that teens do not want to quit smoking. However, convincing data indicate that this is not the case. When asked whether they expected to be smoking in 5 years, only 5% of high school students said yes (95% expected to quit). Unfortunately, quitting is hard, and 75% are still smoking 5 years later. At any one time, approximately 70% of teens say that they want to quit smoking, and 50% of smoking teens actually try to quit each year. Seventy percent of teen smokers report wishing that they had never started smoking.

8. Can teens really become addicted to cigarettes?

Yes. Studies to measure tobacco dependence in adolescents show a wide range of estimates, depending on the population and how dependence is measured. When adolescents try to quit smoking, over one-half report withdrawal symptoms. When asked, most adolescent smokers consider themselves to be addicted to nicotine. They have withdrawal symptoms when they try to quit smoking, it is difficult to quit, and most who quit relapse. Most adolescents who smoke continue to smoke into adulthood.

9. How do I start talking to teens about tobacco?

The Centers for Disease Control and Prevention (CDC) have developed comprehensive guidelines for smoking cessation. The five major steps to counseling in these guidelines are called the **5 A's**. They are based on research with adults but are recommended for adolescents as well:

- **A**sk all teens if they smoke.
- **A**dvise every teen to quit, with a clear, strong, personalized message.
- **A**ssess willingness to try to quit.
- **A**ssist teens in making an attempt if they are ready to try.
- **A**rrange follow-up to prevent relapse or encourage another attempt.

10. If a teen wants to quit, what do I say?

To be a **STAR** in clinic, have the teen do the following:

Set a quit date (ideally within 2 weeks).
Tell family and friends that you want to quit and ask for help and understanding.
Anticipate challenges to quitting and make plans about what to do for each one.
Remove tobacco products from the environment so that it is more difficult to restart.

11. If a teen does not want to quit, should I give a lecture about how bad it is to smoke?

Even adults do not like being told what to do. This is even more true for teens. If you sound like their parents, giving a lecture, the "selective hearing reflex" kicks in, and they may have trouble hearing you. To avoid this reaction, use the **5 R's** of a motivational intervention:

- **R**elevance: try to relate the teen's reason for being in the office to smoking (if the teen is there for a sports physical, talk about improved exercise capacity in nonsmokers).
- **R**isks: ask the teen to identify acute risks (e.g., asthma, aging skin, discolored teeth, bad breath), long-term risks (e.g., heart attacks, cancer), and environmental risks (harming other people).
- **R**ewards: ask the teen to identify the rewards of stopping (e.g., saving money, self-esteem).
- **R**oadblocks: ask the teen to identify barriers to quitting and to think of ways to address them.
- **R**epetition: this intervention should be repeated each time the teen is in clinic and unwilling to make a quit attempt.

The way this technique is done is as important as what is actually said. To increase the chances of this success, you should be empathic, give the teen choices, avoid arguing, and support self-efficacy.

12. I helped one of my patients quit smoking. What do I say at the next visit?

Congratulations! Just like adults, teens have a high rate of relapse. The CDC guidelines suggest the following interventions for every encounter with patients who have quit recently:

- Congratulate them on their success.
- Encourage them to remain abstinent.
- Review the benefits that they are deriving from cessation.
- Discuss the success that they have had (e.g., duration of abstinence, reduction in withdrawal symptoms).
- Review problems encountered or anticipated threats to maintaining abstinence.

13. What can communities do to help teens stop smoking?

The states of California and Massachusetts have been leaders in such efforts. Both started with tax increases on cigarette sales, which both raised the price of cigarettes and funded evidence-based tobacco control programs. In 1989, before the implementation of the programs, the smoking rate in California was approximately equal to that in the rest of the country. However, between 1993 and 1997, the smoking rate varied from 12% to 14% among eighth graders in California, whereas in the rest of the country, the rates steadily increased from 17% to 22% in the same groups. The CDC guidelines for the best practices for comprehensive tobacco control programs include:

- Community programs to reduce tobacco use
- Chronic disease programs to reduce the burden of tobacco-related diseases
- School programs that include a broad-based approach
- Enforcement of tobacco control policies, including restrictions on minors' access and smoking in public places
- Statewide programs to support local community programs
- Counter-marketing attempts to counter protobacco influences
- Cessation programs that are accessible to the entire community
- Surveillance and evaluation system to monitor the program
- Administration and management to facilitate coordination of program components

14. A school principal wants me to help design a plan for the local schools. What should I recommend?

Because children and adolescents spend much of their day in school, this can be an especially effective location to provide tobacco prevention interventions. The CDC developed and published guidelines for effective tobacco-use prevention programs in schools:

- Develop and enforce a school policy on tobacco use.
- Provide instruction about the short- and long-term negative physiologic and social consequences of tobacco use, social influences on tobacco use, peer norms regarding tobacco use, and refusal skills.
- Provide tobacco-use prevention education in kindergarten through twelfth grade. This instruction should be especially intensive in junior high or middle school and reinforced in high school.
- Provide program-specific training for teachers.
- Involve parents or families in support of school-based programs to prevent tobacco use.
- Support cessation efforts among students and all school staff who use tobacco.
- Assess the tobacco-use prevention program at regular intervals.

15. Should teens use nicotine replacement products and/or bupropion hydrochloride (Zyban) to help stop smoking?

In adults, pharmacologic aids can double the cessation rate compared with placebo. The five medications approved by the Food and Drug Administration (FDA) for smoking cessation include bupropion SR and four types of nicotine replacement: patch, gum, inhaler, and nasal spray. The CDC guidelines recommend prescribing medications to aid in cessation for all adults unless there are special circumstances, such as medical contraindications, smoking fewer than 10 cigarettes per day, pregnancy, breast-feeding, or adolescence. Physicians may consider medications for adolescents when there is evidence of nicotine dependence.

At present no good studies have reported the same type of success with medications in teens. Many programs still advocate their use, because in some patients, they seem to help. Current studies may help determine if some teens are helped by medications.

16. If my adolescent patients want to try nicotine replacement, how should they use it?

There are four types of nicotine replacement products: patches, gum, inhaler, and nasal spray. Although there are no absolute contraindications, they are listed as pregnancy category D. Patches are placed on a relatively hairless location, below the neck and above the waist, when patients wake up on their quit day. They should be changed every morning and kept in place all day long. Some patients have a hard time sleeping if they leave the patch on at night and may do better if they take the patch off when they go to bed. The gum is chewed until a "peppery" or "minty" taste emerges; then it is "parked" between the cheek and gum. After about 5 minutes, the flavor decreases; the gum is "chewed" for several seconds and "parked" every 5 minutes for a total of about 30 minutes. The most important advice to give patients using the gum is to use a piece every 1–2 hours because patients tend to chew too few pieces, develop withdrawal symptoms, and give up. Patients must not smoke cigarettes while using nicotine replacement products.

17. What if my patient wants to try Zyban?

Zyban (bupropion SR) has been approved by the FDA for use as a first-line agent for smoking cessation in adults. It has been shown to double abstinence rates compared to placebo. It is contraindicated in patients with a history of seizure disorder or eating disorder and patients who are taking another form of bupropion (such as the antidepressant Wellbutrin). Zyban is started with a dose of 150 mg every morning for 3 days, then increased to 150 mg twice daily. It should be started 1–2 weeks before the quit date and continued for 7–12 weeks afterward.

18. Where can I get more information about teen smoking and cessation?

The above recommendations are summarized from the CDC guidelines, which are available by visiting the Surgeon General's Web site at www.surgeongeneral.gov/tobacco/default.htm or by calling the CDC at 1-800-CDC-1311. These guidelines include additional information about pharmacotherapy and references that form the basis of the guidelines. In addition to the references below, many other web-sites may be useful to you or your adolescent patients. In addition, your local American Lung Association and American Cancer Society can provide more information.

    www.lungusa.org
    www.cancer.org
    www.americanheart.org
    www.cdc.gov/tobacco
    www.communityintervention.com
    www.youthtobacco.com
    www.quitnet.com
    www.smokefreekids.com

BIBLIOGRAPHY

1. Centers for Disease Control and Prevention: Best Practices for Comprehensive Tobacco control Programs-August 1999. Atlanta, U.S. department of Health and Human Services, Centers for Disease Control and Prevention, National Center for Chronic Disease Prevention and Health Promotion, Office on Smoking and Health, 1999 [reprinted, with corrections].

2. Centers for Disease Control and Prevention: Guidelines for school health programs to prevent tobacco use and addiction. MMWR 43(RR-2):1–18, 1994.
3. Colby SM, Tiffany ST, Shiffman S, Niaura RS: Are adolescent smokers ddependent on nicotine? Drug Alcohol Depend 59(Suppl 1):S83–S95, 2000.
4. Fiore MC, Baily WC, Cohen SJ, et al: Treating Tobacco Use and Dependence. Clinical Practice Guideline. Rockville, MD, U.S. Department of Health and Human Services, Public Health Service, 2000.
5. Johnston LD, O'Malley PM, Bachman JG. Cigarette use and smokeless tobacco use decline substantially among teens. University of Michigan News and Information Services, Ann Arbor, MI, 2000. Available: www.monitoringthefuture.org; accessed 05/25/01
6. Mayhew KP, Flay BR, Mott JA: Stages in the development of adolescent smoking. Drug Alcohol Depend 59(Suppl 1):S61–S81, 2000.
7. National Center for Chronic Disease Prevention and Health Promotion Tobacco Information and Prevention Source: Comparative Causes of Annual Deaths in the United States [available online at www.cdc.gov/tobacco/research_data/health_consequences/andths.htm], 2001.

31. TOXICOLOGY AND OVERDOSE

Marcel J. Casavant, M.D.

1. What's the best way to treat the patient with an intentional overdose?

Carefully. Whether suicidal, calling for help, or psychotically self-injurious, such patients present difficult management issues. The physician must remain compassionate while aggressively supporting the patient, aware that the history may be misleading. Although it may not be life-threatening, the intentional ingestion marks a patient at high risk for repeat ingestions or other acts that may be fatal. Intentional ingestions may be a symptom of feared pregnancy, chronic abuse, or depression. Address coexisting issues, such as the lacerated wrists that accompany the overdose or a substance abuse disorder. Certified regional poison control centers are a valuable resource for patients, but they also have information and experience to share with physicians.

2. What is the anticholinergic toxidrome?

The set of physical examination findings that suggest poisoning by an anticholinergic agent. Mad as a hatter (delirium), blind as a bat (dilated pupils and paralysis of accommodation), dry as a bone (dry mucus membranes, absent perspiration), red as a beet (vasodilation), and hot as a hare (hyperthermia) are major clues. In addition, tachycardia, hypertension, urinary retention, and absence of bowel sounds are common.

3. Why do adolescents get the anticholinergic toxidrome?

For the same reasons the rest of us do, though in different frequencies. Jimsonweed ingestion or inhalation and therapeutic or recreational use of medications with anticholinergic side effects (antihistamines, tricyclic antidepressants, antipsychotics) are common reasons.

4. How do we treat patients with anticholinergic toxicity?

Supportive care is usually all that is required. Treat hypertension aggressively: often calming the patient in a quiet room is enough, but benzodiazepines orally or intravenously may help. If hypertension persists, use a vasodilator. Relieve urinary retention with an indwelling urethral catheter; often this step alone calms the patient and relieves hypertension. Gastrointestinal (GI) atony induced by anticholinergics can change the usual rules for GI decontamination. For instance, lavage, even 2 or 3 days after a massive jimsonweed overdose, can still recover large quantities of seeds. On the other hand, multiple doses of charcoal cannot fit into a stomach that has not emptied the first dose and may increase the risk of aspiration. In most cases, a single dose of charcoal suffices. For severe central nervous system toxicity not adequately controlled by benzodiazepines, consider physostigmine. This antidote, however, has dangerous side effects (heart block and asystole, seizures) that are more common when the anticholinergic toxicity is due to tricyclics or other medicines.

5. What is the sympathomimetic toxidrome?

Actually, there are several. The **alpha-adrenergic syndrome** is characterized by hypertension, sometimes with reactive bradycardia. Phenylpropanolamine is one cause. The **beta-adrenergic syndrome** includes tachycardia and often hypertension, although vasodilation in beta-2 stimulation may cause hypotension; tremor is part of the beta toxidrome. Albuterol and theophylline are possible causes, but adolescents are more likely to overdose on caffeine, which is also a beta-2 stimulant. The **mixed sympathomimetic toxidrome** can include any combination of vital sign abnormalities, but usually both pulse and blood pressure are elevated. Hyperthermia, agitation, seizure, coma, and dysrhythmia can occur in any of the sympathomimetic toxidromes. Dry mouth occurs, as in the anticholinergic toxidrome, but the skin is often moist. Check the axillae and palms to distinguish sympathomimetic from anticholinergic toxicity. What about the pupils? Alpha stimulation often causes mydriasis; beta stimulation causes miosis.

6. What type of antihypertensive should be avoided in treating sympathomimetic syndrome?

Because beta stimulation of coronary arteries and peripheral arterioles causes vasodilation, do not use a beta blocker. Beta blockade allows unopposed alpha stimulation, thus raising the blood pressure further!

7. What problems does acetaminophen toxicity cause?

Mostly, just upset stomach, nausea, and vomiting, *if* the patient presents for treatment early after the overdose. Untreated, patients can develop fulminant hepatic failure, which can lead to death or need for a liver transplant. Renal toxicity is reported in about 10% of major overdoses; cardiotoxicity is rare.

8. Why does acetaminophen toxicity remain a common problem in adolescent medicine?

Adolescents, like the rest of us, have ready access to this over-the-counter remedy. Unlike certain other pharmaceuticals, which are packaged in quantities below toxic doses, family-size bottles of acetaminophen at the grocery story contain enough toxin to kill several livers. The "therapeutic window" (ratio of toxic dose to therapeutic dose) is narrow, and many victims underestimate the true toxicity of acetaminophen.

9. How do you treat the patient with an acetaminophen overdose?

Carefully. If the patient presents early, GI decontamination can be accomplished by having the patient drink activated charcoal. A serum acetaminophen concentration is drawn at least 4 hours after the ingestion, and the result is plotted on the Rumack nomogram. You do not need the graph; the treatment line starts at 150 mg/L at 4 hours, then declines with a half-life of 4 hours, i.e., to 75 mg/L at 8 hours, 37.5 mg/L at 12 hours, and so on. If the patient's acetaminophen level is "above the line," treatment with *n*-acetylcysteine should be initiated.

10. What if more than 8 hours have passed since the acetaminophen overdose?

If the patient presents late or the results of a serum acetaminophen concentration cannot be obtained before 8 hours after ingestion, the decision to treat can be based on the estimated dose. If more than 140 mg/kg were ingested, treat the patient. Common wisdom used to say that the antidote does not work if started 16, 20, or 24 hours after the overdose. Now we know that patients treated late do better than patients not treated at all. It is still important to treat the patient who presents more than 16 hours after the overdose.

11. Can we always use the Rumack nomogram to predict acetaminophen hepatotoxicity?

No.

12. When does the Rumack nomogram *not* apply?

It does not work in the first four hours after overdose or for sustained-release acetaminophen products. It works only for single, acute ingestions, not for the young woman who took a handful last night and another handful this morning and a few more immediately before presentation. It also does not help in assessing the young man who took several other drugs with his acetaminophen overdose, particularly if any of these affect the motility of the GI tract. Finally, the nomogram may underestimate the risk to people who have revved-up liver enzymes: alcoholics and patients taking enzyme-inducing medications such as phenobarbital. In all of these cases, have a very low threshold for treating with the antidote, *n*-acetylcysteine.

13. When is it appropriate to stop *n*-acetylcysteine?

The "official" (well-validated, FDA-approved, time-honored) answer is that a full course includes a loading dose (140 mg/kg) followed by 17 maintenance doses (70 mg/kg each) given at 4-hour intervals. Technically, this "official" answer applies only to cases in which the Rumack nomogram applies: acute ingestions of immediate-release acetaminophen, when the time of ingestion is known and no other drugs (especially those that might affect kinetics, such as drugs with anticholinergic properties) are involved.

In certain clinical situations, other criteria may be considered in deciding whether to stop treatment. Some experts may consider stopping therapy when (1) serum acetaminophen concentration is zero or below the lab's threshold of detection; (2) bilirubin and prothrombin time are normal, with transaminases normal or clearly improving; (3) symptoms (vomiting, anorexia) and signs (liver tenderness) have resolved or are clearly resolving; and (4) at least 24 hours of treatment have been administered. To be honest, the "experts" have differing opinions, and some routinely stop *n*-acetylcysteine after 1 or 2 days if there are no signs of hepatotoxicity. Published data to support these shortened regimens are limited, and no other route or duration of *n*-acetylcysteine has been shown to be as safe and effective as the traditional 72-hour course. After an intentional overdose, those 72 hours are also needed for the assessment and stabilization of the psychosocial situation.

14. What occupational toxins injure adolescents?

The answer depends on the adolescent's occupation, of course. Carbon monoxide poisons the garage attendant and those who use gasoline-powered machinery indoors, such as the forklift driver. Chlorine gas affects the pool cleaner. Chlorine or chloramine gases attack the janitor who inappropriately mixes cleaning chemicals. Mercury dust affects the young man who sweeps the broken fluorescent bulbs from the plant floor; lead vapor or dust poisons the plumber's helper and the automotive repair worker; organophosphates, carbamates, and organochlorines attack agricultural workers. Routinely ask your patients about occupational and recreational exposures to toxins.

15. Why not just pump all patients' stomachs after overdose?

Gastric lavage used to be a mainstay of overdose management. In the past decade, however, we came to realize the complications: esophageal and tracheal trauma, pulmonary lavage, charcoal aspiration, charcoal pneumothorax. In addition, it probably does not "teach patients a lesson" as often as previously believed. More importantly, several imperfect studies have shown that overdose patients treated with charcoal alone do as well as those treated with lavage and charcoal. Reserve gastric lavage for patients at risk for dangerous toxicity from a recent ingestion that cannot be treated in a less invasive manner. Lavage may play a role in large, recent ingestions of substances such as iron or lithium, which cannot be adsorbed to charcoal. It is relatively contraindicated in caustic ingestions and most hydrocarbon ingestions. It is absolutely contraindicated in nontoxic ingestions. Here's a secret to save for a special occasion: if you pump a stomach and for some reason want a "tox screen," ask the lab to analyze the gastric aspirate too. Often gastric contents contain the highest concentrations of the ingested substances.

16. When do I order a tox screen?

The tox screen can help answer the question: "What's wrong with this patient?" It is usually more useful when it is positive and less useful when it is negative. Most tox screens are rapid assays for members of 6, 7, or 8 classes of drugs, usually drugs of abuse (cannabinoids, opiates, barbiturates, cocaine metabolites, benzodiazepines) and sometimes a few other agents (e.g., tricyclic antidepressants). "Comprehensive" drug screens generally look for 100–300 drugs—which is hardly comprehensive. The most fascinating part of tox screens is that they vary from institution to institution in the substances for which they test and in sensitivities and specificities. A healthy patient does not need a tox screen, nor does the patient whose signs and symptoms match the toxicity profile of the reported ingestion. But if your patient is sick and you do not know why, but poisoning is on your differential diagnosis, a tox screen may be useful. One more secret: take a minute to call your lab and explain the situation and which toxins could be involved. The technician often can suggest which tests are likely to contribute to the diagnosis.

17. What are the dangers of methanol or ethylene glycol poisoning?

Ethanol, ethylene glycol, and methanol cause intoxication. Methanol is metabolized to formaldehyde and formic acid, and these byproducts can cause blindness and death. Ethylene glycol is metabolized to glycolic, glyoxylic, and oxalic acids. These byproducts injure nerves, kidney, and heart, precipitate calcium, and can cause seizures, dysrhythmias, and death.

18. When should one suspect methanol or ethylene glycol poisoning?

Suspect methanol or ethylene glycol poisoning when the degree of intoxication is higher than expected from the measured serum ethanol level (EtOH) or when the patient is acidotic. Routinely measure the serum osmolality by freezing point depression, and compare the measured value to the predicted serum osmolality:

$$\text{Predicted Osm} = 2\,Na + BUN/2.8 + glucose/18 + [EtOH]\,(mg/dl)/4.6$$

where Na = sodium and BUN = blood urea nitrogen. If the measured osmolality is more than 10 mOsm higher than the predicted osmolality, the patient has unexpected osmols on board; methanol or ethylene glycol should be high on your list. Treatment includes blocking further metabolism of these compounds (use an ethanol drip or fomepizole) and dialysis.

BIBLIOGRAPHY

1. American Academy of Clinical Toxicology and European Association of Poisons Centres and Clinical Toxicologists: Position statements: Gut decontamination. J Tox Clin Tox 35:695–762, 1997.
2. Harrison RJ: Chemicals and gases. Prim Care Clin Office Pract 27:917–982, 2000.
3. Thompson JN, Brodkin CA, Kyes K, et al: Use of a questionnaire to improve occupational and environmental history taking in primary care physicians. J Occup Environ Med 42:1188–1194, 2000.

32. EATING DISORDERS

Martin Fisher, M.D.

1. What eating disorders are seen in adolescents? How are they diagnosed?

The eating disorders seen most commonly in adolescents are anorexia nervosa and bulimia nervosa. People with anorexia nervosa display unhealthy weight loss behaviors; people with bulimia nervosa display binge-eating and purging behaviors; people with both disorders have body image concerns and a fear of gaining weight. Official diagnostic criteria and subtypes for each diagnosis have been established by the American Psychiatric Association as part of the *Diagnostic and Statistical Manual of Mental Disorders* (DSM-IV). People who display evidence of an eating disorder but do not meet all criteria are classified in the DSM-IV as having "eating disorder not otherwise specified" (EDNOS). Studies have shown that large numbers of adolescents fit into the EDNOS category and have a similar degree of psychological disturbance as with those who meet full criteria. Another eating disorder diagnosis described in the DSM-IV, binge-eating disorder, is seen rarely in adolescents.

DSM-IV Diagnostic Criteria for Anorexia Nervosa and Bulimia Nervosa

Anorexia nervosa
A. Refusal to maintain body weight over a minimally normal weight for age and height (e.g., weight loss leading to maintenance of body weight 15% below that expected), or failure to make expected weight gain during period of growth, leading to body weight below 15% of that expected.
B. Intense fear of gaining weight or becoming fat, even though underweight.
C. Disturbance in the way in which one's body weight or shape is experienced, undue influence of body shape and weight on self-evaluation, or denial of the seriousness of current low body weight.
D. In postmenarchal females, amenorrhea, i.e., the absence of at least three consecutive menstrual cycles. (A woman is considered to have amenorrhea if her periods occur only following hormone, e.g., estrogen administration.)

Restricting type: During the episode of anorexia nervosa, the person does not regularly engage in binge eating or purging behavior (i.e., self-induced vomiting or the misuse of laxatives or diuretics).

Binge eating/purging type: During the episode of anorexia nervosa, the person regularly engages in binge eating or purging behavior (i.e., self-induced vomiting or the misuse of laxatives or diuretics).

Bulimia nervosa
A. Recurrent episodes of binge eating. An episode of binge eating is characterized by both of the following:
    1) eating in a discrete period of time (e.g., within any 2-hour period), an amount of food that is definitely larger than most people would consume in a similar period of time in similar circumstances; and,
    2) a sense of lack of control over eating during the episode (e.g., a feeling that one cannot stop eating or control what or how much one is eating).
B. Recurrent inappropriate compensatory behavior to prevent weight gain, such as self-induced vomiting; misuse of laxatives, diuretics, or other medications; fasting; or excessive exercise.
C. The binge eating and inappropriate compensatory behaviors both occur, on average, at least twice a week for 3 months.
D. Self-evaluation is unduly influenced by body shape and weight.
E. The disturbance does not occur exclusively during episodes of anorexia nervosa.

Purging type: The person regularly engages in self-induced vomiting or the misuse of laxatives or diuretics.

Nonpurging type: The person uses other inappropriate compensatory behaviors, such as fasting or excessive exercise, but does not regularly engage in self-induced vomiting or the misuse of diuretics.

From the American Psychiatric Association Diagnostic and Statistical Manual of Mental Disorders, 4th ed. Washington, DC, APA Press, 1994.

2. Describe the epidemiology of anorexia nervosa.

Adolescence is the most common age for the development of anorexia nervosa. Although school-aged children and adults can develop anorexia nervosa, care must be taken to consider alternative diagnoses in nonadolescent age groups. Approximately 90–95% of patients with anorexia nervosa are female. Approximately 0.5% of adolescent females in the United States and Great Britain have anorexia nervosa, with most cases occurring in Caucasian and upper socioeconomic populations. Of late, an increasing prevalence has been noted in other ethnic and racial groups, in adolescents from lower socioeconomic backgrounds, and in developing countries that previously had shown no evidence of the disease.

3. Describe the epidemiology of bulimia nervosa.

Bulimia nervosa occurs more commonly in older adolescents and young adults. As with anorexia nervosa, most patients are female, white, and of higher socioeconomic status. Approximately 1–5% of adolescent females have bulimia; a partial syndrome of vomiting and/or laxative use (without binge-eating) may occur even more commonly, especially in those of college age.

4. Are eating disorders more common now than previously?

A longitudinal study in Rochester, Minnesota, demonstrated that the rate of development of anorexia nervosa increased dramatically in adolescents from the 1930s through the 1980s, while maintaining a steady, low rate throughout the same period in adults. The term *bulimia nervosa* was not used until around 1980; previously the symptoms of bulimia were considered to be only a component of anorexia nervosa. During the past two decades, the prevalence of anorexia and bulimia nervosa has continued to increase, along with a dramatic increase in dieting behaviors in adolescents and young adults as well as in children of junior high school and even elementary school ages.

5. What roles do cultural, psychological and biologic factors play in the etiology of eating disorders?

Cultural norms certainly play a role in the development of eating disorders. Recent examples of societies in which the introduction of Western-style television was followed by the development of eating disorders is the latest evidence of this relationship. Psychological factors, in both the family and the individual, also play a role. Issues of self-esteem and control have been classically studied. Biologic factors, almost surely genetically mediated, have received the most attention of late. Biochemical changes in the brain, perhaps similar to those found in depression, obsessive-compulsive disorder, and addiction, are likely to play a role in onset and continuation of both anorexia and bulimia nervosa. It may well be that weight loss, begun in vulnerable individuals because of an interaction of cultural and psychological factors, may lead to the biochemical changes that then perpetuate eating disorder behaviors.

6. What warning signs should alert the pediatrician to the onset of an eating disorder?

Pediatricians should assess weight and height at all check-ups and follow measurements on a growth chart. Inappropriate or rapid weight loss in any child or adolescent or failure to achieve appropriate increases in weight or height in a growing child or adolescent should raise the suspicion of an eating disorder. Reassurance by the adolescent should not allay the pediatrician's concerns, because most adolescents deny the existence of an eating disorder for as long as possible. Similarly, concerns about the possible onset of an eating disorder by parents and/or school personnel must be taken seriously. In fact, when concerns are raised about obsessions with food and weight or possible vomiting or laxative use, it is the rare situation in which that adolescent does not have an eating disorder, either full-blown or in an early stage. Whenever a suspicion is raised, the pediatrician must explore the situation carefully and follow the adolescent closely until a full determination is made and further steps are taken.

7. Describe the signs and symptoms of anorexia nervosa.

The hallmark of anorexia nervosa is weight loss or failure to make appropriate gains in weight and height in a growing child. Physiologically, the body responds to the amount, speed, and duration of the weight loss as well as to how far below the average weight (for age, sex, and height) the adolescent falls. A rough estimate of the percent below average weight can be determined by using a simple calculation: the average weight for adolescents and young adults is calculated as 100 lb for a female at 5 feet in height, plus 5 lb for each additional inch, and 106 lb for a male at 5 feet in height, plus 6 lb for each additional inch. More recently, body mass index (BMI) also has been used. Adolescents with significant malnutrition can display multiple signs and symptoms, including constipation, dizziness, cold hands and feet, and hair loss; psychological symptoms, including irritability and depression, may become obvious as well.

8. Describe the signs and symptoms of bulimia nervosa.

Most patients with bulimia nervosa display no signs or symptoms of the illness; hence, the person who is vomiting surreptitiously may be quite difficult to detect. Patients with bulimia can be of normal weight, overweight or underweight, and they can undertake purging behaviors (such as vomiting or use of laxatives) from several times a week to several times a day. Some patients may experience dizziness or fatigue after episodes of vomiting or laxative use, and others may be clearly anxious or depressed, but most do not show any specific signs or symptoms and therefore are not detected until family or friends are told or discover their secret.

9. Which laboratory tests should be performed in patients with eating disorders? What abnormalities do they reveal?

The initial laboratory screening tests performed in all patients with eating disorders include a complete blood count, metabolic panel (including electrolytes and liver function tests), urinalysis, and thyroid function tests (generally thyroxine and thyroid-stimulating hormone). Additional tests are performed in patients with amenorrhea (luteinizing hormone [LH], follicle-stimulating hormone [FSH], prolactin, estradiol), an electrocardiogram (EKG) is obtained in patients with bradycardia or significant purging behaviors, and further work-up (such as magnetic resonance imaging [MRI] of the brain or an upper or lower gastrointestinal [GI] series) is considered in patients in whom the etiology is not completely clear. Although laboratory tests are normal in most patients with eating disorders, some important abnormalities may be found. Hypo- or hypernatremia may be detected based on water manipulation by the patient (some patients with eating disorders drink excessively, especially before doctor visits, whereas others drink as little as possible). Vomiting and laxative or diuretic use can cause a hypokalemic, hypochloremic, metabolic alkalosis that at times can result in dangerously low levels of potassium. Malnutrition can cause neutropenia, mild anemia, and, rarely, thrombocytopenia. Malnutrition and purging behaviors can each cause EKG abnormalities, ranging from bradycardia to a prolonged QT interval. Endocrine abnormalities are discussed in question 12 below.

10. What gastroenterologic symptoms do patients with eating disorders experience?

Most patients with eating disorders exhibit gastroenterologic symptoms at some point during the course of their illness. Adolescents with bulimia may have upper abdominal and/or chest pain secondary to irritation of the esophagus, and if acid regurgitation continues long enough, it destroys the enamel of the teeth as well. Gastric emptying and intestinal peristalsis are delayed in patients with anorexia nervosa; symptoms such as abdominal pain, bloating, and constipation are therefore common, either during the starvation phase or even more so with refeeding. Mildly elevated liver function tests may also be seen during starvation or refeeding.

11. Describe the neurologic complications that may be seen in patients with eating disorders.

Neurologic complications are less common. Computed tomography (CT) and MRI studies have shown decreased brain tissue (evidenced as increased size of the sulci) in patients who have lost a significant amount of weight rapidly. Some preliminary evidence indicates that patients also may have subtle cognitive changes that may not be completely reversible. Some patients with severe malnutrition have been reported to develop peripheral neuropathy, which appears to resolve quickly with refeeding, and some patients have had seizures secondary to the hyponatremia that can be caused by excessive water loading.

12. What endocrine abnormalities can be found in patients with eating disorders?

Several endocrine abnormalities are associated with the malnutrition found in anorexia nervosa. Thyroid function is decreased centrally, most likely as a way of decreasing the body's metabolism in the face of insufficient energy intake. This change leads to decreases in pulse, temperature, and EKG voltage. Laboratory values show a low thyroxine (generally in the low-normal range), an even lower triiodothyronine (because of the euthyroid sick syndrome), and a low thyroid-stimulating hormone (because of decreased production from the pituitary). A relative hypercortisolism with loss of diurnal variation is noted in anorexia nervosa, as are decreased LH, FSH and estradiol levels, leading to amenorrhea. Irregular or absent menses also may be seen in some patients with bulimia nervosa.

13. What are the medical consequences of laxative or diuretic use in patients with eating disorders?

Laxative abuse (through fluid and electrolyte losses in chronic diarrhea) and diuretic abuse (through tubular excretion of potassium and hydrogen) can result in the development of a hypokalemic, hypochloremic metabolic alkalosis. Patients who combine vomiting with laxative or diuretic use are at greatest risk of having severe electrolyte disturbances. Adolescents with chronic diuretic use are at risk for the development of renal stones, and those with chronic laxative use may develop rebound edema and significant constipation on cessation of use.

14. Why is ipecac use a concern in patients with eating disorders?

Ipecac, which contains the alkaloid emetine, is used by some patients with bulimia in the same way that it is used to induce vomiting in children with accidental ingestions. Unfortunately, ipecac can cause the development of muscle damage, including an irreversible cardiomyopathy. Several case reports of death due to ipecac use in patients with bulimia nervosa have been reported. It is therefore important to ask about ipecac use and provide appropriate warnings about its potential consequences.

15. What is the effect of anorexia nervosa on bone density?

Adolescents with eating disorders are at risk for the development of osteopenia (bone density > 1 standard deviation below the mean for age) or osteoporosis (> 2.5 standard deviations below the mean). Amenorrhea, which develops when women reach approximately 13–15% below average body weight, is the primary cause, mediated by low estrogen levels. Relative hypercortisolism and other hormonal or metabolic factors also may play a role. Because genetic factors determine baseline bone density levels, duration of amenorrhea is a secondary determinant of the severity of osteopenia/osteoporosis. Since adolescence is the age group during which bone density normally has its greatest increases, development of osteopenia/osteoporosis during the adolescent age group has the potential for significant lifelong implications. Performance of bone density studies is recommended in patients who have had amenorrhea for 6–12 months due to an eating disorder.

16. Are medications useful in the prevention or treatment of bone loss in anorexia nervosa?

Unfortunately, studies indicate that medications, including calcium supplementation and the use of hormonal replacement, are not effective in the prevention or treatment of osteopenia/osteoporosis in anorexia nervosa. Although one study showed a slight benefit with the use of hormonal replacement in patients with severe malnutrition, and many clinicians certainly use this modality, nutritional rehabilitation with resumption of menses is the only effective approach. Even so, it is believed that the bone loss that takes place during the time of malnutrition is never fully recovered. Studies are underway to evaluate the use of biphosphonates in patients with osteopenia/osteoporosis secondary to an eating disorder, but they are not currently indicated for use in adolescents.

17. What is the differential diagnosis of anorexia and bulimia nervosa?
The differential diagnosis of anorexia nervosa includes all of the medical and psychiatric conditions that can cause weight loss. Alternative medical diagnoses must be considered most strongly when the diagnosis of anorexia nervosa is not completely clear (for instance, if the patient totally denies fear of weight gain despite intensive questioning or is out of the usual age range for the development of an eating disorder). It is possible for a person to have one of the medical conditions listed in the table below along with an eating disorder. For instance, studies have shown that adolescents with diabetes mellitus have a higher incidence of eating disorders than the general population, possibly because of the metabolic effects of the illness and the constant attention that adolescents with diabetes mellitus must pay to food and weight issues. Other causes of vomiting must be considered in patients who appear to have bulimia nervosa but deny that vomiting is self-induced. An MRI and/or GI studies may be indicated. Alternative psychiatric diagnoses also must be considered. For instance, an unwillingness to eat sufficiently because of fear of weight gain must be distinguished from an inability to eat because of depression, a fear of eating because of anxiety, or concerns that the food is poisoned because of psychosis.

Differential Diagnosis of Anorexia Nervosa

MEDICAL	PSYCHIATRIC
Inflammatory bowel disease	Affective disorder
Addison's disease	Obsessive-compulsive disorder
Hypo- or hyperthyroidism	Schizophrenia
Diabetes mellitus/insipidus	Substance abuse
Brain tumor	Paranoid disorder
Occult malignancy	Conduct disorder
Infection or inflammation	

18. What is the role of psychiatric comorbidity in patients with eating disorders?
Many, if not most, patients with eating disorders have psychiatric comorbidity, including any of the diagnoses listed in question 17. Although it is clear that depression can precipitate or exacerbate an eating disorder, it is equally clear that malnutrition caused by an eating disorder can precipitate or exacerbate depression. Studies also have shown that patients with obsessive compulsive disorder (OCD) are more likely to have an eating disorder than the general population and that patients with eating disorders are more likely to have OCD than the general population. Other addictive behaviors are also found more commonly in patients with eating disorders, especially those with bulimia. The presence of borderline personality disorder has been found to be one of the most significant prognostic indicators in patients with eating disorders.

19. How is severity of anorexia nervosa determined?
Severity of anorexia nervosa is evaluated based on nutritional, medical and psychological criteria. Calculation of body mass index (BMI) and/or percent below average body weight, determination of amount and speed of weight loss, and evaluation of daily nutritional intake provide an index of nutritional severity. As a general rule, patients who are more than 25% below average weight are strong candidates for hospitalization. Laboratory testing and

determination of cardiovascular stability (including any orthostatic or EKG changes) provide an index of medical severity. In most cases, these tests remain normal despite the presence of significant malnutrition. When they are abnormal, they should prompt consideration of hospitalization. The presence of psychiatric comorbidity and difficulties with family, friends, or school provide an index of psychologic severity. Clinical decisions are made on the basis of the combined nutritional, medical, and psychiatric status.

20. How is severity evaluated in bulimia nervosa?

Each of the factors discussed in question 19 also applies to patients with bulimia nervosa. More specifically, however, evaluation of severity in bulimia is based on the purging behaviors (i.e., vomiting, laxatives, fasting, exercise), the frequency and intensity of binge-eating and purging behaviors, and the presence of laboratory abnormalities. Severity can be more difficult to ascertain in bulimia nervosa than in anorexia nervosa because the clinician is dependent on patient history without an objective criterion such as weight for confirmation. Laboratory abnormalities, which are more common in bulimia, are sometimes the only clue to the severity of the situation.

21. Where are patients with eating disorders treated? By whom?

Most adolescents with eating disorders are treated in outpatient settings. Those with the mildest cases may be treated by a primary care physician, nutritionist, and/or mental health practitioner. Many patients require specialized teams (generally consisting of medical, nutritional, and mental health personnel), which in some settings are coordinated by specialists in adolescent medicine. Patients with more severe disorders require hospitalization, which can take place in an appropriate medical or psychiatric unit. Recently, day programs (3–5 days/week, 6–9 hours/day) and intensive outpatient programs (2–4 days/week, 2–4 hours/day) have been developed to treat patients who require more than regular outpatient care but less than full-time hospitalization.

22. What are appropriate admission and discharge criteria for hospitalization of adolescents with eating disorders?

The Society for Adolescent Medicine has published criteria for admission of patients with eating disorders. These criteria are based on the concept that specific medical and psychiatric factors as well as failure to progress as an outpatient are appropriate reasons for hospitalization. Unfortunately, insurance companies do not necessarily follow the same criteria; clinicians, therefore, may find themselves debating and negotiating with insurance companies to follow these guidelines. No specific guidelines for hospital discharge have been established. As a rule, hospitalization should be long enough to allow sufficient weight gain along with changes in attitude and approach to ensure that subsequent day-program or outpatient care is likely to be successful. Discussions with insurance companies have become a major determinant of the length of inpatient care that can be offered to patients with eating disorders.

Indications for Hospitalization in an Adolescent with an Eating Disorder

Any one or more of the following would justify hospitalization:
1. Severe malnutrition
   Weight < 75% ideal body weight
2. Dehydration
3. Electrolyte disturbances
4. Cardiac dysrhythmia
5. Physiological instability
   Severe bradycardia
   Hypotension
   Hypothermia
   Orthostatic changes

(Table continued on next page.)

6. Arrested growth and development
7. Failure of outpatient treatment
8. Acute food refusal
9. Uncontrollable bingeing and purging
10. Acute medical complications of malnutrition (e.g., syncope, seizures, cardiac failure, pancreatitis)
11. Acute psychiatric emergencies (e.g., suicidal ideation, acute psychosis)
12. Comorbid diagnosis that interferes with the treatment of the eating disorder (e.g., severe depression, obsessive-compulsive disorder, severe family dysfunction)

23. How should nutrition be managed in adolescents with eating disorders?

The patient with anorexia nervosa ultimately must receive enough calories to regain weight, whereas the patient with bulimia nervosa needs to work on restoring normal eating patterns that will lessen the likelihood of binge-and-purge behaviors. Although some in-patients with anorexia nervosa may require enteral (i.e., nasogastric) or parenteral (i.e., hyperalimentation) nutrition, most patients, regardless of setting, are fed orally. Although no two programs use exactly the same methods of accomplishing nutrition goals, as a rule patients are given 3 meals and 2–4 snacks (as supplements or food) per day. Most patients require 2000–3000 calories per day for sustained weight gain, although some patients, especially those with severe malnutrition, may require less for a certain period, and some patients, especially those who are physically active, may require more.

24. What is the refeeding syndrome? How is it managed? How is it avoided?

Patients who are severely malnourished (generally, at least 30% below average body weight for height) are at risk of developing severe complications if they are refed too rapidly. In its mildest form, the refeeding syndrome can include the development of edema (hence fluid should be carefully controlled during the initial refeeding phase) and increased liver function tests (from development of a fatty liver, which resolves over time). In more severe situations, patients may develop hypophosphatemia due to insufficient phosphorus stores in the face of resumption of adenosine triphosphate (ATP) activity in the cells. Hypophosphatemia can lead to cardiac failure, central nervous system depression, and hemolytic anemia. These complications can occur with oral, enteral, or parenteral feeding. The refeeding syndrome is prevented by use of prophylactic phosphorus and by slow refeeding (starting at 800–1000 calories/day and increasing by 100–200 calories/day) in patients who are severely malnourished.

25. What is the role of behavioral modification in the treatment of eating disorders?

Because fear of gaining weight ultimately drives the continuation of eating disorders, especially anorexia nervosa, it may be necessary in many cases to develop behavior modification plans that will force adolescents with eating disorders to accomplish necessary goals. Either positive or negative reinforcement may be used. Plans may vary from the simple restriction of activity in outpatient settings to the complex behavior modification programs used on in-patient units. Fear of hospitalization in its own right may be the incentive that allows some patients to succeed as outpatients.

26. What psychological methods may be used in the treatment of eating disorders?

Although the medical and nutritional aspects of care are crucial for the short-term and intermediate-term outcome of anorexia and bulimia nervosa, for most patients the success of the psychological aspects of care is crucial for long-term outcome. Individual therapy is the mainstay of the psychological treatments for most patients with eating disorders; for some patients, a formal cognitive-behavioral approach is used. Family therapy is especially important for adolescents with eating disorders. Group therapy is used in some settings and may be helpful for many patients. Some patients, however, handle group therapy poorly, becoming involved in negative competition, learning "tricks of the trade," and/or becoming overly identified as a patient with an eating disorder.

27. What is the role of psychopharmacology in the treatment of anorexia nervosa?

Although antidepressant medications (most recently, the selective serotonin reuptake inhibitors [SSRIs]) are used frequently for patients with anorexia nervosa, no evidence indicates that they contribute to improved weight gain. They may be useful, however, in alleviating the depression that can be both a cause and an effect of the eating disorder. Recent studies have shown that antidepressant medications may be useful in prevention of relapse in patients with anorexia nervosa. Some patients with more severe disease have been treated with antipsychotic/antianxiety medications (risperidone or olanzapine) with some success.

28. Describe the role of psychopharmacology in the treatment of bulimia nervosa.

In contrast to anorexia nervosa, antidepressant medications (specifically the SSRIs) have been found to be a useful modality in treatment of bulimia nervosa. Many patients find that the urge to binge and/or purge is decreased by antidepressant treatment, and it is unclear whether this finding is due to a direct effect or is a secondary benefit to the treatment of depression.

29. What is the expected outcome of treatment in adolescents with eating disorders? How does it differ from the outcome in adults?

Several studies have shown that most adolescent patients with anorexia nervosa do well over time. Between two-thirds and three-fourths of adolescents recover completely from anorexia nervosa, despite some increased risk for development of a relapse or another eating disorder later in life. Some adolescents with anorexia nervosa develop a chronic condition, whereas others generally do well but retain vestiges of eating disorder behaviors over the long term. Adults with anorexia nervosa do not have as good a prognosis as adolescents; more patients retain their illness over the long term. Many studies have explored the outcome of bulimia nervosa in adults (with mixed findings), but few data are available about the prognosis for the relatively fewer cases of bulimia nervosa in adolescents.

30. What are the causes of mortality in eating disorders? How frequently do they occur?

Estimates from the adult psychiatric literature cite a mortality rate of 5–10% over the long term. The mortality rate for adolescents is believed to be much lower. By far, the number-one cause of mortality for those with eating disorders is suicide. Other medical causes, including malnutrition, complications of refeeding, and cardiac arrhythmias, are more rare, as is the development of irreversible cardiomyopathy secondary to ipecac ingestion.

31. Describe the current approaches to the prevention of anorexia and bulimia nervosa in adolescents.

One aspect of prevention of eating disorders is case finding. Detecting and treating an eating disorder at an early stage can prevent it from progressing to a later, more intractable stage. Ensuring that families, friends, and school personnel are aware of the signs of an eating disorder and know how to get help is important. Attempts to change the cultural milieu that promotes the development of eating disorders, by working with the press and in schools, are currently under way. There are some questions about the efficacy of these programs, including the questions of whether they have the potential of inadvertently increasing eating disorders.

32. Describe the relationship between eating disorders and other risk behaviors in adolescents.

Patients with eating disorders clearly are at great risk for other mental health disturbances. In addition, studies have shown that adolescents with disordered eating (in school or community samples) have a higher incidence of other health risk behaviors, including smoking, drinking, substance use, and sexual activity. Among patients with fully diagnosed eating disorders, other risk behaviors are more commonly found in those with bulimia nervosa than in those with anorexia nervosa.

BIBLIOGRAPHY

1. American Psychiatric Association: Diagnostic and Statistical Manual of Mental Disorders, 4th ed. Washington, DC, APA, 1994.
2. American Psychiatric Association: Practice guidelines for the treatment of patients with eating disorders (revision). Am J Psychiatry 157(Suppl):1–39, 2000.
3. Becerk AE, Grinspoon SK, Kiblanski A, Herzog DB: Eating disorders. N Engl J Med 340: 1092–1098, 1999.
4. Becker AE, Hamburg P: Culture, the media, and eating disorders. Harv Rev Psychiatry 4:163–167, 1996.
5. Carlat DJ, Cmarago CA Jr, Herzog DB: Eating disorders in males: A report on 135 patients. Am J Psychiatry 154:1127–1132, 1997.
6. Castro J, Lazaro L, Pons F, et al: Predictors of bone mineral density reduction in adolescents with anorexia nervosa. J Am Acad Child Adolesc Psychiatry 39:1365–1370, 2000.
7. Eisler I, Dare C, Russell GFM, et al: Family and individual therapy in anorexia nervosa: A 5-year follow-up. Arch Gen Psychiatry 54:1025–1030, 1997.
8. Fisher M, Golden NH, Katzman DK, et al: Eating disorders in adolescents: A background paper. J Adolesc Health 16:420–437, 1995.
9. Fisher M: Medical complications of anorexia and bulimia nervosa. Adolesc Med State Art Rev 3:487–502, 1992.
10. Fisher M, Schneider M, Pegler C, Napolitano B: Eating attitudes, health risk behaviors, self-esteem, and anxiety among adolescent females in a suburban high school. J Adolesc Health 12:377–384,, 1991.
11. Grinspoon S, Thomas E, Pitts S, et al: Prevalence and predictive factors for regional osteopenia in women with anorexia nervosa. Ann Intern Med 133:790–794, 2000.
12. Howard WT, Evans KK, Quintero-Howard CV, et al: Predictors of success or failure of transition to day hospital treatment for inpatients with anorexia nervosa. Am J Psychiatry 156:1697–1702, 1999.
13. Hsu LKG: Epidemiology of the eating disorders. Psychiatry Clin North Am 19:681–700, 1996.
14. Jones JM, Lawson ML, Daneman D, et al: Eating disorders in adolescent females with and without type 1 diabetes: Cross-sectional study. BMJ 320:1563–1566, 2000.
15. Kaye WH,. Kaplan AS, Zucker ML: Treating eating disorders patients in a managed care environment: Contemporary American issues and a Canadian response. Psychiatry Clin North Am 19:793–810, 1996.
16. Klibanski A, Biller BM, Schoenfeld DA, et al: The effects of estrogen administration on trabecular bone loss in young women with anorexia nervosa. J Clin Endocrinol Metab 80:898–904, 1995.
17. Lucas AR, Beard CM, O'Fallon WM, Kurland LT: Fifty-year trends in the incidence of anorexia nervosa in Rochester, Minn.: A population-based study. Am J Psychiatry 148:917–922, 1991.
18. Palla B, Litt IF: Medical complications of eating disorders in adolescents. Pediatrics 81:613–623, 1988.
19. Robinson E, Bachrach L, Katzman DK: Use of hormone replacement therapy to reduce the risk of oseteopenia in adolescent girls with anorexia nervosa. J Adolesc Health 26:343–348, 2000.
20. Rock CL, Curran-Celentano J: Nutritional management of eating disorders. Psychiatr Clin North Am 19:701–713, 1996.
21. Schebendach J, Nussbaum MP: Nutrition management in adolescents with eating disorders. Adolesc Med State Art Rev 3:541–558, 1992.
22. Solomon SM, Kirby DF: The refeeding syndrome: A review. J Parenteral Enteral Nutr 14:90–97, 1990.
23. Strauss RS: Self-reported weight status and dieting in a cross-sectional sample of young adolescents. Arch Pediatr Adolesc Med 153:741–747, 1999.
24. Walsh BT, Devlin MJ: Eating disorders: Progress and problems. Science 280:1387–1390, 1998.
25. Yager J: Psychosocial treatments for eating disorders. Psychiatry 57:153–163, 1994.

33. MOOD AND ANXIETY DISORDERS

Kathleen L. Lemanek, Ph.D., and Catherine L. Butz, Ph.D.

MAJOR DEPRESSIVE DISORDERS

1. What are the most common affective disorders in adolescents?

Major depressive disorder (MDD) is the most prevalent affective disorder in adolescents. About 80% of adolescents with affective disorders have MDD alone. Another 10% experience a dysthymic disorder without MDD, and the remaining 10% experience both MDD and a dysthymic disorder. Fewer than 1% of adolescents are diagnosed with a bipolar disorder.

2. What is the prevalence of MDD in adolescent males and females?

The prevalence of MDD in adolescents is between 2% and 5% in the general community, slightly less than in adults. By the age of 14 years, girls are twice as likely to be diagnosed with MDD as boys.

3. According to the *Diagnostic and Statistical Manual of Mental Disorders*, 4th edition (DSM-IV), criteria, how is MDD classified?

For a major depressive episode, five or more of the following symptoms must be present during the same 2-week period. At least one of the symptoms is either (1) depressed mood or (2) loss of interest or pleasure

1. Depressed mood (irritable mood may be seen in children or adolescents)
2. Diminished interest or pleasure in almost all activities
3. Weight loss or gain or change in appetite
4. Insomnia or hypersomnia
5. Psychomotor agitation or retardation
6. Fatigue or loss of energy
7. Worthlessness or excessive or inappropriate guilt
8. Diminished ability to concentrate or indecisiveness
9. Recurrent thoughts of death or suicidal ideation

For a diagnosis of a MDD, two or more major depressive episodes must be present, with an interval between episodes of at least 2 consecutive months. The symptoms must cause clinically significant distress or impairment in social, academic/occupational, or other important areas of functioning. Finally, symptoms cannot be attributable to the physiologic effects of substance use or a general medical condition. Separate diagnoses are available for mood disorders due to either one of these conditions.

4. How does dysthymic disorder differ from MDD?

A diagnosis of dysthymic disorder specifies many of the same symptoms, such as poor appetite or overeating, fatigue, and poor concentration. But only two of the six symptoms listed above need to be present. More importantly, a depressed mood must be reported for most days over a 2-year period. For adolescents, depressed mood can be replaced by irritability and be present for at least 1 year. Symptoms must be present for most of the day. No major depressive episode can be present during the first 2 years (1 year for adolescents).

5. Are there differences in the clinical presentation of MDD in adolescents and adults?

Although the same criteria are used to diagnose MDD in adolescents and adults, the pattern of symptoms is somewhat different. Adolescents with MDD are more likely to report feelings of worthlessness, increased guilt, low self-esteem, irritability, and vague somatic complaints. They are less likely to report vegetative symptoms (e.g., weight loss, early morning awakenings) and thoughts of suicide or death than adults. Associated clinical features of depression in adolescents include poor academic performance, cognitive impairment, problematic family relationships, and interpersonal difficulties with peers.

6. Do any disorders frequently coexist in adolescents with MDD?

Disorder	Prevalence of MDD in affected patients
Anxiety disorders	48–71%
Conduct disorder	23–45%
Oppositional defiant disorder	35–79%
Attention deficit–hyperactivity disorder	30–57%
Suicide attempts	73%
Alcohol or drug use or abuse	50–53%

In 80% of cases, MDD occurs *after* the onset of one of the other disorders.

7. Have risk factors been identified for adolescent depression?

Various risk factors place adolescents at risk for experiencing an MDD, including (1) female gender; (2) feelings of low self-esteem or pessimism; (3) stresses such as conflicts with parents, physical illness, or poor school performance; (4) smoking; and (5) past suicidality.

8. Describe the natural history of MDD.

Data from community samples indicate that major depressive episodes last 7–9 months, but symptoms of depression may continue for 1–4 years. Whether estimates are taken from community or clinical samples, about one third to one half of adolescents experience recurrence of a depressive episode. Recurrence and duration of depressive episodes are associated with gender, severity of depression, and family dysfunction. For example, adolescent girls are twice as likely as boys to have recurrent episodes of MDD and to have more severe recurrent episodes. Available data suggest the following:
- 17% of adolescents recover by 16 weeks.
- 48% of adolescents recover by 24 weeks.
- 75% of adolescents recover by 36 weeks.
- 98% of adolescents recover by 5 years.

9. What medications have proved effective for adolescents with MDD?

Four types of antidepressant medications are used in adolescents: selective serotonin reuptake inhibitors (SSRIs), such as sertraline (Zoloft); tricyclic antidepressants (TCAs), such as amitriptyline (Elavil); monoamine oxidase inhibitors (MAOIs), such as phenelzine (Nardil); and a mixed group of medications, including trazodone and bupropion (Wellbutrin). In general, improvement in specific symptoms and overall functioning is evident within 2 weeks of medication administration, although maximal effect may not be seen for 8–12 weeks. Medication is typically administered for 6 months, but symptoms can return if medication is discontinued prematurely. Recent trials with SSRIs reveal some promise in treating MDD in adolescents. Controlled studies indicate that TCAs are not consistently effective and are not superior to placebos.

10. What psychological approaches are effective in treating adolescents with MDD?

Research supports the effectiveness of psychosocial interventions in treating adolescents with depressive symptoms or MDD. Cognitive-behavioral therapy is one of more effective approaches. Specific treatment strategies may include self-monitoring, self-reinforcement, goal setting, challenging irrational thoughts, cognitive restructuring, social skills training, and relaxation training. Family intervention and interpersonal therapy are alternative approaches, but fewer research data support their effectiveness. Treatment sessions usually center on altering family communication, dysfunctional patterns of interaction, and maladaptive relationships among family members. A combination of medication and psychological intervention is recommended in most cases.

ANXIETY DISORDERS

11. What are the most common anxiety disorders? How are they diagnosed?

In simple terms, anxiety results from misinterpretation of environmental stimuli as harmful or dangerous. Misinterpretation leads to fear responses, excessive worry, and/or avoidant behaviors. There are several types of anxiety disorders, some of which appear more commonly in adolescence:

Panic disorder is diagnosed when an adolescent has recurrent panic attacks and worries about having another attack for at least 1 month. Panic attacks are characterized by (1) discreet periods in which sudden onset of fear occurs, (2) a feeling of impending doom, and (3) physiologic symptoms such as shortness of breath, heart palpitations, chest pain or discomfort, choking sensation, sweating, nausea, dizziness, and fear of "going crazy." Panic attacks can coexist with other anxiety disorders. Fifty percent of patients with panic disorder also experience agoraphobia (fear of public places).

Social phobia, also known as social anxiety disorder, involves (1) intense fear of social situations in which one may be exposed to scrutiny, (2) anxiety or panic attacks produced by exposure to social situations, (3) avoidance of social situations, and (4) avoidance or anticipation that interferes with daily activities. The adolescent is aware of his or her excessive fear.

Obsessive-compulsive disorder (OCD) is characterized by (1) recurrent and persistent thoughts and impulses that are considered intrusive and cause distress, (2) recognition of the obsessions and attempts to ignore or suppress them, (3) repetitive behaviors (e.g., hand-washing, checking) that the adolescent is driven to perform in response to the obsession, and (4) behaviors executed to relieve or avoid obsessions, which are excessive and have little to do with thoughts.

Generalized anxiety disorder is diagnosed on the basis of (1) excessive worry about a number of events or activities, occurring most days, for at least 6 months; (2) inability to control worry; (3) three or more of the following symptoms: restlessness, fatigue, poor concentration, irritability, muscle tension, sleep problems; and (4) worry that causes significant distress in functioning.

Other anxiety disorders include: specific phobias, posttraumatic stress disorder, acute stress disorder, and anxiety disorder due to general medical condition.

12. How common is anxiety in children and adolescents?

Studies indicate that 10–20% of children and adolescents suffer from anxiety disorders within any 6-month period. Recently anxiety disorders have been shown to be the most common class of psychiatric disorders affecting children and adolescents. Epidemiologic studies indicate the following prevalence rates in the general population:

Generalized anxiety disorder	2.9–4.6%
Simple phobia	2.4–9.2%
Obsessive-compulsive disorder	1–3.6%
Social phobia	1%
Panic disorder	1%

13. What are the symptoms of an anxiety disorder in adolescent?

Adolescents with anxiety may appear extremely shy, cry frequently, and have fears or persistent worries related to school and peers. School-related anxiety may involve academic failure or test-taking abilities. Patients also may be nail-biters and have a shaky voice and/or rigid posture. Anxious youth may become isolated from friends and avoid participation in school and extracurricular activities. Anxiety disorders can be chronic and persist into adulthood. About 54–65% of adults with anxiety disorders report a history of an anxiety disorder in childhood.

14. What are the risk factors for adolescent anxiety disorder?

Studies have indicated the presence of genetic factors, but familial environment is also a strong predictor. Anxious parents tend to have anxious children. Other risk factors include stressful life events, marital discord, and poverty.

15. What other emotional disorders are commonly associated with anxiety disorders?

Anxiety disorder commonly is associated with other emotional disorders. Studies indicate that 12–50% of children with anxiety also experience depression. Comorbidity for oppositional defiant disorder is 15%; for attention deficit–hyperactivity disorder, 17%. About 50–75% of cases have two concurrent anxiety disorders, such as panic disorder with agoraphobia.

16. How does a practitioner distinguish anxiety from depression?

The comorbidity of anxiety and depression makes it difficult at times to distinguish the two conditions. Typically, the anxiety disorder emerges first, and depressive symptoms or major depressive disorder follows.

Similarly, treatment tends to overlap. Depression, a mood disorder, can be debilitating and significantly affect overall functioning. Symptoms include negative affect, sleep disturbances, appetite disturbances, apathy, and hopelessness. Although depression may be associated with fear responses, they are not as pronounced as in anxiety disorders.

17. What medications are effective in the treatment of anxiety disorders?

Four classes of medications are used with adolescents. SSRIs and TCAs, commonly used as antidepressants, are also effective in treating obsessive-compulsive disorder, panic attacks, and symptoms of agoraphobia. SSRIs are generally preferred for first-line treatment because of their efficacy and more desirable side-effect profile. Benzodiazepines are used for generalized anxiety and panic. Barbiturates are given to adults for the treatment of anxiety but are not commonly prescribed for adolescents. Studies show that over 76% of children and adolescents have a decrease in symptoms 2–6 weeks after beginning medication.

18. What types of psychological therapy are effective in treating anxiety disorders?

Behavioral interventions and cognitive behavioral therapies (CBTs) have been found to be useful in treating anxiety disorders. Behavioral techniques involve direct exposure and relaxation to decrease irrational fears. CBT focuses on identifying irrational thoughts and beliefs that contribute to worry as well as triggers for anxiety. CBT combines thought monitoring with relaxation and imagery as well as direct exposure to the anxiety-inducing object or situation to develop stress management techniques. CBT has been found to significantly decrease anxiety symptoms. Research suggests that symptoms are not present at 1-year follow-up for most patients who are effectively treated.

ADOLESCENT-ONSET SCHIZOPHRENIA

19. According to the DSM-IV, how is adolescent-onset schizophrenia (AOS) classified?

The characteristic symptoms of AOS are basically the same as those for adult schizophrenia. Symptoms are divided into two categories: positive and negative. Positive symptoms include delusions, hallucinations, and disorganized speech or thought processes (e.g., loosening of associations). Negative symptoms pertain to the absence of sociability, appropriate affect (e.g., flattened affect), or energy (e.g., catatonic behavior). Symptoms must be present in some form for at least 6 months, with a 1-month period designated as an active-phase. Impairments or failure to reach age-appropriate expectations in such areas of functioning as school or work, interpersonal relationships, and self-care is evident. In patients with a history of autistic disorder or pervasive developmental disorder, an additional diagnosis of AOS can be made only if delusions or hallucinations are present.

20. Are there gender differences in the prevalence and presentation of AOS?

The prevalence of schizophrenia in the United States is approximately 1%. The prevalence of AOS is about 0.33%; 40% of male patients and 23% of female patients are diagnosed before the age of 19 years. The average age of onset in the United States is approximately 13.9 years. Overall, boys are diagnosed with AOS more often than girls, have an earlier age of onset, and have a poorer premorbid history and worse outcome.

21. What is the clinical outcome or prognosis of AOS?

Outcome for AOS may be measured by the patient's recovery from or decrease in symptoms, educational attainment, social relationships, and independent living. In general, the outcome for AOS is as least as poor as that for adult-onset schizophrenia and perhaps worse for patients whose first hospitalization occurs during adolescence. Although complete remission is seen in about 15–25% of people with AOS, moderate impairment is evident in most patients after the initial hospitalization.

22. Are any medications effective for the treatment of AOS?

There are only a few placebo-controlled studies of the effectiveness of medications in controlling the symptoms of AOS. These studies reveal that neuroleptics, such as thiothixene and thioridazine, are effective in decreasing positive symptoms of AOS compared with placebo. Case reports suggest that risperidone is effective in controlling both positive and negative symptoms of AOS. In general, the available data suggest that neuroleptics are equally effective with AOS and adult-onset schizophrenia.

POSTTRAUMATIC STRESS DISORDER

23. What is posttraumatic stress disorder (PTSD)?

According to the DSM-IV, PTSD in children is characterized by specific symptoms after exposure to an extremely traumatic stressor. The traumatic event may be the direct experience of a situation in which actual or perceived danger, serious injury, or death occurs. PTSD also can result from witnessing injury or death in another person or learning about serious injury or death of a family member or acquaintance. Symptoms associated with PTSD include:
- Reexperiencing of the stressor (e.g., distressing dreams, flashbacks, intrusive thoughts)
- Avoidance of stimuli associated with the trauma
- Hyperarousal (e.g., sleep problems, irritability, hypervigilance, exaggerated startle response)

Symptoms of PTSD must be present for more than 1 month and cause significant distress. Duration of symptoms distinguishes PTSD from an acute stress response.

24. What is the incidence of PTSD?

Studies suggest that 25–60% of children who experience a traumatic event develop PTSD. Some evidence indicates that trauma with a human origin as opposed to a natural disaster has more long-term consequences.

25. What risk factors are associated with PTSD?

Because of the dependent nature of children and young adolescents, they are at greater risk for exposure to trauma. Although many young people are resilient to stressors, 3–58% may experience long-term consequences. Because PTSD is a result of a traumatic event, any such event can be considered a risk factor. In simple terms, PTSD results when people, places, or situations that used to be considered safe become associated with danger and fear. PTSD is commonly associated with personal assault (such as physical or sexual abuse), kidnapping, violent attack on person or property, natural disasters, experiencing or witnessing automobile accidents, and being diagnosed or knowing someone diagnosed with a life-threatening disease. Poor family support also has been shown to correlate with the emergence of symptoms after a traumatic event.

26. What are possible treatments for PTSD?

Individual therapy using cognitive-behavioral interventions has been shown to be effective. Goals of therapy are to help the adolescent make sense of what happened and to manage symptoms of anxiety and depression. Therapy is most effective with family support. Group therapy also has been helpful for groups of children or adolescents who experience the same traumatic event.

BIBLIOGRAPHY

1. American Psychiatric Association: Diagnostic and Statistical Manual of Mental Disorders, 4th ed. Washington, DC, American Psychiatric Association, 1994.
2. Bernstein GA, Borchardt CM, Perwien AR: Anxiety disorders in children and adolescents: A review of the past 10 years. J Am Acad Child Adoles Psychiatry 35:1110–1119, 1996.
3. Davidson JRT, Foa EB (eds): Posttraumatic Stress Disorder: DSM-IV and Beyond. Washington, DC, American Psychiatric Press, 1993.
4. Finn CA: Treating adolescent depression: A review of intervention approaches. Int J Adolesc Youth 8:253–269, 2000.
5. Fleming JE, Offord DR: Epidemiology of childhood depressive disorders: A critical review. J Am Acad Child Adolesc Psychiatry 29:571–580, 1990.
6. Kendall P. (ed): Child and Adolescent Therapy: Cognitive-behavioral Procedures. New York, Guilford Press, 2000
7. Lewinsohn PM, Hops H, Roberts RE, et al: Adolescent psychopathology. I: Prevalence and incidence of depression and other DSM-III-R disorders in high school students. J Abnorn Psychol 102:133–144, 1993.
8. Lewinsohn PM, Rohde P, Seeley JR: Major depressive disorder in older adolescents: Prevalence, risk factors, and clinical implications. Clin Psychol Rev 18:765–794, 1998.
9. Schulz SC, Findling RL, Wise A, et al: Child and adolescent schizophrenia. Psychiatr Clin North Am 21:43–56, 1998.
10. Wagner KD, Ambrosine PJ: Childhood depression: Pharmacological therapy/treatment. J Clin Child Psychol 30:88–97, 2001.
11. Yule W: Post-traumatic stress disorder in children and adolescents. Int Rev Psychiatry 13:194–200, 2001.

34. ATTENTION DEFICIT–HYPERACTIVITY DISORDER

Andrew N. Colvin, Ph.D., John T. Beetar, Ph.D., and Keith Owen Yeates, Ph.D.

1. How is attention deficit–hyperactivity disorder (ADHD) diagnosed?

According to the *Diagnostic and Statistical Manual of Mental Disorders, Fourth Edition* (DSM-IV), the core characteristics of ADHD can be divided into two dimensions: inattention and hyperactivity-impulsivity. Three subtypes of ADHD can be diagnosed based on these dimensions: predominantly inattentive, predominantly hyperactive-impulsive, and the combined subtype. Six of nine core symptoms are required for a diagnosis of the inattentive subtype, and six of nine core symptoms are required for a diagnosis of the hyperactive-impulsive subtype. A diagnosis of the combined subtype requires the presence of 6 of 9 core symptoms from each dimension.

Diagnostic Criteria for Attention Deficit–Hyperactivity Disorder

I. Six or more symptoms of *either* inattention *or* hyperactivity–impulsivity have persisted for at least 6 months to a degree that is maladaptive and inconsistent with development level:
   Inattention
   1. Often fails to give close attention to details or makes careless mistakes in schoolwork, work, or other activities
   2. Often has difficulty sustaining attention in tasks or play activities
   3. Often does not seem to listen when spoken to directly
   4. Often does not follow through on instructions and fails to finish schoolwork, chores, or duties in the workplace (not due to oppositional behavior or failure to understand instructions)
   5. Often has difficulty organizing tasks and activities
   6. Often avoids, dislikes, or is reluctant to engage in tasks that require sustained mental effort (such as homework)
   7. Often loses things necessary for tasks or activities (e.g., toys, school assignments, pencils, books, tools)
   8. Is often easily distracted by extraneous stimuli
   9. Is often forgetful in daily activities
   Hyperactivity–impulsivity
   1. Often fidgets with hands or feet or squirms in seat
   2. Often leaves seat in classroom or in other situations in which remaining seated is expected
   3. Often runs about or climbs excessively in situations in which it is inappropriate (in adolescents or adults, may be limited to subjective feelings of restlessness)
   4. Often has difficulty playing or engaging in leisure activities quietly
   5. Is often "on the go" or often acts as if "driven by a motor"
   6. Often talks excessively
   7. Often blurts out answers before questions have been completed
   8. Often has difficulty awaiting turn
   9. Often interrupts or intrudes on others (e.g., butting into conversations or games)

II. Some hyperactive–impulsive or inattentive symptoms that caused impairment were present before age 7 years

III. Some impairment from the symptoms is present in two or more settings (e.g., school, work, home)

Table continued on following page

Diagnostic Criteria for Attention Deficit–Hyperactivity Disorder (Continued)

IV. Clear evidence of clinically significant impairment in social, academic, or occupational functioning

V. The symptoms do not occur exclusively during the course of a pervasive developmental disorder, schizophrenia, or another psychotic disorder and not better accounted for by another mental disorder (e.g., mood, anxiety, dissociative, or personality disorder)

Adapted from American Psychiatric Association: Diagnostic and Statistical Manual of Mental Disorders, 4th ed. Washington, DC, American Psychiatric Association, 1994.

2. What is the prevalence of ADHD in adolescents?

ADHD is estimated to affect 3–5% of school-age children, and children with ADHD represent 30–40% of children referred for behavioral health services. Children were once thought to grow out of ADHD as they entered adolescence, but it is now recognized that up to 80% of children with ADHD continue to display clinically significant symptoms in adolescence. Moreover, up to 60% of people diagnosed with ADHD in childhood continue to display symptoms as adults. Although the symptoms in adulthood may not meet diagnostic criteria, they are often severe enough to produce functional impairments.

3. How is the presentation of ADHD different in adolescents and children?

Although symptoms of ADHD persist into adolescence, diagnosis is often difficult in this age group. The diagnostic criteria were based on childhood behaviors and do not take into account developmental change in symptom expression. For example, the excessive motor activity seen in ADHD during childhood may be significantly reduced or disappear altogether by the teen years, to be replaced by subjective feelings of restlessness. Attention span and impulse control also may be improved, but adolescents with ADHD often continue to have academic problems due to poor planning and organization. In addition, comorbidities with conduct disorders and mood disorders become more common during adolescence.

4. What disorders other than ADHD can cause problems with attention and disruptive behavior?

- Other disruptive behavior disorders (e.g., oppositional defiant disorder, conduct disorder)
- Learning disabilities
- Mood disorders (e.g., major depression, bipolar disorder, dysthymia)
- Anxiety disorders
- Mild mental retardation
- Sensory problems (e.g., loss of vision or hearing)
- Pervasive developmental disorders (e.g., autism, Asperger's disorder)
- Acute or chronic medical conditions (e.g., lead toxicity, seizure disorders, traumatic brain injury)

5. What disorders or problems commonly occur with ADHD in adolescents?

Oppositional defiant disorder	59%
Conduct disorder	43%
Cigarette use	49%
Alcohol use	42%
Academic failure (grade retention)	29%
Mood disorder (depressed mood)	25%
Anxiety disorder (adult data)	> 25%

6. How is ADHD diagnosed in adolescents?

A medical examination is needed to determine whether the problems with attention and behavioral regulation are due to an acute or chronic illness. Once a medical illness is ruled out, the assessment should focus on the duration of symptoms of ADHD (i.e., were the problems first evident in childhood, or are they of more recent onset?) and the current severity of the symptoms. Broad-band behavior rating forms, such as the Child Behavior Checklist, help to identify coexisting problems. Narrow-band forms, such as Russell Barkley's ADHD Rating Scale, can assess the specific symptoms of ADHD. Finally, psychological testing may help to rule out associated learning or behavior problems.

7. If an adolescent displays symptoms of both bipolar disorder and ADHD, how do you differentiate between the two?

Approximately 59% of adolescents with adolescent-onset bipolar disorder have a concomitant diagnosis of ADHD. The differentiation between the two disorders has been a subject of debate, because problems with attention and behavioral regulation are characteristic of both mania and ADHD. However, when researchers control for the symptoms shared by both disorders, adolescents with bipolar disorder continue to display significant mood problems, suggesting that the ADHD symptoms are not simply a secondary result of mania.

8. Are stimulant medications effective for the treatment of adolescents with ADHD?

Methylphenidate is an effective treatment for ADHD in adolescence. However, standard preparations of the drug, which require teenagers to take the medication several times during the day, often have the unintended effect of nonadherence. Adolescents with ADHD may have difficulty monitoring medication regimens in the more unstructured settings of middle and high schools. New, long-acting formulations of methylphenidate (e.g., Concerta) may improve adherence by eliminating the need for dosing during school hours.

9. What are the common side effects of stimulant medication?
- Loss of appetite   • Irritability
- Poor sleep   • Abdominal pains
- Rebound effects   • Headache

10. Do stimulant medications cause tic disorders?

Although the onset of tics may follow the initiation of stimulant treatment, current evidence does not indicate that stimulants cause tic disorders. However, the use of stimulants may exacerbate tics.

11. Have other treatments been shown to be effective for treating ADHD?

Although medication alone has been shown to be superior to behavioral treatment alone in the Multimodal Treatment Study for ADHD (MTA), children who received only behavioral treatment demonstrated significant improvements in behavior from baseline. Many parents are reluctant to use medication, and noncompliance can interfere with effective medication management. The combination of medication and behavioral treatment was found to be as effective as medication alone and appeared to reduce the need for increased stimulant dosage.

12. Does the use of stimulant medication increase the risk of substance abuse in adolescents with ADHD?

The use of stimulant medication has not been shown to lead to substance abuse in adolescents with ADHD. To the contrary, medication in fact may reduce the chance that teens will develop substance abuse problems. Among adolescents with ADHD who develop substance abuse problems, a comorbid conduct disorder appears to account for the increased rates of substance abuse. In other words, ADHD alone is not sufficient to account for substance abuse in adolescents.

13. Does the use of stimulant medication improve academic performance?

Current research indicates that the use of stimulant medications alone does not have a definite impact on the academic performance of adolescents with ADHD. Indeed, higher-than-optimal doses may have a short-term negative effect on cognitive functioning. Adolescents with

ADHD often have slightly lower overall cognitive ability than their peers and tend to live in families of lower socioeconomic status. Both of these factors influence academic achievement in ways that cannot be eliminated by the use of stimulants. However, recent research has demonstrated that a combination of medication and behavioral treatment can have a positive effect on academic performance, at least in the short term.

14. Is there evidence for neurologic involvement in ADHD?
Although not definitive, recent studies have noted both structural and metabolic differences in certain brain regions. For example, reduced regional cerebral blood flow has been found in the striatum of children with ADHD, and structural differences have been detected in the striatum and frontal lobes. These differences may contribute to the symptoms of ADHD, because frontostriatal circuits are thought to be involved in executive functions such as sustained attention, working memory, and behavioral regulation.

15. What is neurofeedback? Is it effective?
Electroencephalographic (EEG) abnormalities, particularly slowing, have sometimes been found in children with ADHD. Neurofeedback, also called EEG biofeedback, is based on the premise that if children with ADHD learn to normalize EEGs, the symptoms of ADHD will be reduced. Although strong claims have been advanced for the effectiveness of EEG biofeedback, it has not yet received sufficient empirical validation to be considered a treatment of choice.

BIBLIOGRAPHY

1. American Psychiatric Association: Diagnostic and Statistical Manual of Mental Disorders, 4th ed. Washington, DC, American Psychiatric Association, 1994.
2. Barkley RA: Attention-Deficit Hyperactivity Disorder: A Handbook for Assessment and Treatment. New York, Guilford Press, 1998.
3. Barkley RA, Fischer M, Edelbrock CS, Smallish L: The adolescent outcome of hyperactive children diagnosed by research criteria. I: An 8-year prospective follow-up study. J Am Acad Child Adolesc Psychiatry 29:546–557, 1990.
4. Biederman J, Wilens T, Mick E, Spencer T, Faraone SV: Pharmacotherapy of attention-deficit/hyperactivity disorder reduces risk for substance use disorder. Pediatrics 104:1–5, 1999.
5. Faraone SV, Biederman J, Wozniak J, et al: Is comorbity with ADHD a marker for juvenile-onset mania? J Am Acad Child Adolesc Psychiatry 36:1046–1055, 1997.
6. Ingram S, Hechtman L, Morgenstern G: Outcome issues in ADHD: Adolescent and adult long-term outcome. Ment Retard Devel Disabil Res Rev 5:243–250, 1999.
7. Smith BH, Waschbusch DA, Willoughby MT, Evans S: The efficacy, safety, and practicality of treatments for adolescents with attention-deficit/hyperactivity disorder (ADHD). Clin Child Fam Psychol Rev 3:243–267, 2000.

35. SCHOOL AND LEARNING PROBLEMS

John T. Beetar, Ph.D., Andrew N. Colvin, Ph.D., and Keith Owen Yeates, Ph.D.

1. What is a learning disorder/disability (LD)?

An LD is the result of a disruption of central nervous system function that affects the ability to learn how to read, write, or do math. The term also is used to describe deficits in language, visual-spatial, and/or executive functions that impede academic progress. The term is not applicable to learning problems that result from visual or hearing impairments, selected motor handicaps, or mental retardation. LD is not the correct diagnosis when environmental, cultural, or economic disadvantage is considered the primary cause of a student's difficulties. About 5% of public school students are diagnosed as having LDs, with a greater incidence in males.

2. What is dyslexia?

Dyslexia refers to a developmental disability in learning how to read and spell that does not result from mental retardation. The term is used less frequently now than in the past.

3. What are the rules and regulations for students with LDs?

The Individuals with Disabilities Education Act (IDEA) supports special education and related services for students with LDs. IDEA is rooted in Public Law 94-142, enacted in 1975 to establish aid for the education of children with disabilities. IDEA is a federal law that describes the minimal requirements that states must meet to receive federal funds. State laws may vary, and it is helpful to know the specific rules and regulations in your state. Contact the State Department of Education, Office of Special Education to request a handbook written for parents and interested professionals.

4. At what age is an LD diagnosed?

An LD is frequently diagnosed during the elementary school years when academic demands begin to increase. However, teachers and parents may overlook early learning problems, so that LDs may not be diagnosed until middle or high school. Clinicians should consider the possibility of an LD when a student experiences ongoing frustration with particular subjects.

5. How might learning problems be manifested?

- Poor grades
- Lack of motivation
- Difficulty with homework
- Noncompliance
- Truancy
- Depression
- Sleep problems
- Poor appetite
- Frequent somatic complaints
- Inattention
- Social difficulties

6. How are LDs diagnosed?

An LD usually is diagnosed when there is a discrepancy between scores on a standardized intelligence test and academic achievement tests. Research on LDs suggests that the traditional use of IQ–achievement score discrepancies to diagnose LDs probably is not valid. More recent approaches stress core cognitive deficits associated with specific types of learning problems (e.g., poor phonologic and rapid naming skills in reading disorders).

7. How is an LD identified at school?

A team of school professionals generally completes a comprehensive evaluation to assess numerous domains of functioning. A parent may request this type of evaluation. Parents also can ask that a psychologist or neuropsychologist in the local community complete an independent evaluation of their child. Once the evaluation process is completed, the school team and parents meet to discuss the results and to determine whether a child is eligible for services.

8. What can be done for students with LDs?

If a student is determined to be eligible for special education, the school team prepares an individualized education plan (IEP) that documents the services to be provided. The IEP includes goals and methods by which the school intends to help the student reach those goals. A parent must approve the IEP and sign the document along with school officials. Special services may include extra help provided by an LD teacher in either a resource room or the regular classroom. The second approach is often called inclusion services.

9. What does "Section 504" mean?

Section 504 is a civil rights statute that requires schools not to discriminate against children with disabilities and to provide children with disabilities reasonable accommodations. Students who do not meet the criteria for special services under the IDEA definition may do so under Section 504. For example, a student with learning difficulties may not display a discrepancy between IQ and achievement test scores large enough to qualify as learning disabled. Nevertheless, the student may be considered disabled under Section 504 and therefore eligible for assistance.

10. Should a high school student with an LD consider going to college?

Students with LDs often have many cognitive abilities that are average to above average. With the proper support and assistance, they frequently can succeed in higher education. Accommodations can be made for college entrance exams (e.g., extended time limits), and many colleges and universities offer a variety of services to meet the needs of students with LDs. High school guidance counselors are a good resource for information about opportunities in higher education.

11. Do attention deficit and behavior disorders cause an LD?

Attention deficit and behavior disorders do not cause an LD per se. However, many children with an LD also have attention problems and behavioral difficulties, just as many children with ADHD have LDs.

12. What kinds of academic problems do adolescents experience in school?

Adolescence is a time of additional responsibilities, and high school teachers generally expect their students to become increasingly independent in regard to academic work. Although teenagers may want freedom, many students, especially those with learning problems, do not know how to organize their work and time. Thus, they often need instruction in time management and study skills. Classroom teachers and tutors can provide assistance in specific subject areas.

13. What kinds of social problems do adolescents experience in school?

Some teenagers are not prepared for the social demands of adolescence. They may be awkward in social settings and can become the victims of teasing and heckling by peers. To avoid being or feeling different, some teens find it easier to be part of a clique. In that context, pressure to conform to the group's activities generally is strong, even when they are not in the teenager's best interests. Parents and teachers should monitor teenagers' psychosocial adjustment. Poor adjustment can be manifested in diminished appetite, moodiness, withdrawal, irritability, changed sleep patterns, anxiety, disruptive behavior, and lower grades. If emotional or behavioral problems become apparent, referral to a behavioral health professional may be indicated.

14. Do school problems result in family problems?

Many parents learn to advocate effectively for a child with an LD. Other families are not at all adept at dealing with the educational system. Regardless of how well a family addresses a child's learning problems, conflicts frequently arise if parents perceive that the school is not attempting to address their child's special needs. Conflicts also can affect the relationship between a child and his or her parents. State departments of education should have information for parents about local organizations that provide advocacy services. Advocates can assist parents in their dealings with schools and help them secure the proper services for a student in need.

BIBLIOGRAPHY

1. Barkley RA: Attention-Deficit Hyperactivity Disorder: A Handbook for Diagnosis and Treatment. New York, Guilford Press, 1990.
2. Morgan AW, Sullivan SA, Darden C, Gregg N: Measuring the intelligence of college students with learning disorders: A comparison of results on the WAIS-R and the KAIT. J Learn Disabil 30:560–565, 1997.
3. National Information Center for Children and Youth with Disabilities: Questions and Answers about IDEA. (News Digest No. 21, 2nd ed). Washington DC, National Information Center for Children and Youth with Disabilities, 2000.
4. Ohio Coalition for the Education of Children with Disabilities: Section 504 of the Rehabilitation Act of 1973. Marion, OH, Ohio Coalition for the Education of Children with Disabilities, 1998.
5. Siegel L: Issues in the definition and diagnosis of learning disabilities: A perspective on Guckenberger v. Boston University. J Learn Disabil 32:304–319, 1999.

36. ADOLESCENT VIOLENCE AND THE LEGAL SYSTEM

Robert T. Brown, M.D.

1. From what forms of violence do adolescents most often suffer?
The three leading causes of death among adolescents are violent ones: accidents, homicides, and suicides.

2. How many adolescents die from accidents, homicides, and suicides each year?
Among adolescents 15–24 years old, there are 33.6/1000 automobile accident deaths per year. There are approximately 15,000 deaths from accidents per year in this age group, approximately 8000 deaths from homicide, and approximately 5000 suicide deaths per year.

3. What are the risk factors for victimization by violence?
Risk factors are different for the different kinds of violence. For accidents, clearly use of alcohol and/or drugs can increase risk of harm. Marijuana abuse and alcohol abuse are clearly related to risk of victimization. Driving an automobile under the influence is a major contributing factor to violent death and morbidity in adolescents. Putting oneself into situations of risk without thought of potential consequences is another potential antecedent.

4. What are the risk factors for suicide?
Risk factors for suicide include a family history of suicide, substance abuse problems, preexisting psychological morbidity, previous suicide attempts, gay/lesbian sexual orientation, male gender, and access to handguns.

5. What are the warning signs of a possibly suicidal adolescent?
An adolescent who is impulsive and depressed can be suicidal. An adolescent who withdraws from her or his usual group of friends and who becomes socially isolated may be suicidal. An adolescent who has been depressed and has become more and more isolated and who has suicidal ideation and then seems suddenly cheery should be suspected of having decided on a suicide plan. An unexplained, persistent decrease in school performance also should serve as a red flag.

6. What four factors can best determine if an adolescent is at risk for suicide?
Past and present thoughts of suicide; prior self-destructive behavior; and current stressors. If all four are positive, the adolescent has a high risk of suicide.

7. What can the clinician do to help prevent suicide in adolescents?
The key to preventing suicide is to have the topic open for discussion and not to be afraid to ask whether an adolescent is thinking of or planning suicide. Making those who have regular contact with adolescents aware of the possibility of suicide is critical in helping to prevent it. Teachers, youth leaders, coaches, and religious leaders as well as parents should be aware that suicide is a possibility in adolescents, and they should know the warning signs.

8. What community agencies are available to clinicians for help with adolescents who have suffered or who may suffer from violence?
Usually, communities have child protection agencies that are publically funded. In addition, many not-for-profit agencies have effective counseling programs. Psychologists and social workers in hospitals are good resources, as are agencies that tend to the needs of battered

women. Family and juvenile courts are also good resources for these adolescents. For gay, lesbian, bisexual, and transgendered youth, local gay/lesbian alliances and advocacy groups can help with referrals.

9. How many adolescents are sexually abused?

Sexual abuse rates are 2.1/1000 for adolescents 12–15 years old and 1.2/1000 for adolescents 16–17 years old.

10. What are signs of a sexually or physically abused/assaulted adolescent?

An adolescent who has been abused has a higher-than-average risk of running away from home, abusing drugs and alcohol, having significant psychological problems, presenting with nonspecific abdominal pain, having unexplained sexually transmitted infections, and having unexplained physical trauma. Onset of sexual activity before the age of 15 years is a marker for possible coerced sexual activity.

11. How can the clinician detect abuse?

Clinicians must include questions about sexual and physical abuse in the routine history. They should always be suspicious, and they should bring up this topic with all adolescent patients. If these topics are not broached with the adolescent, the problems may never come to light.

12. What resources does the clinician need to help such adolescents?

Social workers, child protective agencies, and other community agencies are available for consultation and advice. Family and juvenile courts also are good resources.

13. Who refers to adolescents as "juveniles"?

A "juvenile" is a correctional system term for any person who is a minor in the eyes of the law.

14. What is the juvenile justice system?

The juvenile justice system is a judicial system that operates separately but parallel to the criminal justice system. It is intended, among other issues, for the disposition of criminal acts by minors; in this age group, the acts are called delinquent rather than criminal. Juveniles are considered to have habilitation potential and not to be totally responsible for their criminal acts. Therefore, they are to be rehabilitated rather than punished even if incarcerated. In the juvenile justice system, perpetrators do not have all of the rights of adult criminals. For example, juveniles do not have the right to bail.

15. How many adolescents are in the juvenile justice system?

Approximately 125,000 adolescents are in residential placement because of delinquency. Girls account for 17% of detained juveniles (short-term) and 12% of committed juveniles (long-term).

16. What is a detention center?

A juvenile detention center is the juvenile justice system's equivalent of a jail, i.e., a short-term incarceration facility. Youths are kept in a detention center until their offense has been considered by the juvenile court and a disposition has been made.

17. What is a reform school?

A "reform" or "training" school is the equivalent of the adult system prison, i.e., a long-term incarceration facility for juveniles. Originally, in the 19th century, such facilities were meant to facilitate "reforming" or "training" girls to be proper women in the eyes of the leaders of conventional society; hence the names. Juveniles generally cannot be kept in a reform school/long-term facility past their 21st birthday. The average length of stay for a juvenile in a long-term facility is 6 months.

18. Why are some adolescents tried in adult courts?

Prosecutors have the prerogative to ask a juvenile court judge to remand a juvenile to the custody of the adult court if the offense is egregiously heinous or if the youth is especially recalcitrant. Some states have enacted statutes with explicit provisions under which juveniles are to be tried as adults, with all the potential consequences of adult incarceration. Most authorities believe that responsibility for remanding cases to the adult justice system should remain with juvenile court judges.

19. What health problems do incarcerated adolescents have?

Juveniles in the justice system frequently have had poor medical care before incarceration and therefore have many health problems that should have received attention earlier. Examples include dental, vision, skin, and other chronic problems. Such youths also suffer from increased incidences of trauma and sexually transmitted infections, including human immunodeficiency virus (HIV). They have multiple psychosocial problems, including depression, conduct disorder, and sexual/physical abuse. They may be at risk for tuberculosis, and they may lack appropriate immunizations for their age.

20. What ensures that adolescents will get the care that they need during incarceration?

While they are incarcerated, youths usually receive care from physicians who have contracts with the detention center or reform school for such services. Some small facilities use community physician offices for the care of inmates. If facilities use the Standards for Juvenile Care of the National Commission on Correctional Health Care, they ensure that proper care is provided to their clients. Ensuring continuity of care after discharge for these high-risk adolescents is a major problem, given that many of them had inconsistent care before incarceration and multiple living arrangements after they are released.

BIBLIOGRAPHY

1. American Academy of Pediatrics: Health care for children and adolescents in the juvenile correctional care system. Pediatrics 107:799–802, 2001.
2. Aubustyn M, Parker S, McAlister Groves B, Zuckerman B: Silent victims: Children who witness violence. Contemp Pediatr 12:35, 1995.
3. Brown RT: Health needs of incarcerated youth. Bull NY Acad Med 70:208–218, 1993.
4. Bureau of Justice Statistics, United States Department of Justice: www.ojp.usdoj.gov/bjs/
5. Chesney-Lind M, Shelden RG: Girls, Delinquency, and Juvenile Justice, 2nd ed. Belmont, CA, Wadsworth, 1998.
6. Durant RH, Pendergast RA, Cadenhead C: Exposure to violence and victimization and fighting behavior by urban black adolescents. J Adolesc Health 15:311–318, 1994.
7. Feinstein RA, Lampkin A, Lorish CD, et al: Medical status of adolescents at time of admission to a juvenile detention center. J Adolesc Health 22:190–196, 1998.
8. Horowitz LM, Wang PS, Koocher GP, et al: Detecting suicide risk in a pediatric emergency department: Development of a brief screening tool. Pediatrics 107:1133–1137, 2001.
9. Kahn DJ, Kazimi MM, Mulvihill MN: Attitudes of New York high school students regarding firearm violence. Pediatrics 107:1125–1132, 2001.
10. Molnar BE, Buka SL, Kessler RC: Child sexual abuse and subsequent psychopathology: Results from the National Comorbidity Survey. Am J Public Health 91:753–760, 2001.
11. Orpinas P, Parcel GS, McAlister A, Frankowski R: Violence prevention in middle schools: A pilot project. J Adolesc Health 17:360–371, 1995.
12. Pratt HD, Greydanus DE: Adolescent violence: Concepts for a new millennium. Adolesc Med State Art Rev 11:103–126, 2000.
13. Standards for Health Services in Juvenile Detention and Confinement Facilities. Chicago, National Commission on Correctional Health Care, 1999.
14. Steinbeck VJ: Factors associated with repeat suicide attempts among adolescents. Aust N Z J Psychiatry 34:437–445, 2000.
15. Talbot M: The maximum security adolescent. New York Times Magazine, Sept. 10, 2000, p 41.

INDEX

Entries in **boldface type** indicate complete chapters.